AF567097

SCOT GERALD FECHTEL, MD, DC, Neurologist, Cascade Neurology, Springfield, Oregon

PRIYA GNANASHANMUGAM, MD, Rheumatology Fellow, University of Washington, Seattle, Washington

MYRON GOLDBERG, PhD, Clinical Associate Professor, Department of Rehabilitation Medicine, University of Washington School of Medicine, Seattle, Washington

MARISOL A. HANLEY, PhD, Research Scientist, Department of Rehabilitation Medicine, University of Washington School of Medicine, Seattle, Washington

TIMOTHY T. HOULE, PhD, Department of Anesthesiology, Wake Forest University School of Medicine, Wake Forest University Health Sciences, Winston-Salem, North Carolina

MARK P. JENSEN, PhD, Professor, Department of Rehabilitation Medicine, University of Washington School of Medicine; Multidisciplinary Pain Center, University of Washington Medical Center-Roosevelt, Seattle, Washington

ALEC L. MELEGER, MD, Director of Pain Medicine Fellowship; Department of Physical Medicine and Rehabilitation, Spaulding Rehabilitation Hospital; Clinical Instructor, Harvard Medical School, Boston, Massachusetts

TRAVIS L. OSBORNE, PhD, Postdoctoral Fellow, Department of Rehabilitation Medicine, University of Washington School of Medicine, Seattle, Washington

STEEN PETERSEN-FELIX, MD, PhD, Department of Anesthesiology, Division of Pain Therapy, Inselspital, Bern, Switzerland

KATHERINE A. RAICHLE, PhD, Postdoctoral Fellow, Department of Rehabilitation Medicine, University of Washington School of Medicine, Seattle, Washington

JAMES P. ROBINSON, MD, PhD, Clinical Associate Professor, Department of Rehabilitation Medicine; Attending Physician, Multidisciplinary Pain Center, University of Washington, Seattle, Washington

KRISTEN BREWER SHERMAN, PhD, Clinical Assistant Professor, Department of Rehabilitation Medicine, University of Washington School of Medicine, Seattle, Washington

CHARLES A. SIMPSON, DC, Vice President, Medical Director, Complementary Healthcare Plans, Inc., Beaverton, Oregon

STEVEN STANOS, DO, Clinical Instructor, Department of Physical Medicine and Rehabilitation, Northwestern University, Feinberg Medical School; Medical Director, Chronic Pain Care Center, Rehabilitation Institute of Chicago, Chicago, Illinois

MARK D. SULLIVAN, MD, PhD, Department of Psychiatry, University of Washington Medical Center Roosevelt Pain Center, Seattle, Washington

CONSULTING EDITOR

GEORGE H. KRAFT, MD, MS, Alvord Professor of Multiple Sclerosis Research Professor, Department of Rehabilitation Medicine; Adjunct Professor of Neurology; Director, Electrodiagnostic Medicine, Western Multiple Sclerosis Center; and Co-Director, Muscular Dystrophy Clinic, University of Washington, Seattle, Washington

GUEST EDITOR

JAMES P. ROBINSON, MD, PhD, Clinical Associate Professor, Department of Rehabilitation Medicine; Attending Physician, Multidisciplinary Pain Center, University of Washington, Seattle, Washington

CONTRIBUTORS

ROGER J. ALLEN, PhD, PT, Associate Professor, Department of Physical Therapy, University of Puget Sound, Tacoma, Washington

LARS ARENDT-NIELSEN, PhD, Professor, Center for Sensory-Motor Interaction, The University of Aalborg, Aalborg, Denmark

KATHLEEN R. BELL, MD, Professor, Department of Rehabilitation Medicine, University of Washington School of Medicine, Seattle, Washington

DONNA BLOODWORTH, MD, Director, Outpatient Physical Medicine and Rehabilitation Clinics, Harris County Hospital District; Associate Professor, Baylor College of Medicine, Houston, Texas

JOANNE BORG-STEIN, MD, Medical Director, Spaulding-Wellesley Rehabilitation Center; Assistant Professor, Department of Physical Medicine and Rehabilitation, Harvard Medical School; Medical Director, Newton Wellesley Hospital Spine Center, Wellesley, Massachusetts

MICHELE CURATOLO, MD, PhD, Professor, Department of Anesthesiology, Division of Pain Therapy, Inselspital, Bern, Switzerland

CARIN E. DUGOWSON, MD, MPH, Associate Professor, Division of Rheumatology; and Adjunct Associate Professor of Epidemiology, University of Washington, Seattle, Washington

DAWN M. EHDE, PhD, Associate Professor, Department of Rehabilitation Medicine, University of Washington School of Medicine, Seattle, Washington

W.B. SAUNDERS COMPANY
A Division of Elsevier Inc.

1600 John F. Kennedy Blvd. • Suite 1800 • Philadelphia, Pennsylvania 19103

http://www.theclinics.com

PHYSICAL MEDICINE AND REHABILITATION CLINICS OF NORTH AMERICA
May 2006
Editor: Debora Dellapena

Volume 17, Number 2
ISSN 1047-9651
ISBN 1-4160-2869-2

The ideas and opinions expressed in *Physical Medicine and Rehabilitation Clinics of North America* do not necessarily reflect those of the Publisher. The Publisher does not assume any responsibility for any injury and/or damage to persons or property arising out of or related to any use of the material contained in this periodical. The reader is advised to check the appropriate medical literature and the product information currently provided by the manufacturer of each drug to be administered to verify the dosage, the method and duration of administration, or contraindications. It is the responsibility of the treating physician or other health care professional, relying on independent experience and knowledge of the patient, to determine drug dosages and the best treatment for the patient. Mention of any product in this issue should not be construed as endorsement by the contributors, editors, or the Publisher of the product or manufacturers' claims.

Physical Medicine and Rehabilitation Clinics of North America (ISSN 1047-9651) is published quarterly by W.B. Saunders, 360 Park Avenue South, New York, NY 10010-1710. Months of publication are February, May, August, and November. Business and Editorial Offices: 1600 John F. Kennedy Blvd., Suite 1800, Philadelphia, PA 19103-2899. Accounting and Circulation Offices: 6277 Sea Harbor Drive, Orlando, FL 32887-4800. Periodicals postage paid at New York, NY and additional mailing offices. Subscription price per year is $160.00 (US individuals), $250.00 (US institutions), $80.00 (US students), $195.00 (Canadian individuals), $320.00 (Canadian institutions), $110.00 (Canadian students), $225.00 (foreign individuals), $320.00 (foreign institutions), and $110.00 (foreign students). Foreign air speed delivery is included in all *Clinics* subscription prices. All prices are subject to change without notice. POSTMASTER: Send address changes to *Physical Medicine and Rehabilitation Clinics of North America*, Elsevier Periodicals Customer Service, 6277 Sea Harbor Drive, Orlando, FL 32887-4800. **Customer Service: 1-800-654-2452 (US). From outside of the US, call 1-407-345-4000.**

Physical Medicine and Rehabilitation Clinics of North America is indexed in *Excerpta Medica, Index Medicus, Cinahl,* and *Cumulative Index to Nursing and Allied Health Literature.*

Printed in the United States of America.

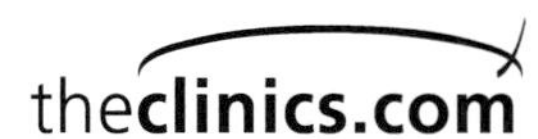

PHYSICAL MEDICINE AND REHABILITATION CLINICS OF NORTH AMERICA

Pain Rehabilitation

GUEST EDITOR
James P. Robinson, MD, PhD

CONSULTING EDITOR
George H. Kraft, MD, MS

May 2006 • Volume 17 • Number 2

SAUNDERS

An Imprint of Elsevier, Inc.
PHILADELPHIA LONDON TORONTO MONTREAL SYDNEY TOKYO

CONTENTS

FORTHCOMING ISSUES

August 2006

Sports Medicine
Gregory A. Strock, MD and
Ralph Buschbacher, MD, *Guest Editors*

November 2006

Performing Arts Medicine
Seneca Storm, MD, *Guest Editor*

RECENT ISSUES

February 2006

New Advances in Prosthetics and Orthotics
Mark H. Bussell, MD, CPO, *Guest Editor*

November 2005

Current Trends in Neuromuscular Research: Assessing Function, Enhancing Performance
Gregory T. Carter, MD, *Guest Editor*

August 2005

Running Injuries
Venu Akuthota, MD and
Mark A. Harrast, MD, *Guest Editors*

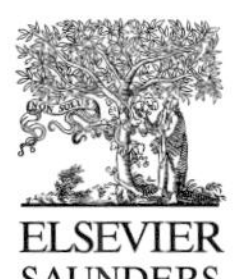

ELSEVIER
SAUNDERS

Phys Med Rehabil Clin N Am
17 (2006) xi–xii

PHYSICAL MEDICINE
AND REHABILITATION
CLINICS OF
NORTH AMERICA

Foreword

Pain Rehabilitation

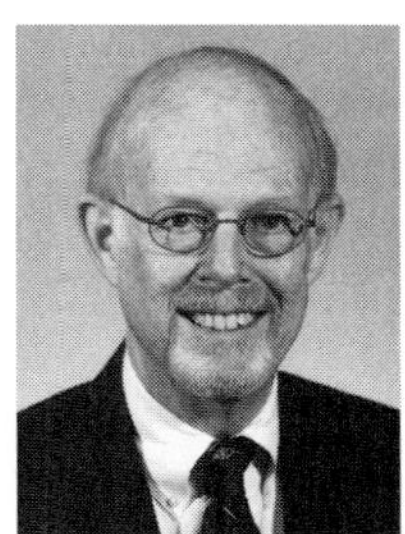

George H. Kraft, MD, MS
Consulting Editor

It has been some time since the *Physical Medicine and Rehabilitation Clinics of North America* published an issue on pain management. The current issue has been in the planning stage for a while, and its publication now is particularly timely, with the advent of the American Board of Medical Specialties (ABMS) pain subspecialty board.

Dr. James Robinson has acquired an outstanding roster of medical pain experts to contribute to this issue. Robinson is both a PhD psychologist and an MD physiatrist and has had a lifelong interest in the management of chronic pain. Jim has long been on the forefront of understanding that pain is more than just a nociceptive condition; it also has a psychologic component, which in many cases of chronic pain can be the major cause of suffering. Dr. Robinson is ideally suited to guest edit this issue.

I believe that this up-to-date issue will hold something of interest for every reader. The largest group of articles provides an in-depth review of medications. Essentially all categories of medications used for pain management are reviewed. Analgesics—both narcotic and nonnarcotic—are, of course, discussed, as are corticosteroids and nonsteroidal anti-inflammatory drugs. Finally, antidepressants, anticonvulsants, muscle relaxants, and spasmolytic medications are reviewed.

Other articles review the neurobiology and epidemiology of pain, as well as pain management in some commonly encountered syndromes: myofacial pain and pain associated with brain injury. The very important psychologic and physical modalities for treatment of pain are reviewed as well. Complementary and alternative management of pain is also discussed.

1047-9651/06/$ - see front matter
doi:10.1016/j.pmr.2005.12.013

Finally, the issue includes articles devoted to the management process itself: evaluation of the patient, planning a treatment strategy, and the role of a multidisciplinary pain treatment center.

Whether in preparation for taking the new ABMS examination, or for use as a text in a pain fellowship, or for looking for strategies for managing complex pain patients, or for seeking out the latest on medications and other treatments, this issue will be indispensable. I believe it will be widely used. Thank you, Jim Robinson, for taking on this task.

George H. Kraft, MD, MS
Department of Rehabilitation Medicine
University of Washington School of Medicine
1959 NE Pacific Street, Box 356490
Seattle, WA 98195-6490, USA

E-mail address: ghkraft@u.washington.edu

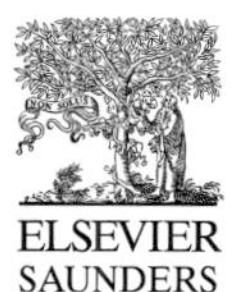

ELSEVIER
SAUNDERS

Phys Med Rehabil Clin N Am 17 (2006) xiii–xix

PHYSICAL MEDICINE AND REHABILITATION CLINICS OF NORTH AMERICA

Preface

Pain Rehabilitation

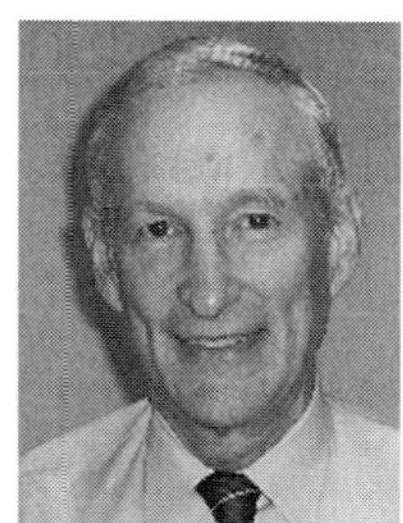

James P. Robinson, MD, PhD
Guest Editor

This issue of the *Physical Medicine and Rehabilitation Clinics of North America* deals with strategies for evaluating and treating chronic pain. Physiatrists need skill in managing chronic pain because they encounter it frequently. Some physiatrists focus their clinical practices on patients who have pain as their major reason for seeking health care. These include physiatrists who work at pain centers and those who focus on the management of spinal disorders. Other physiatrists treat patients who are disabled by conditions that are not necessarily painful, such as spinal cord injury and stroke. For these physicians, pain might be construed as a secondary problem that complicates their attempts to rehabilitate patients. Unfortunately, it is a secondary problem that they are likely to encounter routinely because epidemiologic research demonstrates a high prevalence of chronic pain in most of the patient populations that physiatrists treat (see the article by Ehde and Hanley).

Approaches to pain

Physicians usually provide an eclectic mixture of therapies when they treat patients with chronic pain. Many of the therapies defy any simple classification scheme. For purposes of exposition, though, it is possible to classify most of them into three broad groups: curative/disease modifying, rehabilitative, and palliative.

The curative approach is the simplest to understand and the preferred one when it is applicable. From this perspective, pain is a symptom that, in combination with other symptoms and signs, helps the physician identify

doi:10.1016/j.pmr.2005.12.011

a pathophysiologic process that becomes the target of treatment. In an ideal situation, once the underlying biologic disturbance has been identified and reversed, the patient's symptoms resolve without any additional treatments. Common examples of pain treatment based on the curative perspective include internal fixation and casting for a patient who presents with a painful wrist fracture, appendectomy for a patient who presents with right lower quadrant pain secondary to appendicitis, and angioplasty for a patient who presents with chest pain secondary to cardiac ischemia.

Unfortunately, attempts to relieve pain by curing an "upstream" pathophysiologic process sometimes fail. The reasons for such failure are multiple. Obvious ones include the inability of physicians to identify a pathophysiologic process to account for a patient's pain or their inability to treat the process. A more subtle reason for failure of the curative approach is that chronic pain in some patients may be maintained by alterations in the manner in which the nervous system encodes and processes sensory information rather than by nociception from ongoing tissue injury (see the article by Curatolo and colleagues).

This issue of the *Physical Medicine and Rehabilitation Clinics of North America* focuses on situations in which no curative therapy for pain is available, so that physicians are left with the task of managing the pain. In doing so, they typically use some combination of rehabilitative therapies and palliative therapies.

In a general way, pain rehabilitation is similar to rehabilitation of any medical condition—its goal is to optimize functioning through a combination of physical conditioning, skills training, education, and mobilization of patients' psychologic resources. Many of the patients treated by physiatrists undergo rehabilitative treatment for disorders (eg, spinal cord injury) that may be associated with pain but invariably involve numerous functional deficits unrelated to pain. For these patients, pain rehabilitation becomes a component of the overall rehabilitation program. Thus, for example, a paraplegic who reports shoulder pain as he transfers or uses his wheelchair might experience pain resolution as a result of conditioning to improve his upper body strength and training to improve his transfer techniques. In other settings, pain is the focus of rehabilitative treatment. The best example of this is multidisciplinary pain rehabilitation (see the article by Stanos and Houle).

Rehabilitative therapies influence pain indirectly by addressing secondary effects of the pain (eg, deconditioning) and improving patients' coping skills, whereas palliative therapies focus directly on the pain experience itself. For example, opiates blunt or eliminate the experience of pain without requiring patients to do the kind of work that is demanded by rehabilitative therapies.

Preview

This issue of the *Physical Medicine and Rehabilitation Clinics of North America* describes a variety of palliative and rehabilitative treatments that may be relevant to patients that you treat. It starts (in the article by Curatolo and colleagues) with a review of recent neurobiologic research that supports the role of central hypersensitivity in chronic pain. In a general way, this research supports the conclusion that nociceptive barrages from injured tissues can cause changes in an individual's central nervous system such that his/her subsequent experiences of pain are altered. The concept of central nervous system hypersensitivity provides a possible explanation of the common clinical observation that chronic pain often persists in the absence of on obvious source of ongoing tissue injury.

The article by Ehde and Hanley summarizes epidemiologic research on pain among patients who have various conditions that are typically treated by physiatrists, including spinal cord injury and traumatic brain injury. This research supports two conclusions: (1) that chronic pain has a high prevalence in most of these patient groups and (2) that chronic pain has significant implications for quality of life among the patients.

The article by Fechtel describes strategies for the clinical evaluation of patients who have chronic pain. It highlights the fact that a clinician must adopt a broad perspective when evaluating such patients. Although an evaluation might identify an obvious biomechanical or neurologic cause for a patient's symptoms, Fechtel's article reminds us that the astute clinician must attend to indicators of psychosocial dysfunction as well as biomechanical dysfunction.

The article by Allen addresses pain management therapies that are typically used by physical therapists. It considers the scientific rationale for these physical modalities and the evidence for their efficacy in the treatment of pain. The article does not include a discussion of exercise therapy as a treatment for painful conditions despite the fact that most pain specialists view exercise therapy as extremely valuable for chronic pain patients. This omission reflects my assumption that physiatrists are well versed in exercise therapy.

The articles by Dugowson and Gnanashanmugam, Sullivan and Robinson, Meleger, and Bloodworth deal with pharmacologic agents for the management of pain, including anti-inflammatories, antidepressants, anticonvulsants, muscle relaxants, and opiates. Multiple articles are directed toward pharmacologic therapies because physicians involved in pain management need to have a good grasp of the pros and cons of the many medications that may be helpful in controlling pain.

The article by Osborne and colleagues discusses a range of psychologic therapies that have been developed for this purpose. The broad premise underlying these therapies is that patients who have chronic pain function better if they change behaviors related to their pain and develop appropriate coping strategies and beliefs regarding their pain.

The article by Stanos and Houle is the only article in the issue that focuses on pain rehabilitation. It describes multidisciplinary pain rehabilitation programs in which a variety of rehabilitative interventions are combined to maximize recovery among patients with refractory chronic pain.

The article by Simpson reviews complementary and alternative medicine approaches to the treatment of pain. Physicians who manage pain need to be familiar with these because many patients who have pain choose to undergo complementary and alternative medicine therapies, often in conjunction with allopathic treatments.

Whereas the articles by Dugowson and Gnanashanmugam, Sullivan and Robinson, Meleger, Bloodworth, Osborne and colleagues, Stanos and Houle, and Simpson deal with specific approaches to pain, the articles by Sherman and colleagues, and Borg-Stein focus on specific medical conditions that physiatrists are likely to treat. The article by Sherman and colleagues addresses pain in the context of traumatic brain injury (TBI). As the authors note, chronic pain is a common and vexing problem among TBI patients. Also, the dilemmas that a physician faces when choosing pain treatments for TBI patients are similar to those he/she must face when treating other patient populations with cognitive impairments. The article by Borg-Stein discusses the management of myofascial pain. Myofascial pain is important to physiatrists for two reasons. First, it is felt to have a high prevalence among patients with chronic pain as a primary problem or a secondary one. Second, physiatrists have historically played a major role in the elaboration of theories of myofascial pain and strategies to treat the condition.

What is not covered

This issue of the *Physical Medicine and Rehabilitation Clinics of North America* does not include any systematic discussion of the types of exercise therapy available for patients who have chronic pain or the settings in which exercise therapy might be used. This omission does not imply a disregard of exercise therapy on my part. In fact, I share the widely held view among pain specialists that exercise therapy is absolutely fundamental to effective rehabilitation for most patients who have chronic pain. Rather, the absence of an article on exercise therapy reflects my assumption that that physiatrists are familiar with exercise therapy and routinely try to activate their patients. Thus, this issue is devoted to options that the physiatrist has when patients continue to complain of disabling pain despite having undergone an appropriate trial of exercise therapy.

The issue also does not address therapies that are relevant only to narrow segments of the patient populations that physiatrists are likely to treat. For example, it does not contain a detailed discussion of pharmacologic therapies for migraine headache. Also, it does not include an article on injection therapies, such as facet neurotomies and epidural steroid injections, because these therapies are limited to patients who have spinal pain.

Finally, this issue does not contain a discussion of implantable devices, such as peripheral nerve stimulators, spinal cord stimulators, and intrathecal opiate pumps.

Prototypical cases

To promote continuity across the articles that comprise this issue of the *Physical Medicine and Rehabilitation Clinics of North America*, the authors have been asked to consider how their therapeutic approaches might be used in the treatment of four modal patients. Vignettes describing these patients are given below.

Case 1

A 19-year-old man was involved in an accident while driving a motorcycle. He was not wearing a helmet. He hit his head into a telephone pole during the accident and sustained a skull fracture with intracerebral bleed. He was comatose for 10 days afterward. He did not sustain any other significant injuries in the accident. After his coma resolved, he demonstrated significant cognitive difficulties, along with right-sided paresis and spasticity. He now reports diffuse pain in his right lower extremity. There is no obvious orthopedic reason for this. His right lower extremity pain is thought to be a neuropathic type of pain secondary to his brain injury, with some aggravation caused by his spasticity.

Case 2

A 70-year-old woman has been treated for diabetes mellitus for the past 10 years. She complains of burning pain in both feet. This is severe enough that she reports substantial limitations in her physical activities and severe disruption of her sleep. She has undergone electrodiagnostic testing that demonstrated abnormalities consistent with a diabetic polyneuropathy. The patient's general medical status is noteworthy in that she had a mild myocardial infarction 3 years ago, with subsequent angioplasty. Follow-up evaluations have shown normal left ventricular function and mild to moderate coronary artery stenosis. The patient has a history of hypertension that is adequately controlled with Lisinopril.

Case 3

A 35-year-old woman was rear ended in a motor vehicle accident 1 year ago. She initially complained of fairly diffuse posterior neck pain but reported no discomfort in her shoulder girdle, mid back, or low back and no symptoms suggesting a cervical radiculopathy. A cervical MRI scan was negative for a disk herniation or compromise of neural elements. The patient has been seen by an interventional pain physician, who suspected a facet arthropathy. However, diagnostic medial branch blocks to anesthetize the C5-5 and C6-7 facet joints produced no pain relief, and the interventional pain physician does not think he has more to offer the patient. Since the time of the accident, the patient's pain has gradually spread, so that it now involves essentially the entire spine. On examination, the patient seems to have trigger points involving the upper trapezius and levator scapulae muscles bilaterally. She reports tenderness in 14 of the 18 sites designated by the American College of Rheumatology for the diagnosis of fibromyalgia.

Case 4

A 34-year-old male roofer fell off a roof 1 year ago and sustained an L1 vertebral body fracture. There was no neurologic compromise. An orthopedist recommended against surgical management. The patient was treated conservatively with bracing for several weeks and then went through extensive physical therapy with only modest benefit. Radiographically, his condition stabilized, with no identifiable abnormality other than a 30% loss of height of the L1 vertebral body. He has undergone evaluation by an interventional pain physician. Diagnostic injections including medial branch blocks and discography at the thoracolumbar junction did not delineate any specific pain generator that might be a target for interventional therapy. The patient currently reports severe pain at the thoracolumbar junction. He has no symptoms in his lower extremities.

These cases were selected to represent musculoskeletal pain, neuropathic pain, and fibromyalgia. Complicating factors include cognitive disturbance (Case 1) and cardiovascular disease (Case 2).

As you read the articles in this issue, you will find frequent references to these cases. Also, you will note that most of the authors have amplified the thumbnail sketches given above. Their need to elaborate illustrates the fundamental fact that chronic pain is a product of multiple factors. Consequently, practitioners must go beyond basic medical data to decide how to treat these patients.

A final word

Many physicians find chronic pain difficult and emotionally challenging to treat. Their reticence reflects three basic facts about chronic pain. First, pain is a personal experience that cannot be fully confirmed by a physician or any other third party. Thus, a treating physician frequently experiences uncertainty about how to interpret a patient's pain complaints. This ambiguity becomes especially challenging if the patient demands high doses of opiates to control pain or reports a degree of incapacitation that seems to be excessive relative to the severity of the medical condition. Second, chronic pain reflects the combined influence of a wide range of biologic, psychological, and social factors. Thus, a physician who tries to understand the factors underlying a patient's pain complaints must have expertise in areas other than just the pathophysiology of injuries and diseases. Third, most of the commonly used treatments for chronic pain have not been validated in well-designed studies, and the treatments that have been validated generally demonstrate only modestly beneficial effects. As a result, a physician who treats chronic pain usually cannot practice evidence-based medicine and must be prepared to encounter frequent failures.

The material in this issue does not eliminate the above challenges. In particular, because the various therapeutic approaches described in this issue have essentially never been subjected to head-to-head comparisons, you will not find anything like a simple algorithm to follow when you treat your patients. What the articles do provide is a set of options, along with information about the scientific support for the options and the clinical settings where the options might be considered. Given the widespread gaps in our scientific knowledge regarding the treatment of chronic pain, the orchestration of specific therapies into a coherent treatment program for a chronic pain patient pain still depends on clinical judgment.

I would like to express my appreciation to Dr. George Kraft for asking me to edit this issue of the *Physical Medicine and Rehabilitation Clinics of North America* and to Molly Jay, who has provided the editorial support needed to bring the issue to print. I am especially appreciative of the efforts of the many researchers and clinicians who have taken time from their busy schedules to contribute to the issue. I believe that their cumulative efforts have resulted in an issue that provides conceptual clarity and practical tools for physiatrists.

James P. Robinson, MD, PhD
Department of Rehabilitation Medicine
University of Washington
1959 Pacific Street, Box 356044
Seattle, WA 98195, USA

E-mail address: jimrob@u.washington.edu

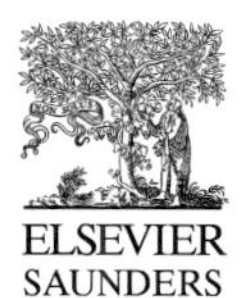
ELSEVIER
SAUNDERS

Phys Med Rehabil Clin N Am
17 (2006) 275–285

PHYSICAL MEDICINE
AND REHABILITATION
CLINICS OF
NORTH AMERICA

Pain in Patient Groups Frequently Treated by Physiatrists

Dawn M. Ehde, PhD*, Marisol A. Hanley, PhD

Department of Rehabilitation Medicine, University of Washington School of Medicine, Box 359740, 325 9th Avenue, Harborview Medical Center, Seattle, WA 98104-2499, USA

Pain is a common problem in persons seen by rehabilitation professionals. Pain may be the primary problem addressed in a rehabilitation setting (eg, musculoskeletal pain), or it may be secondary to other conditions or disabilities (eg, spinal cord injury). This article provides a summary of what is known concerning the scope and impact of chronic pain in rehabilitation populations. This article discusses some methodologic considerations and reviews the prevalence and impact of chronic pain in populations commonly seen by physiatrists and other rehabilitation professionals. This article focuses on the scope of chronic pain in rehabilitation populations that have received less attention in the empirical literature, including patients who have spinal cord injury, traumatic brain injury, multiple sclerosis (MS), and other disabilities. The impact of pain on individuals' functioning and participation in life is reviewed. Issues that affect our understanding of chronic pain in rehabilitation populations are discussed.

Conceptual and methodologic considerations

Before describing the scope of pain in rehabilitation populations, several methodologic and conceptual constraints of the relevant literature must be noted. In this article, we use the term "primary pain problem" to reflect

This article was supported by grant PO1 HD33988, from the National Institute of Child Health and Human Development, National Center for Medical Rehabilitation Research, NIH; grant H133B980017 from the Department of Education's National Institute of Disability and Rehabilitation Research (NIDRR); and CDC grant 1 R49 CE000483-01. Its contents are solely the responsibility of the authors and do not necessarily represent the official view of the NIH, NIDRR, or CDC.

* Corresponding author.

E-mail address: ehde@u.washington.edu (D.M. Ehde).

doi:10.1016/j.pmr.2005.12.009

conditions in which pain is the primary symptom of or defining factor for that disability. Examples of this include back pain, osteoarthritis, and complex regional pain syndrome. We also discuss secondary pain problems, which refers to pain secondary to or co-occurring with another disability, such as spinal cord injury, limb loss, or brain injury.

Although pain is thought to be relatively common among persons seen by physiatrists, there is variability in the literature on its incidence and prevalence. Pain varies in its prevalence based upon the type of disability being considered. Methodologic variability in the literature may also explain some of the discrepancies in rates of pain within various disability groups. For example, even within specific patient populations, studies often differ in the sources from which the samples were drawn (eg, hospital ward, clinic, community, consumer organizations) and in the sampling methodologies used (eg, random, convenience, consecutive cases). Population-based epidemiologic studies of the incidence and prevalence of pain in disability groups are rare, as are studies comparing the relative severity of pain problems in persons who have a disability with nonpatient populations. In addition, for most types of pain seen by rehabilitation professionals, there are few longitudinal studies describing the natural history of pain to guide clinical care or prognosis [1].

How pain is defined and measured varies markedly across studies. The MS pain literature illustrates this. In one community-based study [2], 44% of persons who had MS completing a mail survey were identified as having chronic pain only if they reported having "persistent, bothersome pain" for a 3-month period. This definition is much more restrictive than the definitions used in several other studies of pain in MS, which have used shorter time points, such as 1 month [3] (79% reported pain defined in this way) and different definitions, such as a categorization of "major" and "minor" pain used in one study [4] (42% had "major pain," 20% had "minor pain"). A number of studies [3,5–7] on MS pain have not described the specific questions or measures used to assess the prevalence of pain in their articles. Other studies of MS pain [8–11] excluded persons with headaches from their samples even though headaches and head pain may be secondary to MS disease processes [12]. In addition, acute and chronic pain is not always distinguished in the MS pain literature [13]. Although pain is a common condition in persons who have MS, the literature's considerable variability in samples, methods, and definitions regarding what constitutes pain make it difficult to draw definitive conclusions about the scope of the problem in this population. Similar limitations likely affect our understanding of pain in other rehabilitation patient groups besides MS.

Scope of chronic pain in rehabilitation populations

Pain is a common chronic health condition in the United States and other Western countries. For example, arthritis affects an estimated 21% of adults in the United States and has been described as a leading cause of disability in the United States [14]. The second leading cause of disability in the United States, back/spine problems, is also associated with pain [14]. Pain has been reported to be the most common presenting problem to primary care clinics [15,16]. Although we found no studies reporting the relative frequency with which pain is the primary presenting problem in rehabilitation clinics, given the nature of a physiatric practice, we presume it, too, is common.

Rehabilitation professionals commonly treat such conditions as regional complex pain syndrome, back pain, whiplash injuries, arthritis, and other problems where pain is the primary problem or complaint. The prevalence of these conditions is not reviewed in this article, given the large amount of literature available on these conditions and the focus on secondary pain in this article.

Pain is also a common problem in many adults with a primary disability such as spinal cord injury (SCI), burn injury, stroke, brain injury, and limb loss [1,17]. In some of these populations, an overwhelming number of persons experience pain. For example, as many as 70% to 80% of adults with SCI [1,18], 67% to 85% of adults with AMP [19,20], and 44% to 66% of adults with MS [2,13] report persistent, bothersome pain years after the onset of their disability. Many individuals with these conditions report pain in more than one pain location. The literature suggests that nearly one third of persons who have SCI and limb loss report severe pain [18,19]. Pain in individuals who have such disabilities may have a variety of causes (eg, neuropathic, musculoskeletal). Regardless of its etiology, pain has the potential to compound the disability associated with the disability itself.

The scope and nature of pain in young persons who have physical disabilities has been largely overlooked in the scientific literature [21]. The few studies that exist in this area suggest that pain may be a problem for many young people who have disabilities, including cerebral palsy (CP) [22], limb loss [23,24], and Duchenne muscular dystrophy [25]. Depending on the condition, a variety of factors may place young people with disabilities at risk for pain problems. For example, a recent review of pain in young people who have CP [22] highlighted not only some of the risk factors inherent to the condition (eg, contractures, spasticity, overuse syndromes, nerve entrapments, and orthopedic deformities) but also the frequent, and at times invasive, procedures (surgical, rehabilitative) that may contribute to pain. Further research on the nature, scope, and impact of pain in young persons who have disabilities is essential to improve their overall care.

Impact of chronic pain

The biopsychosocial model of chronic pain, while acknowledging that biological factors are central to the experience of pain, also suggests that the experience of chronic pain is influenced by the cognitive, affective, social, and behavioral domains of life [26]. A large body of literature bears out this hypothesis for primary pain conditions, and a growing number of studies has provided support for the biopsychosocial model in rehabilitation populations [27–31]. For example, Summers and colleagues [32] found that pain severity in persons who have SCI was more closely associated with emotional and cognitive factors than with physiologic factors, such as level of lesion, completeness of injury, and surgical fusion or instrumentation.

Pain interference and disability (general)

In persons who have physical disabilities, pain may present additional obstacles over and above the challenges directly associated with the physical disability. The challenges of pain related to a physical disability have been studied the most in SCI, limb loss, and MS, and to a lesser extent in neuromuscular disorders, CP, and post-polio syndrome. The major finding has been that pain often interferes significantly with life roles and activities, although pain may have a greater impact on some areas of life compared with others. For example, a study of adults who have neuromuscular disease ($n = 193$) found that pain seemed to have a significant impact on mobility, normal work, enjoyment of life, and recreational activities, whereas it had relatively little impact on self-care or relations with other people [33].

Pain may interfere more with daily functioning for some physical disabilities compared with others. Pain seems to have a major impact for a significant subgroup of individuals who have SCI. In one study, substantial subsamples (ranging from 33.6–38.3% of the total sample, $n = 217$) of individuals who had SCI reported that pain interfered with specific domains of life including sleep, exercise, household chores, work, and other daily activities [34]. A German study found that 23% of the sample reported that their daily routine was markedly or almost completely limited by pain [35]. A survey of community residents with SCI [19] found that the proportion of the sample with severe pain-related disability (20% with grade IV on the Chronic Pain Grade) was higher than for patients with headache or with back pain [36]. Similarly, significant subgroups of individuals who have MS report that pain interferes with daily life and activities [2,3,11,12]. One study of patients who had MS found that, of those who had chronic pain, 51% reported mild interference with daily activities, 29% reported moderate interference, and 20% reported severe interference [2]. In contrast, a study of persons who had CP and pain [27] found that patients reported only minor pain interference. Pain in CP seemed to cause less interference with life compared with persons who had SCI [37] or amputation [20], possibly due to a floor effect of the already low functional level for some persons who have CP [38].

Pain may be directly related to the injury or medical condition itself (eg, phantom limb pain after limb loss), or it may be indirectly related to the condition. For example, a person who has paraplegia may develop shoulder pain due to the need to propel a wheelchair. Similarly, a person with a lower limb amputation may develop back pain as a result, at least in part, of biomechanical changes necessitated by the use of a prosthesis for ambulation

[20]. Pain due to secondary or indirect consequences may interfere significantly with participation in activities and impede quality of life (QOL).

Pain interference in specific life roles

Pain may affect a person's ability to work, maintain social relationships, and fulfill other life roles. A survey of members of an SCI self-help association found that a significant number of those who were unemployed reported that pain, rather than paralysis, prevented them from working, and among those who were employed, 85% reported that pain interfered with work [39]. Similarly, studies of individuals who have MS have found that significant subgroups (49% of the sample in one study [7] and 57% in another [12]) report that pain reduced their ability to work or was associated with a greater number of days absent from school or work [40]. However, in other studies, rates of employment did not differ between those who reported pain and those who did not [2,7]. Pain in MS has also been shown to affect social relationships [7] and ability to fulfill roles such as spouse/partner, parent, and friend [12]. Consequences of pain in limb loss include a reduced likelihood of employment and social activities [41,42].

For persons who have physical disabilities, important daily activities may include participating in rehabilitation therapies. More research is needed to understand the impact of pain on rehabilitation, especially research that compares individuals who report pain with those who do not report pain. Pain has been shown to contribute to a decrease in physical performance in persons who have SCI [43] and has been shown to interfere with prosthetic training and walking ability in individuals who have experienced limb loss [44].

Pain interference and fatigue

For some physical disabilities, pain intensity, pain interference, and fatigue are closely linked. The relationship between pain and fatigue has been most thoroughly explored in MS because fatigue is a common and often debilitating symptom of this disease. In one study of persons who have MS, fatigue was the most commonly indicated response to the question asking which factors brought on pain or made it worse [7]. Other studies have found that increased fatigue in MS was significantly associated with higher intensity of pain [11] and greater pain interference [2]. However, these cross-sectional studies cannot determine if pain causes greater fatigue or vice versa; therefore, more research is needed to better understand this relationship in MS and to investigate it in other conditions.

Pain-related fear

Pain may affect functioning directly, or it may influence behavior through mediating variables such as pain-related fear. Living with chronic pain syndromes can be associated with higher levels of stress and anxiety. Pain-related fear has been examined in samples of persons with chronic back pain [45], osteoarthritis [46], and other musculoskeletal pain problems [45] and has been found to be associated with perceived disability [45]. These studies suggest that fear of pain may lead to activity avoidance and resultant physical deconditioning, which may result in greater pain over time. Preliminary evidence supports the significant role of pain-related fear in persons with physical disabilities. For example, in persons who have SCI, fear of activity-related increases in pain was significantly associated with lower observed performance [47]. Individuals whop have intermittent pain episodes, such as some persons with phantom limb pain or residual limb pain after limb loss, may experience anxiety related to their anticipation of the next pain episode. In addition, some individuals who have lower limb loss experience a fear of falling that might increase their general muscle tension. The effects of stress over time and increased muscle tension may exacerbate the perception of pain. We do not know if findings on pain-related fear are applicable to all types of pain problems encountered in rehabilitation settings, but it seems worthwhile to further explore pain-related fear and its impact on rehabilitation goals.

Depression/mental health/QOL impact

The impact of pain on mental health and QOL has been demonstrated for several types of physical disabilities. In persons who have limb loss, a longer duration of amputation-related pain has been associated with increased levels of psychological distress [48], and, consistent with a biopsychosocial model, increases in depression, stress, and anxiety have been associated with intensified PLP episodes [49]. Adults who have CP and pain have been shown to report more dissatisfaction with life and lower mental health scores compared with national norms [50]. Persons who have pain and neuromuscular disorders report significantly poorer QOL relative to national norms [33].

Several studies of physical disabilities have compared subgroups of individuals who have pain with those who do not report pain, providing additional evidence for the impact of pain above and beyond the impact of the disability itself. In several studies of persons who have limb loss, those who experienced pain were more likely to report depressive symptoms [51], anxiety [52], and poorer QOL [53] compared with those who did not report pain. Several studies of individuals who have MS found that those who had pain had significantly poorer mental health compared with those who had no pain [2,12] and that pain severity was a significant predictor of depression [54]; however, other studies found no differences in mental health between pain and no-pain groups [10,55].

The causal relationship between pain and depression is unclear, although several studies support the conclusion that changes in pain intensity in persons with physical disabilities may affect depressive symptoms more than changes in depression affect pain intensity [56,57] and that the relationship between pain and depression may strengthen over time. For example, in persons who have SCI, those who reported increasing pain interference from year 1 to year 2 after injury tended to have lower QOL scores (especially in the domains of overall life satisfaction and mental health) at year 2. In contrast, self-reported QOL tended to increase among those with decreasing pain interference from year 1 to year 2 [57].

Issues that may affect the identification and understanding of persons with chronic pain and disability

What is the impact of cognitive or communication impairments on our understanding and assessment of pain in persons who have disabilities?

Cognitive or communication impairments can occur in some disability conditions associated with pain, such as MS, CP, stroke, and traumatic brain injury. Little research exists concerning the impact of cognitive and communication impairments on pain research, assessment, and treatment. In our experience, the assessment of pain and conduction of pain research in individuals who have such impairments is feasible but at times requires accommodations to mitigate these impairments' effects. For example, in our Program Project research, we have used a number of strategies, such as in-person interviews, collateral interviews, multi-modality assessments, and assistive communication devices to assess pain and deliver pain interventions in persons with cognitive or communication impairments; some of these are described elsewhere [38,50,58]. More research is needed on the reliability and validity of pain measures in groups who have cognitive or communication impairments. Additionally, further research is needed regarding appropriate accommodations for treating and studying pain when cognitive or communication impairments are present.

Is chronic pain any different in rehabilitation populations than in primary pain populations?

Whether chronic pain as a condition secondary to disability is experienced differently than chronic pain as the primary condition remains an open question. Because pain is a uniquely personal experience [59], there is no way to know if the sensation of pain is experienced differently across individuals, pain populations, or types of pain. It seems like a safe conclusion, however, that there may be unique needs in rehabilitation populations, and pain treatment may need to be integrated into various rehabilitation therapies. In addition, a pain problem may not be the only problem or even the most pressing problem when weighed against other concerns, such as mobility issues or bowel/bladder control. It is possible that functional limitations and pain may influence the type of coping strategies that people who have disabilities can use. For example, active coping strategies have been consistently associated with better outcomes [60] and tend to be strongly encouraged in multidisciplinary pain programs, but people who have disabilities may be limited in the extent to which they can make use of certain active coping strategies, such as exercise and increased activity. One study found that persons who have CP and pain, compared with persons who have nondisability-related chronic pain, were less likely to use physical coping strategies and more likely to use cognitive strategies, such as diverting attention and reinterpreting pain sensations [27]. This issue may warrant further exploration to design interventions appropriate for promoting coping in persons with functional limitations or to adapt coping interventions for persons who have progressive conditions, such as MS.

What is the relevance of the biopsychosocial model for understanding pain in rehabilitation populations?

In understanding pain in rehabilitation patients, it is important to consider carefully the biological causes for or contributors to pain. For some patients and some conditions, assessing and treating pain at the biological level may be sufficient. However, in many cases, conceptualizing pain from a broader biopsychosocial model may increase one's understanding of the problem and offer additional targets for treatment. Pain has the potential to affect psychosocial functioning, and there is growing evidence that psychosocial variables may affect pain severity and adjustment to pain. Certain coping responses, such as resting and catastrophizing, have been shown to be predictive of poorer adjustment to pain in several different samples of persons who have disabilities, including CP [27], SCI [47], and limb loss [28,29]. More research, especially longitudinal research, is needed to better understand the multidirectional relationships among pain, biological factors, and psychosocial functioning.

Summary

This article highlights the significant prevalence and impact of pain in persons who have disabilities and points to the need for additional research in this area. Theory-driven research examining biopsychosocial models of and treatments for chronic pain are the important next steps in this area. The extensive literature on persons in whom pain is the primary disability provides a useful basis for such research. Pain may be one of several problems facing rehabilitation professionals in their care of persons with disabilities. Nonetheless, given the suffering associated with it, pain warrants careful assessment and, as indicated, intervention.

References

[1] Ehde DM, Jensen MP, Engel JM, et al. Chronic pain secondary to disability: a review. Clin J Pain 2003;19:3–17.

[2] Ehde DM, Gibbons LE, Chwastiak L, et al. Chronic pain in a large community sample of persons with multiple sclerosis. Mult Scler 2003;9:605–11.
[3] Svendsen KB, Jensen TS, Overvad K, et al. Pain in patients with multiple sclerosis: a population-based study. Arch Neurol 2003;60:1089–94.
[4] Goodin DS. Survey of multiple sclerosis in northern California. Northern California MS Study Group. Mult Scler 1999;5:78–88.
[5] Kassirer MR, Osterberg DH. Pain in chronic multiple sclerosis. J Pain Symptom Manage 1987;2:95–7.
[6] Rae-Grant AD, Eckert NJ, Bartz S, et al. Sensory symptoms of multiple sclerosis: a hidden reservoir of morbidity. Mult Scler 1999;5:179–83.
[7] Warnell P. The pain experience of a multiple sclerosis population: a descriptive study. Axone 1991;13:26–8.
[8] Solaro C, Brichetto G, Amato MP, et al. The prevalence of pain in multiple sclerosis: a multicenter cross-sectional study. Neurology 2004;63:919–21.
[9] Moulin DE, Foley KM, Ebers GC. Pain syndromes in multiple sclerosis. Neurology 1988;38:1830–4.
[10] Indaco A, Iachetta C, Nappi C, et al. Chronic and acute pain syndromes in patients with multiple sclerosis. Acta Neurol (Napoli) 1994;16:97–102.
[11] Beiske AG, Pedersen ED, Czujko B, et al. Pain and sensory complaints in multiple sclerosis. Eur J Neurol 2004;11:479–82.
[12] Archibald CJ, McGrath PJ, Ritvo PG, et al. Pain prevalence, severity and impact in a clinic sample of multiple sclerosis patients. Pain 1994;58:89–93.
[13] Ehde D, Osborne TL, Jensen MP. Chronic pain in persons with multiple sclerosis. Phys Med Rehabil Clin N Am 2005;16:503–12.
[14] CDC. Prevalence of disabilities and associated health conditions among adults-United States, 1999. Morb Mortal Wkly Rep 2001;50:120–5.
[15] Turk DC, Melzack R, editors. Handbook of pain assessment. 2nd ed. New York: Guilford Press; 2001.
[16] Deyo AR. Low-back pain. Sci Am 1998;1998:48–53.
[17] Benrud-Larson LM, Wegener ST. Chronic pain in neurorehabilitation populations: prevalence, severity, and impact. Neuro Rehabilitation 2000;14:127–37.
[18] Turner JA, Cardenas DD, Warms CA, et al. Chronic pain associated with spinal cord injuries: a community survey. Arch Phys Med Rehabil 2001;82:501–9.
[19] Ehde DM, Czerniecki JM, Smith DG, et al. Chronic phantom sensations, phantom pain, residual limb pain, and other regional pain after lower limb amputation. Arch Phys Med Rehabil 2000;81:1039–44.
[20] Czerniecki JM, Ehde DM. Chronic pain after lower extremity amputation. Crit Rev Phys Med Rehabil 2003;15:309–32.
[21] Engel JM. Physical therapy and occupational therapy for pain management in children. Child Adolesc Psychiatr Clin N Am 1997;6:817–28.
[22] McKearnan KA, Kieckhefer GM, Engel JM, et al. Pain in children with cerebral palsy: a review. J Neurosci Nurs 2004;36:252–9.
[23] Krane EJ, Heller LB. The prevalence of phantom sensation and pain in pediatric amputees. J Pain Symptom Manage 1995;10:21–9.
[24] Wilkins KL, McGrath PJ, Finley GA, et al. Phantom limb sensations and phantom limb pain in child and adolescent amputees. Pain 1998;78:7–12.
[25] Engel JM, Kartin D, Jaffe KM. Exploring chronic pain in youths with duchenne muscular dystrophy: a model for pediatric neuromuscular disease. Phys Med Rehabil Clin N Am 2005;16:1113–24.
[26] Novy DM, Nelson DV, Francis DJ, et al. Perspectives of chronic pain: an evaluative comparison of restrictive and comprehensive models. Psychol Bull 1995;118:238–47.
[27] Engel JM, Schwartz L, Jensen MP, et al. Pain in cerebral palsy: the relation of coping strategies to adjustment. Pain 2000;88:225–30.

[28] Hanley MA, Jensen MP, Ehde DM, et al. Psychosocial predictors of long-term adjustment to lower-limb amputation and phantom limb pain. Disabil Rehabil 2004;26:882–93.

[29] Jensen MP, Ehde DM, Hoffman AJ, et al. Cognitions, coping and social environment predict adjustment to phantom limb pain. Pain 2002;95:133–42.

[30] Turner JA, Jensen MP, Warms CA, et al. Catastrophizing is associated with pain intensity, psychological distress, and pain-related disability among individuals with chronic pain after spinal cord injury. Pain 2002;98:127–34.

[31] Hill A, Niven CA, Knussen C. The role of coping in adjustment to phantom limb pain. Pain 1995;62:79–86.

[32] Summers JD, Rapoff MA, Varghese G, et al. Psychosocial factors in chronic spinal cord injury pain [see comments]. Pain 1991;47:183–9.

[33] Jensen MP, et al. Chronic pain in persons with neuromuscular disease. Arch Phys Med Rehabil 2005;86:1155–63.

[34] Widerstrom-Noga EG, Felipe-Cuervo E, Yezierski RP. Chronic pain after spinal injury: interference with sleep and daily activities. Arch Phys Med Rehabil 2001;82:1571–7.

[35] Stormer S, Gerner HJ, Gruninger W, et al. Chronic pain/dysaesthesiae in spinal cord injury patients: results of a multicentre study. Spinal Cord 1997;35:446–55.

[36] Von Korff M, Ormel J, Keefe FJ, et al. Grading the severity of chronic pain. Pain 1992;50:133–49.

[37] Turner JA, Cardenas DD. Chronic pain problems in individuals with spinal cord injuries. Semin Clin Neuropsychiatry 1999;4:186–94.

[38] Schwartz L, Engel JM, Jensen MP. Pain in persons with cerebral palsy. Arch Phys Med Rehabil 1999;80:1243–6.

[39] Rose M, Robinson JE, Ells P, et al. Pain following spinal cord injury: results from a postal survey. Pain 1988;34(1):101–2.

[40] Vickrey BG, Hays RD, Harooni R, et al. A health-related quality of life measure for multiple sclerosis. Qual Life Res 1995;4:187–206.

[41] Millstein S, Bain D, Hunter GA. A review of employment patterns of industrial amputees–factors influencing rehabilitation. Prosthet Orthot Int 1985;9:69–78.

[42] Pezzin LE, Dillingham TR, MacKenzie EJ. Rehabilitation and the long-term outcomes of persons with trauma-related amputations. Arch Phys Med Rehabil 2000;81:292–300.

[43] Te R, et al. Psychosocial predictors of physical performance in disabled individuals with chronic pain. Clin J Pain 2003;19:18–30.

[44] Carabelli RA, Kellerman WC. Phantom limb pain: relief by application of TENS to contralateral extremity. Arch Phys Med Rehabil 1985;66(7):466–7.

[45] Vlaeyen JW, Linton SJ. Fear-avoidance and its consequences in chronic musculoskeletal pain: a state of the art. Pain 2000;85:317–32.

[46] Heuts P, et al. Pain-related fear and daily functioning in patients with osteoarthritis. Pain 2004;110:228–35.

[47] Rudy TE, Lieber SJ, Boston JR, et al. Psychosocial predictors of physical performance in disabled individuals with chronic pain. Clin J Pain 2003;19:18–30.

[48] Hill A. The use of pain coping strategies by patients with phantom limb pain. Pain 1993;55: 347–53.

[49] Arena JG, Sherman RA, Bruno GM, et al. The relationship between situational stress and phantom limb pain: cross-lagged correlational data from six month pain logs. J Psychosom Res 1990;34:71–7.

[50] Engel JM, Jensen MP, Hoffman AJ, et al. Pain in persons with cerebral palsy: extension and cross-validation. Arch Phys Med Rehabil 2003;84:1125–8.

[51] Sherman RA, Sherman CJ, Bruno GM. Psychological factors influencing chronic phantom limb pain: an analysis of the literature. Pain 1987;28:285–95.

[52] Sherman RA, Sherman CJ, Parker L. Chronic phantom and stump pain among American veterans: results of a survey. Pain 1984;18:83–95.

[53] van der Schans CP, Geertzen JH, Schoppen T, et al. Phantom pain and health-related quality of life in lower limb amputees. J Pain Symptom Manage 2002;24(4):429–36.

[54] Sullivan MJL, Edgley K, Mikail S, et al. Psychological correlates of health care utilization in chronic illness. Can J Rehabil 1992;6:13–21.

[55] Stenager E, Knudsen L, Jensen K. Acute and chronic pain syndromes in multiple sclerosis. Acta Neurol Scand 1991;84:197–200.

[56] Cairns DM, Adkins RH, Scott MD. Pain and depression in acute traumatic spinal cord injury: origins of chronic problematic pain? Arch Phys Med Rehabil 1996;77(4):329–35.

[57] Putzke JD, Richards JS, Hicken BL, et al. Interference due to pain following spinal cord injury: important predictors and impact on quality of life. Pain 2002;100:231–42.

[58] Ehde D, Jensen MP. Feasibility of a cognitive restructuring intervention for treatment of chronic pain in persons with disabilities. Rehabil Psychol 2003;49:254–8.

[59] Dudgeon BJ, Gerrard BC, Jensen MP, et al. Physical disability and the experience of chronic pain. Arch Phys Med Rehabil 2002;83:229–35.

[60] Boothby JL, Thorn BE, Stroud MW, et al. Coping with pain. In: Gatchel RJ, Turk DC, editors. Psychosocial factors in pain. New York: The Guilford Press; 1999. p. 343–59.

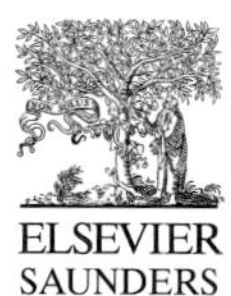

ELSEVIER
SAUNDERS

Phys Med Rehabil Clin N Am
17 (2006) 287–302

PHYSICAL MEDICINE
AND REHABILITATION
CLINICS OF
NORTH AMERICA

Central Hypersensitivity in Chronic Pain: Mechanisms and Clinical Implications

Michele Curatolo, MD, PhD[a,*],
Lars Arendt-Nielsen, PhD[b],
Steen Petersen-Felix, MD, PhD[a]

[a]*Department of Anesthesiology, Division of Pain Therapy, Inselspital, 3010 Bern, Switzerland*
[b]*Center for Sensory-Motor Interaction, The University of Aalborg, Fr. Bajers Vej 7D3, 9220 Aalborg, Denmark*

In the last two decades, animal studies have consistently demonstrated the occurrence of profound changes in the central nervous system (CNS) after peripheral injury. These changes are responsible for enhanced neuronal excitability and enhanced pain [1]. Studies in healthy volunteers have shown that experimentally induced peripheral injury or inflammation determines exaggerated pain response, which results from increased excitability of the CNS (ie, central hypersensitivity) [2]. Chronic pain patients display features of central hypersensitivity, as demonstrated by several clinical investigations [3–6].

The purposes of this article are (1) to provide insights into the mechanisms underlying central hypersensitivity, (2) to review the published evidence on the presence of central hypersensitivity in chronic pain, (3) to highlight reflections on the possible clinical relevance of central hypersensitivity, and (4) to offer a perspective of possible prevention and treatment of central hypersensitivity. This article represents an update of our previous article on central hypersensitivity in patients who have chronic pain after whiplash injury [7]. Here, the scope is enlarged to include chronic pain conditions in general.

Mechanisms of central hypersensitivity

This section presents the preclinical evidence on the presence and mechanisms of central hyperexcitability and neuronal plasticity.

* Corresponding author.
E-mail address: michele.curatolo@insel.ch (M. Curatolo).

doi:10.1016/j.pmr.2005.12.010

Peripheral sensitization

Tissue injury leads to an inflammatory response with release of potassium ions, substance P, bradykinin, prostaglandins, and other substances [8]. These substances may induce a sensitization of peripheral receptors with changes in the response characteristics of primary afferent fibers [9]. They may activate normally inactive or "silent" nociceptors [10]. Bradykinin reduces the activation threshold of heat nociceptors, an effect that is mediated by cyclooxygenase products [11]. The sensitized nociceptors can then be activated at normal body temperature, which can explain spontaneous inflammatory pain [12]. The inflammatory response induces gene expression in the dorsal root ganglion, resulting in an increased synthesis of peripheral receptors, which contributes to the increased sensitivity of the nociceptor [13]. After long-lasting nociceptive stimulation, Aβ-fibers may start synthesizing receptors that are normally found only in C-fibers, thereby simulating a phenotype shift, with the Aβ-fiber adopting C-fiber characteristics [14]. These sensitizing events mediate primary hyperalgesia (ie, a reduced threshold for eliciting pain and enhanced pain to suprathreshold stimuli within the injured area) [15]. Peripheral sensitization results in an increased nociceptive input to the spinal cord.

Peripheral sensitization can be induced experimentally in healthy volunteers by topical capsaicin [16]. Capsaicin acts at the vanilloid receptor, an excitatory ion channel expressed by nociceptors, which contributes to the detection and integration of pain-producing chemical and thermal stimuli [17].

Spinal cord plasticity

Prolonged afferent nociceptive input may induce a reversible increase in the excitability of central sensory neurons [1], mostly via activation of the N-methyl D-aspartate (NMDA) receptor [18,19]. Activation of NMDA receptors is linked to expression of cyclooxygenase-2 (COX-2) in the spinal cord, and there is evidence that COX-2 inhibitors prevent central sensitization in the animal [20]. COX-2 expression is not confined to the neural structures connected to the site of inflammation but involves the whole spinal cord and the supraspinal centers [21]. This phenomenon seems to be mediated by humoral factors rather than by neural transmission of the peripheral input into the spinal cord [21]. It may be responsible, at least in part, for a generalized hypersensitivity to peripheral stimulation such that pain is experienced in response to stimulation of tissues that are at a distance from the site of injury.

An expansion of the receptive field (the cutaneous area that, when stimulated, elicits a response from a single spinal neuron) of individual dorsal horn neurons has been documented [22]. Afferent input from areas adjacent to the normal receptive field may be able to depolarize the hyperexcitable dorsal horn neuron. As a result, a peripheral stimulus activates a higher number of dorsal horn neurons, and hyperalgesia may also be evoked in areas outside the injured region. A method to study receptive fields in humans using the withdrawal reflex after electrical stimulation of the foot sole has been recently developed [23]. A first clinical study has shown expansion of receptive fields in persons who have spinal cord injury, probably as a result of loss of inhibitory descending control or increased sensitivity of the spinal reflex loop (Fig. 1) [23].

The glial cells, which were earlier regarded as purely supportive, have become implicated in exaggerated pain states [24]. They may be activated by peripheral injury and can contribute to central hyperexcitability.

Additional profound structural changes include destruction of inhibitory interneurons and aberrant excitatory connections [1]. Destruction of inhibitory interneurons, which has been observed after nerve injury, contributes to hyperexcitability and is prevented by NMDA-antagonists [25]. After nerve injury, Aβ-fibers that normally terminate in the deep dorsal horn may sprout to establish functional synaptic contacts in superficial dorsal horn layers where nociceptive C-fibers terminate [26]. This is one of the possible explanations for the induction of pain sensations after stimulation of Aβ-fibers by innocuous stimulation, such as light touch (allodynia). Peripheral nerve injury induces upregulation of the calcium channel alpha-2-delta subunit at the dorsal root ganglion and postsynaptically in the spinal dorsal

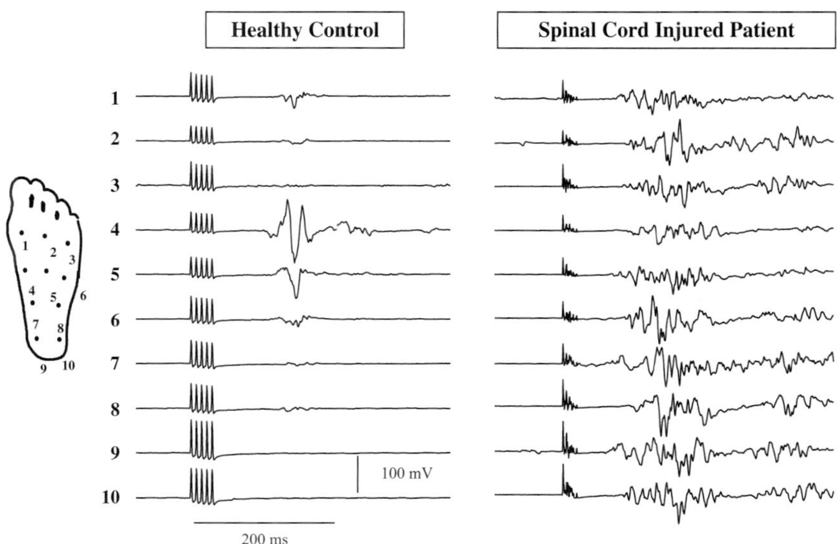

Fig. 1. Receptive field model used in a study on patients who have spinal cord injury. The figure shows the results in one healthy control subject and a patient. Ten electrodes were applied at the sole of the foot (left drawing), and the electromyographic response at the muscle tibialis anterior after electrical stimulation of each site at an intensity of 1.4 times the reflex threshold is shown. In the healthy subject, the reflex was elicited after stimulation of only two sites (4 and 5); in the patient, the reflex could be evoked by stimulating the whole foot sole. This indicates expansion of the reflex receptive fields. (Courtesy of Lars Arendt-Nielsen, Aalborg, Denmark.)

horn, which is associated with development and maintenance of allodynia [27].

Nerve injury also produces depression of the inhibitory mechanisms within the spinal cord (ie, reduction in the concentration of gamma-aminobutyric acid [GABA]), a decrease in the number of GABA- and opioid receptors, and an increase in the concentration of cholecystokinin, with consequent amplification of the nociceptive signal being transmitted to higher centers [28].

Supraspinal modulation

Spinal cord hyperexcitability elicited by trauma, inflammation, or surgery is influenced by descending facilitatory and inhibitory pathways [29]. Most of the research on this issue has focused on descending inhibition. The periaqueductal gray and endogenous opioid peptides play a central role in the inhibition of spinal cord neuronal responses [30]. Noxious stimulation induces the release of encephalin, an endogenous opioid, at supraspinal and spinal levels [31,32]. Further inhibitory modulation is exerted by serotonergic [33] and noradrenergic descending systems [34,35].

The clinician is frequently confronted with the hypothesis that psychological mechanisms may be responsible for pain amplification. Therefore, pain facilitation may have high clinical relevance. Recently, some of the mechanisms involved in descending facilitation have been clarified. Earlier research on brain modulation of pain concentrated on descending inhibitory pathways. However, the descending facilitatory pathways may be important in maintaining hyperexcitability [36]. Serotonin seems to be involved in descending inhibition and facilitation of pain. There is evidence that the increase in pain sensitivity after peripheral tissue damage is regulated by neurokinin-1–expressing neurons within the spinal cord that project to higher brain areas [37]. After receiving information from these spinal cord neurons, the involved brain areas activate descending pathways that excite 5-hydroxytryptamine-3 (5-HT3) receptors in the spinal cord. This 5-HT3 activation contributes to spinal cord hyperexcitability [38]. Such a spino-brain-spinal loop includes areas of the brain involved in emotional and affective responses to pain [37]. These data provide additional explanation for the widespread pain hypersensitivity after peripheral lesion, a common phenomenon in chronic pain patients [5,39]. The activity of these pathways involving the 5-HT3 receptors could be driven by anxiety and fear, which are frequently observed in pain patients. These data may represent the physiologic basis for an amplification of the pain experience in patients who have psychologic distress. Furthermore, these findings explain the analgesic effect of inhibitors of the 5-HT3 receptor, such as ondansetron or tropisetron, in chronic pain states in humans [40,41].

There is clear evidence that tissue trauma or inflammation leads to a reversible increase in the excitability of the CNS through regional neuronal and systemic humoral mechanisms. Potentially irreversible changes have been documented, particularly after nerve injury. The peripheral sensitization and the hyperexcitability of dorsal horn neurons reduce the threshold for eliciting Aδ- and C-fiber pain. Aβ-fiber–transmitted mechanical stimuli, which do not produce pain under normal conditions, may activate the hyperexcitable dorsal horn neurons, ultimately resulting in pain sensation (allodynia) [1,42]. These alterations are likely to substantially contribute to persisting pain.

Central hypersensitivity in chronic pain patients

Methods to investigate central hypersensitivity in patients

In patients, direct measurements of activity in spinal cord or brain neurons cannot be made. Therefore, it is impossible to provide direct evidence for neuronal hyperexcitability. However, hypersensitivity can be investigated indirectly by quantitative sensory tests. Typically, a standardized and quantifiable sensory stimulus is applied at a peripheral tissue. The stimulus intensity is increased gradually until the subject perceives the stimulus as painful. The intensity at which the stimulus perception turns to pain is defined as the pain detection threshold. The intensity at which the pain is perceived as intolerable is defined as the pain tolerance threshold. Alternatively, a standardized painful stimulus is applied, and the intensity of the evoked pain is recorded. Using these methods, hypersensitivity is detected when sensory stimulation evokes pain at stimulus intensities that do not induce pain in normal subjects (lower pain threshold) or when a standardized painful stimulus evokes stronger pain in patients than in normal subjects. An additional possibility is to study the map of the pain areas after intramuscular injection of a painful substance (eg, hypertonic saline) (Fig. 2) [43]. Other methods to explore the sensory system are available, but a detailed description is beyond the scope of this article. The interested reader can find more information in review articles [44,45].

Considering the methods described in this article, a central question is whether hypersensitivity to sensory stimulation is the result of peripheral or central mechanisms. Peripheral sensitization is limited to the site of injury or inflammation. At this level, quantitative sensory tests cannot distinguish peripheral from central hypersensitivity. However, whenever pain hypersensitivity is observed after sensory stimulation of healthy areas, its cause must be a hyperexcitability of the CNS (central hypersensitivity). There is no evidence that peripheral mechanisms could account for higher pain sensitivity in healthy tissues. Therefore, it is generally accepted that sensory stimulation of healthy tissues explores the excitability state of the CNS.

Evidence for central hypersensitivity in chronic pain patients

There is consistent evidence that groups of patients who have chronic pain after whiplash injury have lower pain thresholds than groups of healthy

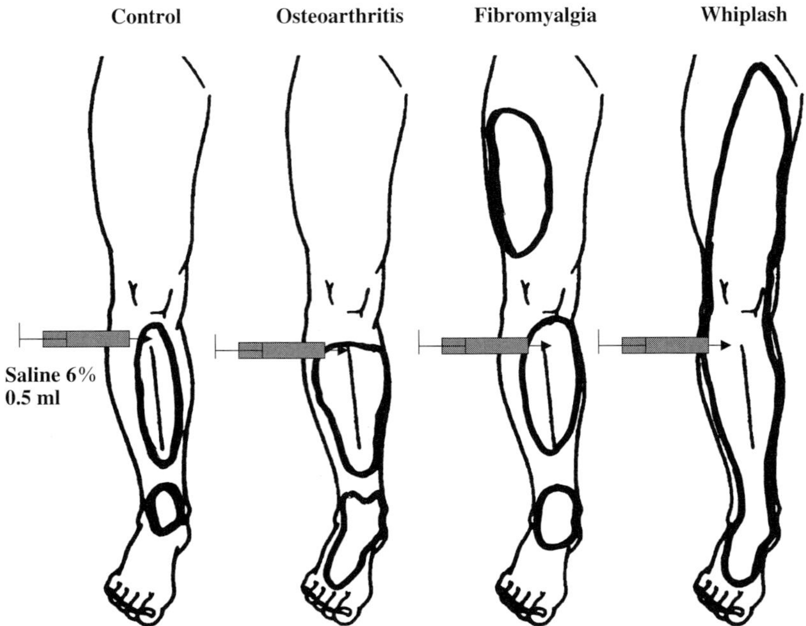

Fig. 2. Pain maps after intramuscular injection of hypertonic (6%) saline 0.5 mL into the tibial anterior muscles of individual subjects. Notice the wider areas of referred pain in patients compared with the healthy subject, strongly indicating central hypersensitivity. (Courtesy of Lars Arendt-Nielsen, Aalborg, Denmark.)

subjects [39,46–48]. The absence of tissue damage at the site of testing (eg, the leg in patients suffering from neck pain) suggests central sensitization of nociceptive pathways as the cause of the pain hypersensitivity. Whiplash patients and patients who have other chronic pain syndromes display a spread of pain sensation to much wider body areas after intramuscular injection of hypertonic saline compared with healthy control subjects, which strongly suggests central hypersensitivity [5,47,49]. The results of psychophysical studies were confirmed by electrophysiologic investigations that provided objective evidence for spinal cord hypersensitivity in whiplash and fibromyalgia patients [3,50]. The presence of generalized hyperalgesia 1 month after a whiplash injury seems to be a predictor of persistence of symptoms 6 months after the trauma [51]. It is unclear whether central hypersensitivity is per se a determinant of poor recovery, independent of the severity of the primary tissue lesion. Sensory abnormalities are not the only predictors of persistence of symptoms: Initial disability, older age, and psychologic distress seem to be associated with poor recovery [52].

The trapezius region has a lower pain threshold than the region of the anterior tibia muscle and a lower threshold for repeated stimulation inducing short-lasting pain hypersensitivity (temporal summation) [53]. This may explain the high frequency of chronic pain at the neck and shoulder region in that the stimulus threshold to induce pain and related central plasticity changes may be lower in these than in other body areas. Additional regional pain syndromes in which central hypersensitivity has been documented are osteoarthritis [5], tension-type headache [54], temporomandibular joint pain [55], pain in endometriosis [6] and postmastectomy pain [56]. Central hypersensitivity has also been observed in patients who have fibromyalgia [3,49,50], a poorly understood pain syndrome in which a disturbance of the central processing of sensory input is increasingly accepted as at least one of the pathophysiologic mechanisms explaining symptoms.

Taken together, the evidence shows that patients who have various types of chronic pain display pain hypersensitivity after sensory stimulation of healthy tissues, most likely resulting from an alteration of the central processing of sensory input. The central hypersensitivity is not confined to the areas of the CNS that are connected to the painful region; it is probably generalized. Central hypersensitivity is probably a common feature of all chronic pain syndromes.

Determinants of central hypersensitivity in chronic pain patients

It is impossible to perform direct measurements of CNS activity in patients. Most of the explanations of chronic pain are based on animal data and surrogate assessments on healthy volunteers or patients. This approach has limitations. First, in basic research it is possible to perform assessments before and after an injury or the onset of inflammation. Therefore, changes of the assessed outcomes can be attributed to the induced noxious event. Conversely, the cause–effect relationship between a peripheral lesion and exaggerated pain responses cannot be established in patients with certainty because there is no recording of the sensory function before appearance of the lesion. The possibility that the low pain thresholds recorded in patients were also present in the same individuals before the peripheral event cannot be ruled out. Second, studies on experimentally induced central hypersensitivity, in animals or in healthy volunteers, cannot reproduce the complexity of the pain experience in patients. Third, unlike chronic pain, experimentally induced nociception is of short duration. Therefore, the pathophysiology of hypersensitivity states in patients is likely to differ substantially from the one evoked experimentally. Despite these limitations, most data from basic research are consistent with phenomena observed in patients and reasonably explain many of the abnormal pain responses typical of chronic pain.

Tissue damage

Trauma-induced tissue damage can determine the neuronal plasticity changes that underlie central hypersensitivity. An important question arises: Can central hypersensitivity persist after resolution of tissue damage and explain chronic pain? Or rather, is it the case that central hypersensitivity amplifies nociception from a diseased tissue but disappears after injury heals and no nociceptive input arrives at the spinal cord? It is difficult to address this question in patients, mainly because it is impossible to rule out peripheral damage with certainty even using advanced diagnostic tools.

In certain circumstances, it can be stated that central hypersensitivity disappears or loses clinical relevance when the nociceptive input from the diseased tissue is blocked distal to the spinal cord. This is the case of regional pain syndromes that can be treated effectively by peripheral interventions. For instance, radiofrequency lesion of the nerves that supply the zygapophysial joints produces complete pain relief in patients with zygapophysial joint pain [57], indicating that tissue damage is the most important determinant of the pain complaints in these patients. Because central hypersensitivity is present in whiplash patients [3], it can be argued that it amplified pain arising from the peripheral focus but was not the primary determinant of pain. In a study on painful osteoarthritis of the hip [58], abnormally low pain thresholds normalized after surgery, indicating that central hypersensitivity was maintained by chronic nociceptive pain. On the other hand, hyperalgesia of the skin of patients who have pain caused by renal or ureteral calculosis normalized after removal of the calculi, but hyperalgesia of subcutaneous and muscular tissues did not completely normalize, indicating persisting neuroplasticity changes [59]. The clinical relevance of this possible persisting hyperalgesia despite successful pain treatment remains uncertain. Infiltration of tender points in patients who have neck pain after whiplash injury affected central hypersensitivity detected at areas close to the site of pain but not at areas distant to it (the leg) in the short term [60]. These results suggest that different mechanisms underlie hyperalgesia localized at areas surrounding the site of injury and hyperalgesia generalized to distant body areas. Central hypersensitivity responsible for hyperalgesia at the neck may be a dynamic condition, modulated by changes in nociceptive input from the periphery. Conversely, short-term changes in nociceptive input may not affect generalized central hypersensitivity, which determines hyperalgesia at areas far distant from the neck. It can be hypothesized that expression of COX-2 in the whole CNS [21], cortical mechanisms, and activation of descending facilitatory pathways [37] may play an important role in the determination of generalized hypersensitivity and would not respond rapidly to changes in nociceptive input.

In summary, tissue damage is a determinant of central hypersensitivity in patients. Whether central hypersensitivity in the absence of peripheral damage is the cause of pain in patients remains uncertain.

Supraspinal modulation: psychologic factors

There is experimental support for the influence of cognitive and behavioral alterations on injury-induced central sensitization [29]. Furthermore, experimentally induced anxiety lowers pain thresholds [61]. Therefore, psychologic distress may have a role in the determination of central hypersensitivity in patients.

The possibility that central hypersensitivity has a pure psychogenic origin cannot be ruled out but has almost no experimental support. Central hypersensitivity may be the mechanism by which somatic and psychologic factors find their common neurobiologic correlate. We propose that tissue and nerve damage produce central hypersensitivity as a result of the plasticity of the CNS. The psychologic distress that results from the chronic pain condition contributes to central hypersensitivity, thereby producing further amplification of pain (Fig. 3).

Brain plasticity

Recent research has increasingly dealt with brain mechanisms of pain processing in humans. This is mostly the result of the availability of new brain imaging techniques, such as positron emission tomography [62], single photon emission tomography [63], and functional MRI [64]. A review of this research is beyond the scope of this article, but some important achievements obtained by using imaging methods deserve mention.

The cortical representation of body areas can undergo alteration. Reorganization of the cortical body map has been demonstrated in patients who have phantom limb pain [65], low back pain [66], and complex regional pain syndrome [67]. There is a strong correlation between extent of cortical reorganization and intensity of phantom limb pain [68]. Treating phantom limb pain with opioids can reduce the cortical reorganization [69].

Using MRI brain scan data, Apkarian and colleagues [70] have recently shown that chronic back pain is associated with decreased prefrontal and thalamic gray matter density. The magnitude of this decrease is equivalent to the gray matter volume lost in 10 to 20 years of normal aging. The decreased volume is related to pain duration, indicating a 1.3 cm^3 loss of gray matter for every year of chronic pain.

These phenomena suggest that profound plasticity changes can occur at high brain centers in chronic pain conditions, but their clinical implications, particularly in relation to hypersensitivity states, are unclear.

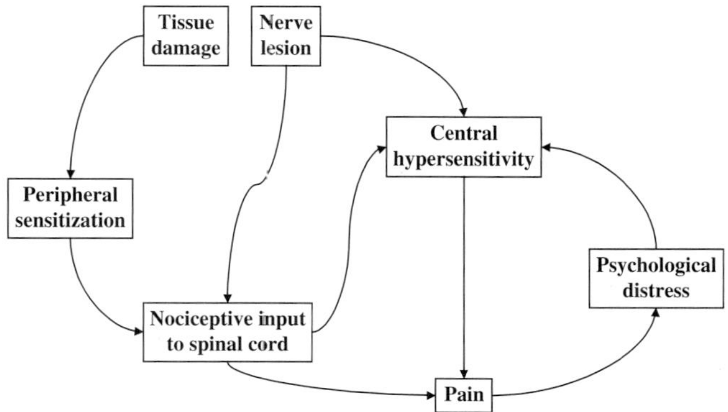

Fig. 3. Possible role of central hypersensitivity in the pathophysiology of chronic pain.

Therapeutic options

Theoretically, central hypersensitivity can be prevented or treated by the following approaches: (1) block or reduction of the nociceptive input from the injured areas, (2) specific pharmacologic intervention on the spinal cord mechanisms underlying central hypersensitivity, or (3) pharmacologic or psychologic interventions acting at a supraspinal level and the descending modulatory system.

Peripheral modulation

If ongoing nociceptive input from a diseased tissue is the main determinant of central hypersensitivity, interventions aiming at treating tissue damage or preventing nociceptive impulses from arriving at the spinal cord could also produce resolution of central hypersensitivity. However, with few exceptions [57], there is no way to provide a long-lasting block of peripheral nociceptive afferents in most chronic pain conditions. Moreover, in many patients who have chronic pain, the anatomic source of pain cannot be identified with certainty.

Nevertheless, even if no causal treatment that can produce resolution of symptoms and disability is available, preventing or treating central hypersensitivity is expected to reduce symptoms by preventing amplification of nociceptive input. One way of attenuating hypersensitivity is to reduce nociceptive input to the spinal cord neurons by pharmacologic interventions that affect the encoding and transmission of nociceptive signals. For instance, nonsteroidal antiinflammatory drugs and opioids act partly by reducing prostaglandin synthesis at peripheral tissues and presynaptic inhibition of transmitter release in the spinal cord, respectively. The κ-opioid receptor seems to be upregulated after visceral inflammation, and κ-opioid receptor agonists have been shown to be effective as peripheral analgesics in preclinical studies [71,72]. A novel κ-opioid receptor agonist, administered systemically, produced profound peripheral analgesia without causing side effects [72]. Certain anticonvulsants, such as carbamazepine, act at sodium channels [73] that are upregulated in neuropathic pain [74], thereby attenuating ectopic discharges to the spinal cord. Capsaicin applied locally acts at the vanilloid receptor that is responsible for heat-induced pain [75]. Long-term application of capsaicin has been shown to desensitize the nociceptor, leading to pain relief in neuropathic [76] and possibly musculoskeletal [77] pain conditions. These interventions may provide unspecific attenuation of central hypersensitivity, in that the postsynaptic exposure of spinal neurons to excitatory transmitters is reduced.

Spinal cord modulation

Because of the involvement of COX-2 in central sensitization, nonsteroidal anti-inflammatory drugs may have a role in the treatment of hypersensitivity states. NMDA-antagonists may provide specific treatment of central hypersensitivity, given the involvement of the NMDA receptor in the generation of neuronal hyperexcitability [19]. Although the use of the NMDA-antagonist ketamine is limited by its unfavorable side effect profile, low intravenous doses are well tolerated and effective in acute pain [78,79]. Oral ketamine has been used in few investigations on neuropathic pain syndromes, with inconsistent results [80,81]. There is some evidence that ketamine and opioids are mostly effective when used in combination, given the effect of the two drugs on different spinal cord mechanisms: Opioids act presynaptically on the initial neuronal response, whereas NMDA-antagonists inhibit the following neuronal hyperexcitability [82]. The chronic use of ketamine is problematic because of side effects, poor bioavailability after oral administration [83], potential drug abuse, and lack of long-term clinical data. A possible approach is the development of antagonists of the NMDA-receptor that act on the NR2B subunit because there is preclinical evidence that such drugs may have a lower potential for producing side effects while keeping the analgesic effect [84].

Antagonists of the NMDA receptor acting on its glycine site inhibited central hypersensitivity in animal studies [85,86]. The same was observed with antagonists of G-protein–coupled metabotropic glutamate receptors [87]. These drugs could therefore represent new classes for the treatment of hypersensitivity states. Antagonism of spinal inhibitory mechanisms mediated by glycine and γ-aminobutyric acid receptors induces central sensitization [88,89]. Therefore, imbalance of these mechanisms may be involved in the development of central hypersensitivity and might be treated by drugs acting at inhibitory spinal receptor sites. The above investigations are at a preclinical stage.

It has recently been demonstrated that sodium-channel expression is upregulated not only in the peripheral nerve but also in spinal sensory neurons after peripheral nerve injury, which can contribute to neuropathic pain [90]. This is also a possible site of action of carbamazepine [73]. Gabapentin [91] and pregabalin [92] may attenuate central hypersensitivity by acting at the calcium channel alpha-2-delta-1 subunit that is upregulated after nerve injury.

Supraspinal modulation

Because of a possible role of cognitive and behavioral factors in postinjury central sensitization [29], psychologic treatments have a potential to attenuate central hypersensitivity. We are not aware of investigations that have addressed this issue.

Descending opioidergic [93], serotoninergic [94], and noradrenergic [94] pathways modulate nociceptive transmission in the spinal cord and could therefore attenuate central hypersensitivity. Thus, opioids, antidepressants, and α_2-adrenoreceptor antagonists could reduce central hypersensitivity by enhancing descending inhibition. The use of inhibitors of the 5-HT3 receptors may attenuate generalized central hypersensitivity because of the role of mechanisms involving these receptors in anxiety-driven hypersensitivity states [37]. Clinical studies have shown an effect of inhibitors of the 5-HT3 receptors on fibromyalgia [40] and neuropathic pain [41].

The data reported here show that there are potentially useful modalities for the treatment of hypersensitivity states. Some of these therapies are used in clinical practice but have not been subjected to rigorous scientific scrutiny. Others are at a preclinical stage. The sparse published evidence and the clinical experience show, at best, a quantitatively modest efficacy of the currently available treatment modalities.

Summary

The available literature consistently shows increased pain sensitivity after sensory stimulation of healthy tissues in patients who have various chronic pain conditions. This indicates a state of hypersensitivity of the CNS that amplifies the nociceptive input arising from damaged tissues. Experimental data indicate that central hypersensitivity is probably induced primarily by nociceptive input arising from a diseased tissue. In patients, imbalance of descending modulatory systems connected with psychologic distress may play a role.

There is experimental support in animal studies for the persistence of central hypersensitivity after complete resolution of tissue damage. This is particularly true for neuropathic pain conditions, whereby potentially irreversible plasticity changes of the CNS have been documented in animal studies. Whether such changes are present in musculoskeletal pain states is at present uncertain. Despite the likely importance of central hypersensitivity in the pathophysiology of chronic pain, this mechanism should not be used to justify the lack of understanding on the anatomic origin of the pain complaints in several pain syndromes, which is mostly due to limitations of the available diagnostic tools.

Treatment strategies for central hypersensitivity in patients have been investigated mostly in neuropathic pain states. Possible therapy modalities for central hypersensitivity in chronic pain of musculoskeletal origin are largely unexplored. The limited evidence available and everyday practice show, at best, modest efficacy of the available treatment modalities for central hypersensitivity. The gap between basic knowledge and clinical benefits remains large and should stimulate further intensive research.

References

[1] Woolf CJ, Salter MW. Neuronal plasticity: increasing the gain in pain. Science 2000;288: 1765–9.

[2] LaMotte RH, Shain CN, Simone DA, et al. Neurogenic hyperalgesia: psychophysical studies of underlying mechanisms. J Neurophysiol 1991;66:190–211.

[3] Banic B, Petersen-Felix S, Andersen OK, et al. Evidence for spinal cord hypersensitivity in chronic pain after whiplash injury and in fibromyalgia. Pain 2004;107:7–15.

[4] Staud R, Vierck CJ, Cannon RL, et al. Abnormal sensitization and temporal summation of second pain (wind-up) in patients with fibromyalgia syndrome. Pain 2001;91:165–75.

[5] Bajaj P, Graven-Nielsen T, Arendt-Nielsen L. Osteoarthritis and its association with muscle hyperalgesia: an experimental controlled study. Pain 2001;93:107–14.

[6] Bajaj P, Madsen H, Arendt-Nielsen L. Endometriosis is associated with central sensitization: a psychophysical controlled study. J Pain 2003;4:372–80.

[7] Curatolo M, Arendt Nielsen L, Petersen-Felix S. Evidence, mechanisms and clinical implications of central hypersensitivity in chronic pain after whiplash injury. Clin J Pain 2004; 20:469–76.

[8] Rang HP, Bevan S, Dray A. Chemical activation of nociceptive peripheral neurones. Br Med Bull 1991;47:534–8.

[9] Treede R-D, Meyer RA, Raja SN, et al. Peripheral and central mechanisms of cutaneous hyperalgesia. Prog Neurobiol 1992;38:397–421.

[10] Schmidt R, Schmelz M, Forster C, et al. Novel classes of responsive and unresponsive c nociceptors in human skin. J Neurosci 1995;15:333–41.

[11] Petho G, Derow A, Reeh PW. Bradykinin-induced nociceptor sensitization to heat is mediated by cyclooxygenase products in isolated rat skin. Eur J Neurosci 2001;14:210–8.

[12] Liang YF, Haake B, Reeh PW. Sustained sensitization and recruitment of rat cutaneous nociceptors by bradykinin and a novel theory of its excitatory action. J Physiol 2001;532: 229–39.

[13] Michael GJ, Priestley JV. Differential expression of the mRNA for the vanilloid receptor subtype 1 in cells of the adult rat dorsal root and nodose ganglia and its downregulation by axotomy. J Neurosci 1999;19:1844–54.

[14] Neumann S, Doubell TP, Leslie T, et al. Inflammatory pain hypersensitivity mediated by phenotypic switch in myelinated primary sensory neurons. Nature 1996;384:360–4.

[15] LaMotte RH, Thalhammer JG, Torebjörk HE, et al. Peripheral neural mechanisms of cutaneous hyperalgesia following mild injury by heat. J Neurosci 1982;2:765–81.

[16] Culp WJ, Ochoa J, Cline M, et al. Heat and mechanical hyperalgesia induced by capsaicin: cross modality threshold modulation in human c nociceptors. Brain 1989;112:1317–31.

[17] Caterina MJ, Schumacher MA, Tominaga M, et al. The capsaicin receptor: a heat-activated ion channel in the pain pathway. Nature 1997;389:816–24.

[18] Woolf CJ, Thompson SWN. The induction and maintenance of central sensitation is dependent on n-methyl-d-aspartic acid receptor activation: implications for the treatment of post-injury pain hypersensitivity states. Pain 1991;44:293–9.

[19] Dickenson AH, Sullivan AF. Evidence for a role of the NMDA receptor in the frequency dependent potentiation of deep rat dorsal horn nociceptive neurones following c fibre stimulation. Neuropharmacology 1987;26:1235–8.

[20] McCrory CR, Lindahl SG. Cyclooxygenase inhibition for postoperative analgesia. Anesth Analg 2002;95:169–76.

[21] Samad TA, Moore KA, Sapirstein A, et al. Interleukin-1beta-mediated induction of Cox-2 in the CNS contributes to inflammatory pain hypersensitivity. Nature 2001;410:471–5.

[22] McMahon SB, Wall PD. Receptive fields of rat lamina 1 projection cells move to incorporate a nearby region of injury. Pain 1984;19:235–47.

[23] Andersen OK, Finnerup NB, Spaich EG, et al. Expansion of nociceptive withdrawal reflex receptive fields in spinal cord injured humans. Clin Neurophysiol 2004;115:2798–810.

[24] Watkins LR, Milligan ED, Maier SF. Spinal cord glia: new players in pain. Pain 2001;93: 201–5.

[25] Azkue JJ, Zimmermann M, Hsieh TF, et al. Peripheral nerve insult induces NMDA receptor-mediated, delayed degeneration in spinal neurons. Eur J Neurosci 1998;10:2204–6.

[26] Mannion RJ, Woolf CJ. Pain mechanisms and management: a central perspective. Clin J Pain 2000;16:S144–56.
[27] Li CY, Song YH, Higuera ES, et al. Spinal dorsal horn calcium channel alpha2delta-1 subunit upregulation contributes to peripheral nerve injury-induced tactile allodynia. J Neurosci 2004;24:8494–9.
[28] Woolf CJ, Mannion RJ. Neuropathic pain: aetiology, symptoms, mechanisms, and management. Lancet 1999;353:1959–64.
[29] Dubner R, Ren K. Endogenous mechanisms of sensory modulation. Pain 1999;(Suppl 6): S45–53.
[30] Fields HL. Sources of variability in the sensation of pain. Pain 1988;33:195–200.
[31] Chapman V, Diaz A, Dickenson AH. Distinct inhibitory effects of spinal endomorphin-1 and endomorphin-2 on evoked dorsal horn neuronal responses in the rat. Br J Pharmacol 1997;122:1537–9.
[32] Millan MJ, Czlonkowski A, Millan MH, et al. Activation of periaqueductal grey pools of beta-endorphin by analgetic electrical stimulation in freely moving rats. Brain Res 1987; 407:199–203.
[33] Solomon RE, Gebhart GF. Mechanisms of effects of intrathecal serotonin on nociception and blood pressure in rats. J Pharmacol Exp Ther 1988;245:905–12.
[34] Yeomans DC, Clark FM, Paice JA, et al. Antinociception induced by electrical stimulation of spinally projecting noradrenergic neurons in the a7 catecholamine cell group of the rat. Pain 1992;48:449–61.
[35] Archer T, Jonsson G, Minor BG, et al. Noradrenergic-serotonergic interactions and nociception in the rat. Eur J Pharmacol 1986;120:295–307.
[36] Suzuki R, Rygh LJ, Dickenson AH. Bad news from the brain: descending 5-HT pathways that control spinal pain processing. Trends Pharmacol Sci 2004;25:613–7.
[37] Suzuki R, Morcuende S, Webber M, et al. Superficial NK1-expressing neurons control spinal excitability through activation of descending pathways. Nat Neurosci 2002;5:1319–26.
[38] Green GM, Scarth J, Dickenson A. An excitatory role for 5-HT in spinal inflammatory nociceptive transmission; state-dependent actions via dorsal horn 5-HT(3) receptors in the anaesthetized rat. Pain 2000;89:81–8.
[39] Curatolo M, Petersen-Felix S, Arendt-Nielsen L, et al. Central hypersensitivity in chronic pain after whiplash injury. Clin J Pain 2001;17:306–15.
[40] Farber L, Stratz TH, Bruckle W, et al. Short-term treatment of primary fibromyalgia with the 5-HT3-receptor antagonist tropisetron: results of a randomized, double-blind, placebo-controlled multicenter trial in 418 patients. Int J Clin Pharmacol Res 2001;21:1–13.
[41] McCleane GJ, Suzuki R, Dickenson AH. Does a single intravenous injection of the 5HT3 receptor antagonist ondansetron have an analgesic effect in neuropathic pain? A double-blinded, placebo-controlled cross-over study. Anesth Analg 2003;97:1474–8.
[42] Coderre TJ, Katz J, Vaccarino AL, et al. Contribution of central neuroplasticity to pathological pain: review of clinical and experimental evidence. Pain 1993;52:259–85.
[43] Graven-Nielsen T, Arendt-Nielsen L, Svensson P, et al. Quantification of local and referred muscle pain in humans after sequential i.m. injections of hypertonic saline. Pain 1997;69: 111–7.
[44] Curatolo M, Petersen-Felix S, Arendt-Nielsen L. Sensory assessment of regional analgesia in humans: a review of methods and applications. Anesthesiology 2000;93:1517–30.
[45] Curatolo M, Petersen-Felix S, Arendt-Nielsen L. Assessment of regional analgesia in clinical practice and research. Br Med Bull 2004;71:61–76.
[46] Sheather Reid RB, Cohen ML. Psychophysical evidence for a neuropathic component of chronic neck pain. Pain 1998;75:341–7.
[47] Koelbaek Johansen M, Graven-Nielsen T, Schou Olesen A, et al. Generalised muscular hyperalgesia in chronic whiplash syndrome. Pain 1999;83:229–34.
[48] Moog M, Quintner J, Hall T, et al. The late whiplash syndrome: a psychophysical study. Eur J Pain 2002;6:283–94.

[49] Sörensen J, Graven Nielsen T, Henriksson KG, et al. Hyperexcitability in fibromyalgia. J Rheumatol 1998;25:152–5.
[50] Desmeules JA, Cedraschi C, Rapiti E, et al. Neurophysiologic evidence for a central sensitization in patients with fibromyalgia. Arthritis Rheum 2003;48:1420–9.
[51] Sterling M, Jull G, Vicenzino B, et al. Sensory hypersensitivity occurs soon after whiplash injury and is associated with poor recovery. Pain 2003;104:509–17.
[52] Sterling M, Jull G, Vicenzino B, et al. Physical and psychological factors predict outcome following whiplash injury. Pain 2005;114:141–8.
[53] Ashina S, Jensen R, Bendtsen L. Pain sensitivity in pericranial and extracranial regions. Cephalalgia 2003;23:456–62.
[54] Bendtsen L, Jensen R, Olesen J. Decreased pain detection and tolerance thresholds in chronic tension-type headache. Arch Neurol 1996;53:373–6.
[55] Svensson P, List T, Hector G. Analysis of stimulus-evoked pain in patients with myofascial temporomandibular pain disorders. Pain 2001;92:399–409.
[56] Gottrup H, Andersen J, Arendt-Nielsen L, et al. Psychophysical examination in patients with post-mastectomy pain. Pain 2000;87:275–84.
[57] Lord SM, Barnsley L, Wallis BJ, et al. Percutaneous radio-frequency neurotomy for chronic cervical zygapophyseal-joint pain. N Engl J Med 1996;335:1721–6.
[58] Kosek E, Ordeberg G. Abnormalities of somatosensory perception in patients with painful osteoarthritis normalize following successful treatment. Eur J Pain 2000;4:229–38.
[59] Giamberardino MA, de Bigontina P, Martegiani C, et al. Effects of extracorporeal shock-wave lithotripsy on referred hyperalgesia from renal/ureteral calculosis. Pain 1994;56:77–83.
[60] Herren-Gerber R, Weiss S, Arendt Nielsen L, et al. Modulation of central hypersensitivity by nociceptive input in chronic pain after whiplash injury. Pain Med 2004;5:366–76.
[61] Rhudy JL, Meagher MW. Fear and anxiety: divergent effects on human pain thresholds. Pain 2000;84:65–75.
[62] Petrovic P, Ingvar M. Imaging cognitive modulation of pain processing. Pain 2002;95:1–5.
[63] Di Piero V, Ferracuti S, Sabatini U, et al. A cerebral blood flow study on tonic pain activation in man. Pain 1994;56:167–73.
[64] Davis KD. The neural circuitry of pain as explored with functional MRI. Neurol Res 2000; 22:313–7.
[65] Karl A, Birbaumer N, Lutzenberger W, et al. Reorganization of motor and somatosensory cortex in upper extremity amputees with phantom limb pain. J Neurosci 2001;21:3609–18.
[66] Flor H, Braun C, Elbert T, et al. Extensive reorganization of primary somatosensory cortex in chronic back pain patients. Neurosci Lett 1997;224:5–8.
[67] Maihofner C, Handwerker HO, Neundorfer B, et al. Patterns of cortical reorganization in complex regional pain syndrome. Neurology 2003;61:1707–15.
[68] Flor H, Elbert T, Knecht S, et al. Phantom-limb pain as a perceptual correlate of cortical reorganization following arm amputation. Nature 1995;375:482–4.
[69] Huse E, Larbig W, Flor H, et al. The effect of opioids on phantom limb pain and cortical reorganization. Pain 2001;90:47–55.
[70] Apkarian AV, Sosa Y, Sonty S, et al. Chronic back pain is associated with decreased prefrontal and thalamic gray matter density. J Neurosci 2004;24:10410–5.
[71] Sengupta JN, Snider A, Su X, et al. Effects of kappa opioids in the inflamed rat colon. Pain 1999;79:175–85.
[72] Vanderah TW, Schteingart CD, Trojnar J, et al. Fe200041 (d-phe-d-phe-d-nle-d-arg-nh2): a peripheral efficacious kappa opioid agonist with unprecedented selectivity. J Pharmacol Exp Ther 2004;310:326–33.
[73] Ambrosio AF, Soares-Da-Silva P, Carvalho CM, et al. Mechanisms of action of carbamazepine and its derivatives, oxcarbazepine, BIA 2-093, and BIA 2-024. Neurochem Res 2002;27:121–30.
[74] Craner MJ, Klein JP, Renganathan M, et al. Changes of sodium channel expression in experimental painful diabetic neuropathy. Ann Neurol 2002;52:786–92.

[75] Caterina MJ, Leffler A, Malmberg AB, et al. Impaired nociception and pain sensation in mice lacking the capsaicin receptor. Science 2000;288:306–13.
[76] Sindrup SH, Jensen TS. Efficacy of pharmacological treatments of neuropathic pain: an update and effect related to mechanism of drug action. Pain 1999;83:389–400.
[77] Frerick H, Keitel W, Kuhn U, et al. Topical treatment of chronic low back pain with a capsicum plaster. Pain 2003;106:59–64.
[78] Adriaenssens G, Vermeyen KM, Hoffmann VL, et al. Postoperative analgesia with i.v. patient-controlled morphine: effect of adding ketamine. Br J Anaesth 1999;83:393–6.
[79] Aida S, Yamakura T, Baba H, et al. Preemptive analgesia by intravenous low-dose ketamine and epidural morphine in gastrectomy: a randomized double-blind study. Anesthesiology 2000;92:1624–30.
[80] Haines DR, Gaines SP. N of 1 randomised controlled trials of oral ketamine in patients with chronic pain. Pain 1999;83:283–7.
[81] Fitzgibbon EJ, Hall P, Schroder C, et al. Low dose ketamine as an analgesic adjuvant in difficult pain syndromes: a strategy for conversion from parenteral to oral ketamine. J Pain Symptom Manage 2002;23:165–70.
[82] Chapman V, Dickenson AH. The combination of nmda antagonism and morphine produces profound antinociception in the rat dorsal horn. Brain Res 1992;573:321–3.
[83] Yanagihara Y, Ohtani M, Kariya S, et al. Plasma concentration profiles of ketamine and norketamine after administration of various ketamine preparations to healthy japanese volunteers. Biopharm Drug Dispos 2003;24:37–43.
[84] Malmberg AB, Gilbert H, McCabe RT, et al. Powerful antinociceptive effects of the cone snail venom-derived subtype-selective NMDA receptor antagonists conantokins G and T. Pain 2003;101:109–16.
[85] Quartaroli M, Carignani C, Dal Forno G, et al. Potent antihyperalgesic activity without tolerance produced by glycine site antagonist of N-methyl-D-aspartate receptor GV196771A. J Pharmacol Exp Ther 1999;290:158–69.
[86] Quartaroli M, Fasdelli N, Bettelini L, et al. GV196771A, an NMDA receptor/glycine site antagonist, attenuates mechanical allodynia in neuropathic rats and reduces tolerance induced by morphine in mice. Eur J Pharmacol 2001;430:219–27.
[87] Neugebauer V, Chen PS, Willis WD. Role of metabotropic glutamate receptor subtype mGluR1 in brief nociception and central sensitization of primate STT cells. J Neurophysiol 1999;82:272–82.
[88] Sivilotti L, Woolf CJ. The contribution of GABAA and glycine receptors to central sensitization: disinhibition and touch-evoked allodynia in the spinal cord. J Neurophysiol 1994;72:169–79.
[89] Russo RE, Nagy F, Hounsgaard J. Inhibitory control of plateau properties in dorsal horn neurones in the turtle spinal cord in vitro. J Physiol 1998;506:795–808.
[90] Hains BC, Saab CY, Klein JP, et al. Altered sodium channel expression in second-order spinal sensory neurons contributes to pain after peripheral nerve injury. J Neurosci 2004;24:4832–9.
[91] Luo ZD, Calcutt NA, Higuera ES, et al. Injury type-specific calcium channel alpha 2 delta-1 subunit up-regulation in rat neuropathic pain models correlates with antiallodynic effects of gabapentin. J Pharmacol Exp Ther 2002;303:1199–205.
[92] Fink K, Dooley DJ, Meder WP, et al. Inhibition of neuronal Ca(2+) influx by gabapentin and pregabalin in the human neocortex. Neuropharmacology 2002;42:229–36.
[93] Yu XM, Hua M, Mense S. The effects of intracerebroventricular injection of naloxone, phentolamine and methysergide on the transmission of nociceptive signals in rat dorsal horn neurons with convergent cutaneous- deep input. Neuroscience 1991;44:715–23.
[94] Li P, Zhuo M. Cholinergic, noradrenergic, and serotonergic inhibition of fast synaptic transmission in spinal lumbar dorsal horn of rat. Brain Res Bull 2001;54:639–47.

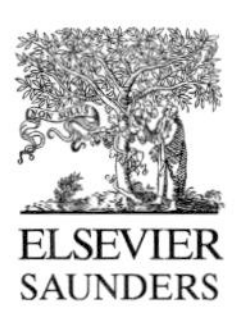
ELSEVIER
SAUNDERS

Phys Med Rehabil Clin N Am
17 (2006) 303–314

PHYSICAL MEDICINE
AND REHABILITATION
CLINICS OF
NORTH AMERICA

Patient Evaluation and General Treatment Planning

Scot Gerald Fechtel, MD, DC

Cascade Neurology, 960 North 16th Street, Springfield, OR 97477, USA

How does one approach the patient with complaints of chronic pain? What are the questions that need to be addressed? How does one go about answering those questions? The purpose in this article is to guide the clinician in evaluating each patient, eliciting meaningful data, and developing an initial plan of treatment.

Pain is the most complex human health dilemma approached by modern medicine. Although many life-threatening conditions have yielded to the scientific method, with reductions in human disease burden, patients with chronic pain rarely experience complete alleviation of their symptoms despite research that has produced an abundance of information about pain physiology, the pain signaling system within spinal cord and brain, and the pharmacology of pain.

The clinical experience of pain encompasses nociception, anxiety, social disorganization, sleep impairment, depression, frustration, and encounters with caring and compassionate health care workers (and those who are not). It often leads to severe financial and occupational burdens and litigation and can destroy a previously successful life. This is not the care of a simple medical illness; it requires of the clinician a commitment to comprehensive evaluation, reasonable treatment planning, and steadfast follow-up.

In a recent publication, Miaskowski [1] noted that Ahles and colleagues [2] were the first to develop a multidimensional model applicable to the pain experience. They noted five dimensions of the pain experience: (1) physiologic, (2) sensory, (3) affective, (4) cognitive, and (5) behavioral. The physiologic dimension was the source of, or initiator of, the pain input to the central nervous system (CNS). The sensory dimension describes the quality, location, and intensity of the experience. The affective dimension describes

E-mail address: sfechtel@earthlink.net

doi:10.1016/j.pmr.2005.12.008 ***pmr.theclinics.com***

the emotional component: anxiety and depression. The cognitive portion describes the impact of the pain on thought processes and the impact of the experience upon the self-concept of the patient and consequently the "meaning" of the pain. Finally, the behavioral aspect describes the impact of the experience on the patient's physical activity and medication use. This initial model was developed in reference to cancer pain. Later, McGuire [3] added a sociocultural dimension and suggested that this broadened model was applicable to the whole of human pain experience.

To effectively "manage" an individual patient's pain, we must address each of these parts of the pain experience. What are the questions the clinician must address to improve the pain patient's experience? The first is, Where does the pain come from? Is it nociceptive? Is it central? Is it a combination of both?

What maintains the pain? Is it chronic nociception from articular damage, an unstable joint, or physiologic aberration? Are there adaptive responses the patient is using that exacerbate the pain? Are medications interfering with recovery? Are there unspoken biases or cultural preconceptions that are inhibiting recovery? What role does the CNS play? Current research in the process of central sensitization is leading to new directions in thought about musculoskeletal pain. Are there issues of secondary gain; release from unpleasant family, occupational, or other societal duties? What about the secondary effects of pain? Decreased physical activity, weight gain, and exacerbation of other unrelated medical issues complicate the treatment process.

Observation of the patient yields other clues. The physical examination can challenge etiologic hypotheses, provide data to suggest ancillary investigations, and move the clinician toward at least initial answers to these questions.

There are many tools that can assist in gathering initial information. The Visual Analogue Scale [4] is useful and easy to administer. More focused inventories, such as the Beck Depression Inventory [5], give further insight. Functional assessments such as the Oswestry Low Back Pain Disability Questionnaire [6] give more specific information. The Minnesota Multiphasic Personality Inventory [7] requires more time and more professional interpretation and yields background information about the patient and perhaps their adaptive strategies in approaching illness. There are many such tools available. Having tools the clinician is comfortable with easily at hand facilitates information gathering when office time is limited.

In gathering the history directly, the quality of pain perceived can be helpful. Although no single pain descriptor is reliable as an indicator of the etiology of pain, reports of "burning," "electric," "tingling," or "numb" sensations can point to the peripheral nervous system. "Dull" or "aching" sensations often implicate the joints or soft tissues, especially when exacerbated by movement. Poorly localized pain directs us to the CNS. Indescribable pain suggests that psychological issues may be paramount.

Duration of pain and changes in intensity and geography over time provide valuable insight into the patient's psychological status. Pain that is unrelenting, present throughout the day, and recalcitrant to multiple interventions may reflect more "suffering" than nociception. Long-term treatment of such conditions with antinociceptive approaches rarely improves function.

Other elements of a patient's history may be relevant. Has there been a prior similar injury? If so, what was the outcome? How long was the recovery period? Were there any problems during the treatment? What about other medical illnesses? The role of diabetes and thyroid issues in complicating recovery is clinical fact. Does the family history document similar problems in other family members? Is there a hint of a genetic disorder that may complicate or predispose to injury? A social history may suggest exposures that could play a role in further delaying or complicating recovery (eg, exposure to industrial chemicals, previous or current nutritional deprivation, or exposure to blood products and recreational chemicals).

There are many physical examination techniques devoted to providing information about the source of pain. Each of the physical examination strategies is tailored to individual regions of the body. No single test provides definitive proof of a specific etiology. An examination strategy that attempts to address all of the tissues involved in a given body region is required. Mechanisms to challenge the muscles, tendons, ligaments, transiting nerves, and blood vessels need to be developed. There are excellent textbooks of physical examination methods available to the clinician.

The physical examination can be best understood as a process of observation of the parts of a patient that are relevant to the reported pain experience. Attention to the way a patient moves brings a great deal of information: Is movement restricted or fluid? Are restrictions regional or global? Is it accompanied by pain behavior? Pain behavior can be appropriate or pathologic in itself. A person intent upon impressing the examiner with the severity of their pain experience has little psychological room to allow symptomatic improvement. Stoicism can also impair the examiner's understanding of the patient's problem.

How does the patient relate to the examiner? This is a question taught in the mental status examination, but it is useful for the pain clinician. What if a person presents in a recalcitrant fashion, one that is uninvolved, rude, or suggests such a rigid belief system that it is unlikely that there is any possibility of change? These observations should guide the clinician in planning how to approach the patient for physical and medical treatments.

Assessment of the vital signs remains an important tool. A patient with an infection or catastrophic hypertension may be a pain emergency. The next most critical examination should include palpation of the involved soft tissues for texture, temperature, and tenderness. Orthopedic examination demonstrates the ranges of motion of relevant joints. It should dynamically stress the supporting muscles and tendons of the involved region. If muscle is the source of pain, the pain should be worse with movement of the muscle. Tendons and their attachments can generate pain and can be differentiated from other musculoskeletal pain sources.

Some sense of vascular function must be obtained. Ischemia can generate pain through several mechanisms. Peripheral vascular compromise can generate pain, but some research suggests that neurologic claudication can be a factor in the low back [8]. Impaired blood flow to working muscle can directly provoke pain, as can vascular insufficiency to the nerve root. This "central" or neurogenic claudication is difficult to prove and to treat.

Although many patients report symptoms suggestive of neurologic dysfunction, their sensation, strength, and reflexes are often normal. These must be tested in sufficient detail for the clinician to be certain that function is normal. Sensation should be probed with at least two modalities in all areas of concern. Do not overlook the autonomic system. Sweat patterns and skin health can guide the remainder of the examination.

The 0- to 5-point muscle strength scale [9] is useful for the assessment of peripheral nerve–injured soldiers, but it is not helpful without additional observation in the pain patient. Effort is the key to understanding muscle strength presentation. If the patient puts forth suboptimal effort, is that failure because of depression, fear, pain, or deception? Only if you are convinced that sufficient effort has been expended can a conclusion about muscle strength be useful. Look for a pattern of muscle impairment that can be explained by local injury, peripheral nerve, root, or cord level dysfunction.

The most commonly studied reflexes are those of the muscle unit, the so-called myotactic or deep tendon reflexes. Individual performance varies. Pattern is the important observation. The observation that all reflexes are unusually brisk or unusually dull may be important only in a larger context. If the patient is hypothyroid or has other deficiency diseases, this may explain the observed tendon response. For patients who seem to have globally increased reflexes, the clinician must consider upper motor neuron diseases and must be comfortable in assessing for them. Often these patients do not harbor more worrisome disease. Remembering the bell curve of normal can reduce your concern about these outliers.

The fibromyalgia literature has promoted palpation of tissue texture as a way of understanding some soft tissue pain. The "trigger" and "tender" point in muscle is a way of describing pain sources in the musculature [10]. Observation of joint anatomy for deformity and function is needed. The ability to discern joint effusion or bursal edema is important. The chiropractic literature has debated the role of joint kinematics in spine-related pain. The ability to perceive failure of intersegmental spine joints to move in their normal modes helps guide the assessment of focal sources of nociception.

Another useful orthopedic trick is remembering that the joint above and below the area of concern can contribute to its pain and pathology.

Similarly, recalling that jaw clenching, tooth grinding, and temporomandibular joint dysfunction can contribute to neck pain and headache can assist the clinician in sorting out these complex problems.

The psychological status of the patient is not documented only by written inventories or scales. The observant clinician notes how the patient presents himself and how the patient interacts during the history taking and examination process. Patterns of resistance to substantive questions in discussion of the history, depression, or sometimes deception can be noted. When such concerns arise, additional physical examination trials can be performed to clarify (eg, performing tests of the same tissue through a different means, observing the patient when distracted, and repeating the examination with an eye to patient consistency). Consideration of formal psychological or perhaps neuropsychological examination is appropriate under these circumstances. Waddell [11] has published much in the arena of psychological impact upon recovery and pain.

Imaging is a source of much confusion in pain. Data can be distorted into positive or negative bents. Degenerative joint disease observed in the spine can be derided as irrelevant or blamed for clinically unrelated pain. The limits of each imaging modality must be recalled. When considering bone, it is useful to recall that immediate postinjury plain radiographs may miss a nondisplaced fracture. Seventy-two hours postinjury may be required for sufficient calcium to be removed for the fracture line to become visible. Similarly, CAT imaging does not see the posterior cranial fossa with adequate detail for the evaluation of subtle lesions. Movement artifact can obscure even the most appropriate images. If there is concern about degenerative disease and its role in a patient's current pain complaints, ancillary investigations can be performed. The role of nuclear bone scan in supporting the notion of active arthritic changes in focal pain is well established. Provocative disk injections can identify a nociceptive source for back pain in well-selected patients. The role of magnetic resonance scanning in pain is always expanding.

Electrophysiologic evaluation of peripheral nerve and muscle function remains a useful tool. The ability to sort out a peripheral polyneuropathy from a local nerve injury and to discriminate muscle disease from that of the nerve assists in the pain evaluation. The limitations of the study must be kept in mind. In pain patients, pain fibers (small unmyelinated C fibers) are not evaluated. A "normal" nerve conduction and EMG report does not rule out neuropathic pain.

Just as the role of vital signs in the assessment of a patient may be undervalued, so is assessment of systemic body function. Discovering that a pain patient has diabetes, low thyroid function, or hepatitis C guides treatment and rehabilitation efforts.

This article does not attempt to reproduce the expertise of the many available textbooks but attempts to integrate all of the elements a clinician is required to bring to the assessment of an individual pain patient. The principal weapon the physician brings to the clinical battle is a disciplined thought process. Keeping in mind the complexities of neurophysiology, injury pathophysiology, and human psychology provides the clinician a framework to develop a strategy to approach each patient. Here, prototypical cases presenting common scenarios encountered in the clinic are addressed. Because successful treatment of pain patients relies upon this thought process, these cases are presented as one might experience them in the clinic to highlight that point.

Case 1

A 19-year-old man was involved in a motorcycle rollover without a helmet. He has emerged from a 10-day coma and suffered skull fracture and intracerebral bleed. He complains of right lower extremity pain.

Applying our multidimensional pain understanding, we would start with the physiologic assessment. Orthopedic examination demonstrates no focal musculoskeletal lesion. There are no fractures. There is a full range of motion of all joints in the lower extremity. Vascular function is intact with normal skin temperature and turgor. Capillary refill is normal. There is no excessive play in any of the joints to manual stress. On neurologic examination modest, global, right-sided paresis and spasticity are noted. This is documented by increased tone in the right upper and lower extremity and increased deep tendon reflexes. His muscle strength on the right is a 4+ of 5; the left side is normal at 5+ of 5. Sensory testing is intact but documents dysesthesia to light touch and pin with brisk increase in burning pain and delayed resolution of the increase.

Cognitive functioning is impaired. Neuropsychologic examination documents memory impairments, depression, and emotional lability consistent with a traumatic brain injury. Neuroimaging demonstrates an improving left-sided intracerebral hemorrhage involving the left thalamus. His skull fracture is stable after neurosurgical evacuation of the hemorrhage.

The pain is described as diffuse in location and not affected by movement of the limb. The quality of the pain is burning with a "twisting" component. The intensity of the pain is reported to be so severe that it interferes with walking and sleep. The nursing staff reports that the pain is worsening his depression and that he perseverates on it to such an extent that he does not accomplish his daily rehabilitation goals.

The unit social worker notes that this 19-year-old high school dropout has a long drug and alcohol history and no family support. He smokes two packs of cigarettes a day. His pregnant 18-year-old girlfriend lives with her abusive mother. He has been employed in a string of laboring and retail jobs for the last 2 years, all without health or disability insurance.

The family reports that this patient has been healthy all of his premorbid life and is without other medical illnesses. He had been an average student with no prior involvement in the legal system.

Do we have sufficient information to develop a treatment plan for his pain?

Yes. This seems to be a central pain state, with the etiology of the pain the left thalamic injury. The pain may be aggravated by his spasticity on the right side. Pharmacologic interventions to address this may require membrane-stabilizing agents, antidepressants, and antispasmodic agents. Education of the patient about the source of his pain is required. Addressing the cognitive difficulties is required. Social work intervention to help him reestablish a self-supporting lifestyle and adjusting life goals is required. Developing an integrated treatment plan to address these goals is the purpose of the evaluation. Accessing the roles that multiple providers of psychological and physical assistance might play is the conundrum. Will these interventions be effective in reducing the perceived pain? Probably. Will they stop his pain? Not likely.

Case 2

A 70-year-old hypertensive woman with a 10-year history of diabetes mellitus complains of bilateral burning pain in her feet.

Our odyssey begins with observation in this case. This is an age-appropriate 70-year-old woman. She has a modest thoracic kyphosis that does not interfere with her gait. She shuffles modestly. There is moderate evidence of osteoarthritis with marked Heberden's nodes in all fingers of her hands. There is modest atrophy of intrinsic muscles of the hands. She seems to have less atrophy in the feet, but small calf musculature is present. Orthopedic examination of the lower extremities demonstrates modest laxity of knee-supporting ligaments and reduced hip range of motion. Neurologic examination produces reduced light touch and pin below the knees symmetrically. There is no evidence of abnormal response to sensory testing. She has proximal weakness with the iliopsoas testing 4 of 5 for strength bilaterally. The distal muscles are similarly weak. Deep tendon reflexes are 2+ at the adductor muscles with modest spread. The patellar tendon reflex is trace bilaterally, and the Achilles' reflexes are unelicitable with and without reinforcement. The lower-extremity skin demonstrates fragility, poor turgor, poor capillary refill, and evidence of venous stasis. She has 1+ pitting edema to the midcalf.

Previous imaging has shown advanced degenerative changes in the lumbar spine with moderate foraminal narrowing, disk thinning, and bulging at multiple low lumbar levels. Electrophysiologic examination demonstrates prolonged nerve conduction in the few lower-extremity superficial nerves that can be tested without electromyographic changes. There are no changes suggestive of radiculopathy.

The pain is described as burning in character. It is worse at night or with walking more than 50 feet. Occasionally she complains that it feels like she is walking on gravel, particularly if barefoot. Her feet vary from hot to cold at night, making it difficult to be comfortable while trying to sleep. She complains of significant daytime drowsiness and some impairment of her short-term memory.

The medical history provided evidence of previous myocardial infarction, approximately 3 years prior, leading to successful angioplasty. There is no evidence of restenosis of those vessels. Lisinopril has been regularly used and was successful in maintaining reasonable blood pressures at repeated family doctor office visits. Oral agents have been used to control the blood sugars, but the patient's glucose diary records fairly frequent evening sugars in the 300s and morning glucose levels often in the 200s. A recent full physical and laboratory examination by the referring family physician demonstrated no anemia; normal thyroid function; and normal electrolyte, kidney, and liver functions. There was no evidence of autoimmune disease, and serum proteins were normal. There was no history of contact with industrial or agricultural chemicals.

The daughter attending our examination is a 45-year-old attorney. She reports that her mother is visiting less with the grandchildren, seems to be avoiding family contact, and does not seem to be attending to her household chores with the same vigor that the daughter is used to. There seems to be no financial stress, although the patient's husband died 2 years prior.

Do we have sufficient information to generate a successful treatment plan?

Yes. This seems to be a case of diabetic polyneuropathy with sensory and motor losses. The pain is neuropathic. Treatment is complicated by the cardiac disease and the medications required. A commonly used medication for this condition, amitriptyline, may be contraindicated in this instance. There may be difficulty tolerating other neuropathic pain medications, such as gabapentin, because of side-effects such as dizziness. Attention to better glucose control offers the possibility of reduced progression of the neurologic injury but cannot be expected to improve function. Concern about depression in this patient is warranted. Physical therapy consultation may be warranted to address gait safety. Home health assessment of this patient's living quarters is indicated to address items such as night lights in the bedroom, slick walking surfaces, and other impediments to safe walking. Stairs at home and high bathtub walls may affect this patient's safety. A treatment plan that integrates all of these elements and that includes frequent follow-up in the clinic to assess progress, tolerability of medications and other treatments, and the patient's ability to continue successful self-care must be implemented.

Case 3

A 35-year-old woman was involved in a motor vehicle accident 1 year prior. Initial pain was centered in the posterior neck. The pain has generalized into whole spine discomfort. Recently, diagnostic medial branch blocks to the C4-5 and C6-7 facets bilaterally produced no significant relief of the neck pain.

Observation of this patient shows a woman who looks about 10 years older than her stated age. She seems tired and dejected. There is poor eye contact and an increased latency to respond during the history taking. Vocal volume is low and moderately monotonous. Her skin is normal, and there is no dependent edema. Capillary refill is rapid and complete. Palpation discloses hypertonicity of a number of muscle groups including paraspinals, trapezius, and gluteals. The muscles have embedded tender points that do not trigger radiating pain but are surprisingly painful with modest palpatory pressure and reproduce much of her discomfort. Fourteen of the 18 sites required by the American College of Rheumatology definition of fibromyalgia are positive for pain and tissue texture changes consistent with "tender points." Range of motion of all spine joints is modestly reduced by pain complaints. Maneuvers to challenge spine integrity are painful only when they stretch muscles. Compression and traction directed to the cervical spine give only local discomfort. Sciatic stretch tests provoke only low back pain at 60°. Sensation is nondermatomally reduced, but there is no dysesthesia. Muscle strength is symmetrical and full when she gives good effort, but this provokes complaints of discomfort. Deep tendon reflexes are normal. Observation, distraction, and simulation tests do not suggest nonorganic pain concerns.

Previous spinal imaging demonstrates only age-appropriate degenerative changes, without evidence of disk herniation or significant foraminal encroachment. Laboratory tests are normal, without evidence of anemia, electrolyte, liver, or kidney abnormalities. Thyroid function is normal. Serum proteins are normal.

The history is of gradually increasing intensity and spread of pain complaints. Her sleep has been markedly interrupted by pain and positioning issues since the accident. Before that there was no problem with rest or energy. She now finds it difficult to complete a day at work and has been missing occasional days. Her housework is suffering, with complaints from the family. It has been difficult, especially during the last 6 months, to participate in family-related gatherings. When asked about depression, she tearfully acknowledges occasional suicidal thoughts but has never developed a suicidal plan.

Is this a case of chronic sprain of the spine after a motor vehicle accident? No. Although the initial trauma may have been a sprain to the spine supporting soft tissues, this presentation is fibromyalgia. This complex and controversial disorder requires multidisciplinary treatment planning. Attention to pain, depression, and sleep disorder is required. The goal is one of reactivating this patient to improve activity tolerance, muscular endurance, and daytime energy. No single modality of treatment is successful, but a carefully tailored and monitored schedule of interventions may result in reduced pain perception and enhanced lifestyle and satisfaction.

Case 4

While working, a 34-year-old man slipped from a roof and fell 25 ft 1 year ago. Initial evaluation disclosed an L1 vertebral body fracture that was stable. There was neither spinal canal nor neurologic compromise. Orthopedic evaluation counseled nonsurgical management. He was not a vertebroplasty candidate. Over the past year he has complained of severe pain localized to the thoracolumbar junction. Recent diagnostic blocks and discography failed to identify a specific pain generator.

We have all evaluated this patient once or twice. He wore a stained T-shirt, rumpled jeans, scuffed shoes, and a well-loved baseball cap scrunched on his head, with the ensemble capped by a long since worn out back brace girdling his abdomen. He initiates the conversation by informing us that he has been a roofer for 10 years and that his back is worn out. He started roofing after military service in the army, which he joined after high school. There was no service connected injury or disability. He played football in high school successfully and with out injury.

Examination shows an age-appropriate man with a little bit of extra abdominal insulation. His standing posture shows a flat spine with some paravertebral muscular splinting focal to the thoracolumbar junction. The shoulders are a bit rounded. He ambulates with a minimum of spine mobility. His cervical spine has normal range of movement. He actively resists thoracolumbar spine flexion and extension. Rotational challenge to the thoracolumbar spine encounters considerable moaning and groaning, again with resistance. When prone, he can partially relax the paraspinal muscles but only with repeated exhortations. Otherwise the muscles are rigid. There is no loss of sensation in the paraspinal skin or in the lower extremities. His strength in all muscle groups tested is normal. Reflexes are normal in the legs and unelicitable in the abdominal region. His chest expansion is 1 in.

Imaging demonstrates a healed compression fracture with the loss of 30% of the anterior vertebral body height. The posterior vertebral structure is stable with no compromise of the central canal or neuroforamina. A bone scan is equivocal. Previous imaging is consistent, with no underlying concern about cord compromise. There are no laboratory abnormalities.

When trying to qualify his pain sensation, he is only able to report that "it just hurts, real bad!" He is sleeping better and awakens somewhat refreshed on most mornings. His wife is not complaining about his mood swings as much lately, by his report. His employer would like him to come back to work, but he is worried about going back to roofing.

What are the goals of rehabilitation in this case? Can we expect to stop his pain? Will control of his pain get him back to work as a roofer? It is likely that a combination of antiinflammatory, muscle relaxing, and analgesic medications will reduce his perceived pain. Exercise retraining to develop a pattern of movement that minimizes muscular stress and enhances muscular endurance may help. Questions of functional recovery can be answered, in this case, with some evidence. Hazel and colleagues [12] followed 25 patients who had compression fracture without neurologic deficit for a minimum of 9 years. With only one exception, all patients functioned as well as uninjured subjects of comparable age. In a study of childhood vertebral compression fracture, Zambelli and colleagues [13] noted that at 10-year follow-up, two thirds of the patients reported some persistent pain, and half of the patients reported daily pain. We can counsel this patient that he can expect some persistent pain but that he can also expect to be able to function in some physical capacity. Whether he can return to work in roofing is a question that only time will answer. Our treatment plan must include medications, physical measures, occupational rehabilitation, and education about chronic pain and its impact upon physical and emotional functioning if we expect to improve his life.

Summary

Treating pain patients is difficult. The usual problems encountered in providing coherent and effective treatment for any chronic medical illness are compounded in painful conditions by time, society's choices, and the cultural role of the patient. Effective treatment of these patients depends on the persistence of the clinician. We must persist in requiring a complete history to understand the patient and his or her problem. We must persist in performing a thorough physical examination to uncover sufficient understanding of the patient's physiology. We must persist in developing a comprehensive treatment plan to cover all of the intervening concerns. We must persist in following the patient in the clinic to make sure that the plan is completed and that complications that arise are dealt with efficiently. This can lead to considerable satisfaction and frustration.

There remain many unanswered questions in the evaluation of pain patients and of pain itself. How accurate is physical examination in providing information about a given patient that is relevant to treating pain? Can physical examination reliably elicit a nociceptive focus for a specific individual's chronic pain experience? Is all long-term pain a smorgasbord of nociceptive, central sensitization, and neuromodulatory mechanisms? Can acute pain be more consistently aborted to minimize the development of chronic pain? Over the next few years, as our expanding knowledge of neuropharmacology, neurophysiology, and pain modulation in the CNS combines with better understanding of pain psychology and sociology, we clinicians will expect to have happier and more productive patients.

References

[1] Miaskowski C. Principles of pain assessment. In: Pappagallo M, editor. The neurological basis of pain. New York: McGraw-Hill; 2005. p. 195–207.

[2] Ahles TA, Blanchard EB, Rickdoschel JC. The multidimensional nature of cancer-related pain. Pain 1983;17:277–88.
[3] McGuire DB. The multidimensional phenomenon of cancer pain. In: McGuire DB, Yarbro CH, editors. Cancer pain management. Philadelphia: Saunders; 1987. p. 1–4.
[4] Revill SI, Robinson JD, Rosen M, et al. The reliability of a linear analogue for evaluating pain. Anaesthesia 1976;31:1191–8.
[5] Richter P, Werner J, Heerlein A, et al. On the validity of the Beck Depression Inventory: a review. Psychopathology 1998;31:160–8.
[6] Fairbank JC, Pynsent PB. The Oswestry Disability Index. Spine 2000;25:2940–52.
[7] Arbisi PA, Butcher JN. Psychometric perspectives on detection of malingering of pain: use of the Minnesota Multiphasic Personality Inventory-2. Clin J Pain 2004;20:383–91.
[8] Porter RW. Spinal stenosis and neurogenic claudication. Spine 1996;21:2046–52.
[9] John J. Grading of muscle power: comparison of MRC and analogue scales by physiotherapists. Medical Research Council. Int J Rehabil Res 1984;7:173–81.
[10] Alvarez DJ, Rockwell PG. Trigger points: diagnosis and management. Am Fam Physician 2002;65(4):653–60.
[11] Waddell G, McCulloch JA, Kummel E, et al. Nonorganic physical signs in low-back pain. Spine 1980;5:117–25.
[12] Hazel WA Jr, Jones RA, Morrey BF, et al. Vertebral fractures without neurological deficit. A long-term follow-up study. J Bone Joint Surg Am 1988;70(9):1319–21.
[13] Zambelli PY, Dutoit M, Genton N. Dorso-lumbar spinal compression fractures in the child. Follow-up at the termination of development. Helv Chir Acta 1991;58(1–2):119–22.

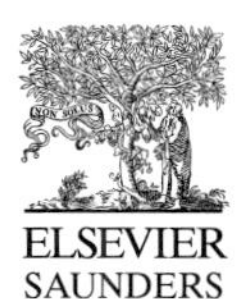

ELSEVIER
SAUNDERS

Phys Med Rehabil Clin N Am
17 (2006) 315–345

PHYSICAL MEDICINE
AND REHABILITATION
CLINICS OF
NORTH AMERICA

Physical Agents Used in the Management of Chronic Pain by Physical Therapists

Roger J. Allen, PhD, PT

Department of Physical Therapy, University of Puget Sound, 1500 North Warner, CMB 1070, Tacoma, WA 98416, USA

The primary role of physical therapy in the treatment of patients suffering from chronic pain is to prescribe, facilitate, and pace therapeutic activities for functional physical restoration [1–4]. Within their sphere of practice, physical therapists have at their disposal and the expertise to administer a wide choice of physical agents (frequently referred to as physical modalities) that may be used to attenuate pain [5–8].

Physical agents may influence pain by resolving inflammation [7,8], facilitating tissue repair [7,8], activating temporary analgesia [8,9], altering nerve conduction [8], providing a counterirritant [8], modifying muscle tone or collagen extensibility [8], reducing the probability of maladaptive central neuropathic changes developing into chronic pain-generation loci [10–12], or otherwise providing palliative relief from pain sensations [6]. In a physical therapy setting, agents are rarely used in isolation; rather, they are used to enhance the effectiveness of other therapeutic interventions directed at functional restoration [4,13].

When prescribing physical agents for the treatment of chronic pain, two essential patient-specific issues must be considered. First, although agents may be useful in a variety of ways for treating chronic pain, they are frequently implemented for temporary attenuation of pain sensations [5,7]. Administering physical agents for passive palliative relief to patients with chronic pain is controversial [4] and should be considered on an individual case basis. For a given patient, providing temporary relief via physical agents may create a therapeutic window of opportunity for the therapist to mobilize tissue or address movement impairments [4]. For others, palliative treatment may psychologically reinforce a maladaptive cycle of pain behavior or generate disincentives for the patient to approach pain

E-mail address: rallen@ups.edu

1047-9651/06/$ - see front matter
doi:10.1016/j.pmr.2005.12.007

management in an active or functional manner. This may hinder progress toward functional recovery [4].

The second consideration relates to supposition regarding the locus of pain generation and appropriately matching the physical agent's effects with what affects the pathology or symptoms arising from that pain generation site or process. As an example, an agent such as pulsed ultrasound, whose therapeutic value is to aid in the resolution of inflammation at local tissue, is of little or no value for treating central thalamic pain. In chronic pain cases, the pain generation site may shift over time [11,14–19]. Dorsal horn or cortical neuroplastic changes may result in chronic central pain generation after an inciting distal lesion [11,16,17]. New secondary pain generation sites may also develop from excessively restricted mobility [14,15,18,19]. The original lesion may have resolved, with the current pain complaint now being generated by secondary structural and pathophysiologic changes associated with lack of active motion [14,15]. The applied physical agent must address the specific source of pain generation, neurologically interrupt pain transmission by operating on peripheral nerve conduction or central gating mechanisms, or provide an effective counterirritant. When nociceptive pain is being generated by damaged or inflamed tissue, locally effective agents may be applied. If pain symptoms are largely being generated by neuropathic or central neuroplastic remodeling components, then only agents capable of influencing neural transmission or central processing are likely to be beneficial.

To articulate the strength and quality of evidence supporting the use of physical therapy agents for specific indications, a rating system was developed by Canadian task force groups, proposing a hierarchy of three grades (grades I–III) [7,20,21]. Applications of physical agents with evidence from controlled studies on human volunteers, published in peer-reviewed journals, regardless of level of randomization or blindness, are rated "grade I"; noncontrolled human studies are "grade II"; and human case studies are "grade III" [7]. This article uses this rating system, as applied by Belanger [7], as a first-order approximation of the quality of evidence for each physical agent genre.

Superficial thermal agents: heat and cold

Thermotherapy

Thermotherapy in rehabilitation is the therapeutic application of superficial mild heat to increase circulation, enhance healing, increase soft tissue extensibility, and control pain. Heat may be delivered to superficial tissues via conduction (eg, hot packs, paraffin dips, microwavable rice-filled cloth bags, electric heating pads), convection (eg, hydrotherapy, fluidotherapy), or radiation (eg, infrared lamps for treating dermal ulcers and psoriasis) [8]. In the context of pain management, potential therapeutic benefits of superficial heat are due to its effects on metabolic, neuromuscular, and hemodynamic activity.

Although the therapeutic mechanisms attributable to superficial heat primarily influence tissue healing and acute nociceptive pain generation, thermotherapy may have utility in the comprehensive treatment of chronic pain. With mild increases in tissue temperature, the oxygen–hemoglobin dissociation curve shifts to the right, making more oxygen available for tissue repair. Increases in enzymatic activity increase oxygen uptake by the cell, thus enhancing healing [8]. Increased skeletal muscle temperature (to 42°C) has been reported to decrease firing rates of gamma and type II muscle spindle efferents while increasing Golgi tendon organ type Ib fiber firing rates [22–24]. This may reflexively reduce skeletal muscle tone and spasm by lowering alpha motor neuron firing rates [25]. Reducing skeletal muscle activity may be useful in breaking the pain-spasm-pain exacerbation cycle [26].

Superficial heat has been reported to elevate nociceptive threshold [27]. Although it does not travel over large-diameter fibers, the afferent thermoreceptive message of superficial heating has been hypothesized to produce inhibitory modulation of dorsal horn pain gates [8] or to provide a counterirritant stimulus to cortically compete with pain perception. Pain may be significantly influenced indirectly via local vasomotor effects and increased blood flow. Cutaneous thermoreception directly results in the release of bradykinin, leading to local vasodilation in the heated area [28]. After synapsing in the dorsal horn, input from thermal receptors inhibits sympathetic vasomotor efferents in the intermediolateral gray area, thereby decreasing neurogenic vasoconstriction [8]. In addition to the decrease in sympathetic vasomotor outflow, local vasodilation and increased vascular perfusion may influence pain by decreasing tissue ischemia [29], helping to resolve hyperalgesia, thus returning nociceptors to normal firing thresholds and clearing the region of exacerbating metabolites such as prostaglandins. Although increases in blood flow of up to 30 ml per 100 g of tissue have been reported [22], these effects primarily influence cutaneous blood vessels and the tissue regions they supply with less evident vasodilation in deep muscle vasculature due to the minimal ability of superficial agents to carry increased temperature to deep structures [8].

Superficial heat, in the form of hot packs, paraffin, and hydrotherapy, has been broadly evaluated for effectiveness in treating rheumatoid arthritis. Although six controlled studies have found it a beneficial adjunct [30–34], two have found it ineffective [35,36], with the possibility of heat harming the condition through increased collagenase activity damaging compromised articular cartilage [37]. Uncontrolled grade II comparative studies report beneficial effects of superficial heat for chronic low back pain [38–42], neck and shoulder pain [43], and trigger point pain in the neck and back [44].

Contraindications to thermotherapy include applying heat over regions of acute injury, inflammation, hemorrhagic areas, malignancy, impaired sensation, and thrombophlebitis; hemorrhagic areas; abdomens of pregnant women; or patients manifesting relevant cognitive impairments [7,8]. Precautions should be taken when applying heat over areas with impaired circulation, edema, or superficial metal implants or open wounds; with patients manifesting poor thermal regulation, cardiac insufficiency, or acute inflammatory disorders [37]; or with hypotensive patients or patients prone to syncope when heating large body areas [7,8].

Cryotherapy

In a rehabilitation context, cryotherapy withdraws heat from the body through the use of mild superficial cooling agents. Cryotherapy is used to control pain, edema, and inflammation; to enhance movement; and to attenuate spasticity [8]. The body surface may be exposed to cold though conduction (eg, cold packs, ice massage, cryopressure garments combining cold with compression, bags of frozen corn), convection (eg, cold whirlpool immersion, contrast baths), or evaporation (eg, vapocoolant sprays). The therapeutic effects of cold generally result from its actions on metabolic, neuromuscular, and hemodynamic processes [8].

The application of cold may decrease nociceptive input and pain perception through local and central nervous system mechanisms. In response to cold, the vasoconstrictive response decreases the release of local vasodilating substances, which decreases nociceptor sensitization [26]. Due to metabolic axonal changes, for every 1°C drop in interstitial temperature, nerve conduction velocity of somatosensory afferent fibers drops approximately 2 m/s, with A-delta fibers being the most sensitive to cold-mediated attenuations in velocity [22]. Cold application for 10 to 15 minutes may go beyond immediate changes and produce pain reductions for more than 1 hour [8]. Continued analgesia may be caused by conduction blocking of A-delta nociceptive fibers, inhibitory gating of pain by thermoreceptive fibers, and the maintenance of subnormal deep tissue temperature for 1 to 2 hours after cold exposure [8,45]. Prolonged application of cold has also been demonstrated to produce reversible total nerve conduction blocks [46]. Cold application theoretically interrupts the pain-spasm-pain cycle, reducing muscle spasm and extending pain relief after tissue temperature has recovered to normal values [8]. Finally, by applying vapocoolant sprays over skeletal muscle, so-called "cryostretch" is possible [8,47,48]. Immediate analgesia is afforded by evaporative cooling reduces muscle spasm and allows muscle with excess neurogenic tone to be stretched for increased range of motion [48,49].

Although the existing literature strongly supports the efficacy of cryotherapy in the management of acute trauma, cryotherapy may play a role in treating chronic pain conditions. Two uncontrolled comparative studies [47,50] and case studies [51,52] have reported cryotherapy to be a beneficial adjunct in treating muscle spasms and myofascial pain. Comparative grade II studies found cryotherapy to be a beneficial adjunctive tool in the management of low back pain [41,53], chronic headache [54,55], trigeminal neuralgia [56], and chronic osteoarthritis [57].

Contraindications to cryotherapy include cold urticaria; cold intolerance or hypersensitivity; Raynaud disease or phenomenon; cryoglobulinemia or paroxysmal cold hemoglobinuria; and deep open wounds, regenerating peripheral nerves, areas of circulatory compromise or peripheral vascular disease, and skin areas of impaired somatosensory discrimination [7,8].

Therapeutic ultrasound

In contrast to superficial agents, deep-heating agents are capable of producing temperature elevations at tissue depths of 3 cm or greater through conversion of a nonthermal energy source into heat within tissue [8,58]. One of the most commonly used deep-heating agents is ultrasound, with several authors reporting it to be the most widely used physical agent available to clinicians [7,59,60]. Therapeutic ultrasound is clinically used in three forms: continuous, for raising deep tissue temperature; pulsed, for activating nonthermal physiologic effects; and as a phonophoresis driving agent for transdermal delivery of topical medication [7,8].

Unlike ultrasound used for medical imaging, therapeutic ultrasound is used to deliver energy to deep tissue sites, via propagation of ultrasonic waves, to produce increases in tissue temperature or nonthermal physiologic changes [6,58]. Rather than transmitting ultrasonic waves through tissue and then processing a returning echo to generate an image of underlying structures, therapeutic ultrasound is one-way energy delivery. Via a reverse piezoelectric effect, a crystal sound head transmits acoustic waves typically at 1 or 3 MHz and at amplitude densities of between 0.1 and 3 w/cm^2 [3,8]. Although still comfortably in the ultrasonic range, this is a lower frequency than that used for imaging but is a notably higher wattage.

Ultrasonic energy causes soft tissue molecules to vibrate from exposure to the compression and rarefaction caused by the acoustic wave. Increased molecular motion leads to microfriction between molecules, and frictional heat is generated, thus increasing tissue temperature [7]. In addition to heat generation through microfriction, heat may be generated at specific tissue interfaces due to changes in sonic impedance within the tissue. Different tissue types have varying abilities to attenuate ultrasonic acoustic waves [58]. When passing from tissue of low sonic impedance to one of high impedance (such as from muscle to bone), heat is generated at the interface through shearing and reflection of the wave [22]. This is true at the periosteum, where continuous application of ultrasound can produce periosteal pain due to differential heating [22]. Referred to as ultrasound's "thermal effects," this heating is reported to produce increased collagen extensibility, increased nerve conduction velocity, altered local vascular perfusion, increased enzymatic activity, altered contractile activity of skeletal muscle, and increased nociceptive threshold [22,29,58,61].

Administering ultrasound discontinuously at a specified duty cycle of on–off pulses produces cavitation and streaming [7,8,58]. The cyclic drop in pressure created by acoustic waves causes normally present minute gas pockets in the tissue to develop into microscopic bubbles, or cavities. With therapeutic ultrasound, stabile acoustic cavitation results, whereby the microbubbles pulsate without imploding. This pulsation leads to microstreaming of fluid around the pulsating bubbles [7,58]. When occurring around cells, this process is reported to alter cell membrane activity, vascular wall permeability, and facilitate soft tissue healing [7,58,63]. Increases in skin and cell membrane permeability from pulsed ultrasound are thought to be partially responsible for the ability of ultrasound to deliver medication to deep tissue sites transdermally.

Pulsed ultrasound has been reported to produce a variety of effects. Some of these are contradictory, such as improved blood flow and increased vasomotor activity [64,65]. Many ultrasound effects may be intensity dependent, with physiologic reversals occurring at different dosing levels [58]. Although usually used for nonthermal effects, pulsed ultrasound produces a concomitant therapeutic effect, meaning that heating and nonthermal effects occur simultaneously [7,66].

Clinical indications for continuous ultrasound relate to the usefulness of deep tissue heating. The heating of collagen increases its extensibility by altering its tertiary molecular bonding. This makes ultrasound a useful aid for therapists treating scar tissue, joint contractures, tissue adhesions, and maladaptive shortening of connective tissue [7,8,58], all of which could be structural contributors to chronic pain [14,15]. Pain reduction via increased nociceptive threshold may be achieved with continuous ultrasound [7,8,22,58]. Proposed mechanisms for increased nociceptive thresholds include counterirritation, heat activation of large diameter afferent fibers, or alteration of nociceptive receptor sensitivity [58]. In numerous studies, varying in rigor, ultrasound has been reported effective in treating pain from a variety of origins including soft tissue lesions [67], muscle spasms [68], tendonitis [69], myofascial trigger points [58], carpal tunnel syndrome [70], back pain [71], epicondylitis [72], complex regional pain syndrome (CRPS) [73], and phantom limb pain [74].

Although the mechanisms remain unclear, pulsed ultrasound has long been used for treating acute and chronic inflammation [75,76] and to promote tissue healing [58]. A further application of pulsed ultrasound for treating pain and inflammation is via phonophoresis. A preparation of a steroid (eg, dexamethasone) or analgesic (eg, lidocaine) is used as the coupling medium between the soundhead and skin surface [8,58]. Pulsed ultrasound transdermally drives the medication deep into tissue by altering the permeability of the stratum corneum and then deep cell membranes [8,77]. Although administered for local tissue effects, drugs delivered through phonophoresis become systemic, and their systemic contraindications must be considered [8].

Controlled grade I studies have found ultrasound to be useful in the treatment of soft tissue lesions [67], shoulder pain [79], shoulder adhesive capsulitis [80], and pain associated with prolapsed intervertebral discs [71]. For osteoarthritis [81,82], carpal tunnel syndrome [70,83], shoulder calcific tendonitis [69,84], and elbow epicondylitis, grade I investigations are divided into those that report benefits from ultrasound and those that do not. Available grade I studies assessing ultrasound's usefulness for treating postextraction dental pain [85,86], shoulder peritendinitis [87], perineal postlabor pain [88,89], and subacromial bursitis [90] report no significant beneficial effects over controls.

Contraindications to ultrasound include directing acoustic energy over malignant lesions, pregnant abdomens, plastic implants, hemorrhagic regions, cemented areas of prosthetic joints, ischemic regions, insensate areas, infected lesions, electronic implants (including neurostimulators), areas that have been exposed to radiotherapy within the past 6 months, fractures, epiphyseal growth plates in skeletally immature patients, thrombotic areas, orbits of the eyes, gonads, and spinal cord after laminectomy [7,8]. The most common adverse effect is periosteal pain from continuous ultrasound [8], although some authors feel this is the indicator that therapeutic temperature has been reached in deep tissue [22].

Although efficacy evidence for therapeutic application of ultrasound is mixed, ultrasound is widely used by physical therapists as an adjunct to the management of pain and inflammation [3,91,92]. Aside from possible placebo effects, its therapeutic actions are almost exclusively at the tissue level. This makes it a potential tool for nociceptive pain but of limited or no use for central pain or chronic pain exacerbated by neuroplastic remodeling. Prescribing its use for patients with chronic pain should result from reasonable evidence that the pain is, at least in part, generated by an active lesion at the nociceptive level.

Diathermy

Diathermy is the use of shortwave (wavelength 3–30 m, frequency 10–100 MHz) or microwave (wavelength 0.001–1 m, frequency 300 MHz to 300 GHz) electromagnetic radiation to produce heat within body tissue through conversion [8]. The United States Federal Communications Commission has assigned 13.56, 27.12, and 40.68 MHz for medical applications of shortwave and 2450 MHz for microwave medical applications [7,8]. Shortwave diathermy (SWD) is typically generated using the 27.12-MHz band [7,8].

Diathermy has potential advantages over other agents used to heat subcutaneous tissue. First, diathermy can produce heat at deeper tissue levels than superficial agents [8]. Second, it can heat larger areas than other penetrating agents (eg, ultrasound) [8]. Third, shortwave radiation does not experience a transmission impedance change while passing from soft tissue to bone, as does sound energy. Therefore, unlike ultrasound, it is not reflected by bone and does not cause differential heating at tissue interfaces or present risk of periosteal burning [8].

Microwave diathermy (MWD) has two disadvantages limiting its potential use. Unlike SWD, MWD reflects when encountering even slight variations in soft tissue density, thus producing shearing, standing waves, and local hot spots in relatively superficial tissue [8]. The high frequency of MWD, combined with its high reflectivity at tissue interfaces, means that MWD tends to bring superficial tissues to intolerably high temperatures before therapeutically useful temperature increases are achieved at the deeper target tissue levels. For this reason, the clinical use of MWD has been nearly abandoned in most countries in favor of SWD and ultrasound [7].

Shortwave energy can be delivered as continuous electromagnetic radiation (continuous shortwave diathermy [CSWD]) for deep heating of soft tissue or in pulsed form (pulsed shortwave diathermy [PSWD]) to induce nonthermal effects [7]. As electromagnetic energy is delivered to the tissue via CSWD, increased average molecular kinetic energy leads physiologically to thermal heating effects of vasodilation, increased rate of nerve conduction, increased collagen extensibility, acceleration of enzymatic activity, changes in skeletal muscle strength, and possibly increased nociceptive threshold [8]. In contrast with superficial heating, which produces physiologic heating effects within a few millimeters of the dermis, CSWD may be used to produce these effects within deep muscle [8].

By pulsing the delivery of shortwave energy with low amplitude, short-duration pulses at a low-duty-cycle SWD do not generate sustained increases in tissue temperature due to dissipation of transient heat from vascular perfusion of the area [8]. However, as with ultrasound, when pulsed energy is applied at subthermal levels, a number of nonthermal changes occur [93]. Although the mechanisms of nonthermal effects are speculative, they are broadly attributed to modified ion binding, which affects cellular functions of protein synthesis and ATP production [7,94–96]. The influence of electromagnetic fields on ion binding has been reported to produce a cascade of physiologic responses that may include growth factor activation in fibroblasts and neurons, macrophage activation, and alterations in myosin phosphorylation [8,97].

There is evidence that PSWD application for 40 to 45 minutes increases microvascular perfusion of local tissue in normal subjects and adjacent to ulcer sites in patients with diabetic ulcers [8,98,99]. Increased local perfusion has the capability to increase oxygenation of deep tissue, decrease anaerobic metabolism, enhance nutrient availability, and assist phagocytosis [8]. Although it is most probable that CSWD and PSWD produce thermal and nonthermal effects, a result of either mode of application is increased cellular metabolism and functioning, which may have implications for the promotion of healing [7].

Due to its ability to heat large areas of deep tissue, potential indications for the clinical use of CSWD include augmentation of healing, decreased joint stiffness in large areas such as the hip or diffuse spinal regions, and increased joint range of motion when combined with stretching [8]. Possible clinical indications for the use of nonthermal PSWD include pain control via edema reduction and enhanced healing of soft tissue wounds (eg, burns, pressure ulcers, and surgical wounds), peripheral nerve lesions, and fractures [8]. The possible clinical benefit of SWD to beneficially address these conditions must be considered not only on its demonstrated effects but also on the strength of clinical efficacy evidence.

Most of the recent literature on clinical efficacy of SWD evaluates potential tissue healing effects, with a few available studies addressing SWD application in chronic pain management. Pulsed electromagnetic fields (PEMF) have been reported to be a useful therapy for nonunion fractures [100,101], failed arthrodeses [102], and osteonecrosis [103]. Another form of PEMF, magnetotherapy, has been applied to treat chronic pain of various origins [104–106], venous ulcers [107,108], and tendonitis [109,110]. Although both are pulsed delivery of electromagnetic radiation, PEMF and PSWD are not synonymous [7]. Two studies found significant decreases in neck pain and increases in range of motion in patients who had cervical spine injuries after using PSWD for 3 weeks compared with a placebo device [111,112]. Two early (1959 and 1964) grade I controlled studies [113,114] reported beneficial results treating osteoarthritis with SWD, whereas three more recent investigations did not find SWD therapy to produce significant reductions in osteoarthritic pain intensity over control subjects [115–117]. Three controlled investigations failed to demonstrate significant benefits of SWD in treating ankle sprains [118–120]. A single uncontrolled study reported positive outcomes using PSWD treating post-traumatic algoneurodystrophy (CRPS) [121]. A single available controlled study found SWD beneficial for managing low back pain [122].

The nature of the radiant energy that allows SWD to increase tissue temperature gives rise to special precautions and contraindications. Some materials absorb disproportionate amounts of electromagnetic energy, such as metals, fat, and tissue with high free water concentrations [8]. Other materials (eg, drops of perspiration) act as lenses, focusing the energy. High absorption and focusing may lead to hazardous increases in adjacent tissue temperature [7,8]. Burning or fire could be caused by the presence of metal implants, pacemakers, neurostimulators, or copper-bearing intrauterine contraceptive devices within the body or any metal outside the patient's body (eg, jewelry, coins, clothing zippers) or in close proximity to the patient within the shortwave radiant field (eg, metal parts in a treatment table, zippers in pillow cases) [7]. The immediate environment must be cleared of metal and electronic or magnetic equipment. "Well, the first time I lit a patient on fire with diathermy..." began a therapist's anecdote relating how she had forgotten about the metal zipper of the inner pillowcase beneath the patient's head.

Special precautions must be taken when treating obese patients, when treating high adipose regions, or under circumstances when the patient begins perspiring [8] and over moist wound dressings or ischemic areas [7]. Because of variation in absorbency, some tissue areas may be burned while others are spared [8]. The patient's skin must be kept dry during treatment to prevent scalding from hot perspiration [8].

Contraindications to SWD include pregnancy, malignancy, and applying SWD over insensate skin regions. Because of potential damage due to heat generation, CSWD should not be applied over the eyes, testes, or epiphyseal growth plates in skeletally immature patients.

Although SWD has good tissue penetration properties and the ability to heat or deliver pulsed energy to deep structures, it is rarely used in the treatment of pain. This is because of the many ways that patients can be harmed via soft tissue burns. Using a pharmacologic analogy, its therapeutic index is uncomfortably low compared with other physical agents. Most clinics have abandoned its use, and it is a rare physical therapy facility that has the equipment available and in use with therapists adequately trained and experienced in its application. Recent promotion of the clinical use of SWD is for wound-healing applications.

Laser

Laser therapy uses light that is monochromatic, coherent, and highly directional [8]. Proposed uses for laser therapy in physical rehabilitation settings include the promotion of wound healing and pain management [7,8]. Although laser therapy has been widely used in Europe for more than a decade [123], it was not until February of 2002 that the US Food and Drug Administration approved the therapeutic use of laser therapy for the temporary relief of pain.

Special properties of laser light allow the potential for direct delivery of electromagnetic light energy to tissue depths slightly below the dermis and possible indirect physiologic effects at deeper levels [8,124]. The ability of laser light to penetrate is a function of tissue type and the laser's wavelength and resistance to scatter [125]. The most commonly used wavelengths for clinical application of laser light range from 600 to 1300 nm, allowing a direct tissue penetration depth of 1 to 4 mm [8]. A second variable parameter of laser light affecting its clinical use is power or wattage [7,8]. Cold lasers with output powers of less than 500 mW, at a power density of about 50 mW/cm^2, have been used in rehabilitation settings to theoretically promote healing and manage pain via photobiomodulation of chromophores within the affected tissue. The term "low-level laser therapy" (LLLT) is used to describe the therapeutic application of cold lasers to facilitate photobiomodulation [7,125,126]. The most frequently used lasers for LLLT are semiconductor diode types (904-nm gallium-arsenide lasers or gallium-aluminum arsenide lasers) with wavelengths that may vary based on aluminum content [7].

Although the physiologic effects of low-wattage lasers are not well established or understood, there is consensus in the literature that LLLT can induce photobiomodulation effects [7,126,127]. As laser light penetrates the skin, its photons are absorbed by cellular chromophores (light-absorbing molecules) that undergo photobiomodulation via influence over respiratory chain enzymes in the form of photobiostimulation or photobioinhibition according to the Arndt-Schultz law of photobiologic activation [7,125]. This asserts a dose-response interaction effect whereby low dosages trigger a photobiostimulation response and higher dosages trigger a photobioinhibition response [125]. Wound-healing effects are attributed to photobiostimulation, whereas pain management has been reported to be a function of photobioinhibition [7]. Photobiomodulation effects via cold laser on calcium channels have been reported to cause increased fibroblast, macrophage, and lymphocyte activity [128–132].

For temporary analgesia, the effect of LLLT on nerve conduction velocity has been addressed by numerous grade I controlled studies. Some have shown small increases or decreases in peripheral nerve conduction velocity with corresponding slight changes in distal latencies [133–136], whereas others report finding no effect [137,138]. The ability of LLLT to influence nerve conduction velocity in a clinically significant way seems uncertain at this time. That is not to say that LLLT modulation of pain from peripheral nerve involvement could not be influenced via another, as yet uncertain, mechanism.

The two primary indications for LLLT are wound healing and pain management. Efficacy studies related to both applications yield varied results. Of 17 English language studies reviewing the clinical impact of LLLT on cutaneous wounds and ulcers, 14 have demonstrated beneficial outcomes. Of three grade I controlled studies on wound healing, two conducted before 1992 using He-Ne lasers [139,140] reported no benefit over control subjects, whereas a more recent work published in 1999 [141] reported a beneficial effect, citing the importance of appropriate candidate selection for LLLT.

The effect of LLLT has been addressed in numerous studies of varying quality for a wide spectrum of conditions that generate pain. For many disorders, outcomes of controlled studies are decidedly split between those that show some clinically significant beneficial effect over control subjects and those that do not. Regarding arthritic conditions, four [142–145] of seven [142–148] controlled studies reported beneficial results for patients with rheumatoid arthritis, and five [149–153] of seven [149–155] studies yielded positive therapeutic responses for osteoarthritic conditions. Two controlled studies addressing the ability of LLLT to relieve pain secondary to trigger point stimulation reported beneficial results [156,157], whereas the treatment of myofascial pain per se displays a different clinical picture, with three studies [158–160] reporting no significant effect over controls. Three [161–163] of four [161–164] studies assessing the impact on teninopathies report no beneficial findings, with regional epicondylitis showing a positive response to therapy in one [165] of five [165–169] grade I controlled studies.

Regarding pain originating from a specific locus, controlled studies reporting LLLT benefits have been published regarding trigeminal pain [170,171], postherpetic pain [172], perioral herpes pain [173], and postsurgical abdominal pain [174]. Laser therapy has not demonstrated significant benefits in available grade I studies concerned with ankle pain [175], temporomandibular joint disorder [176], muscle soreness [177,178], plantar fasciitis [179], chondromalacia [180], or orofacial pain [181].

The foremost contraindication to the use of LLLT is exposure of the eye to laser light. Additional contraindications include exposing any of the following regions to low-level laser light: locally to endocrine glands [8]; photosensitive skin areas; hemorrhagic areas; any area within 4 to 6 months after radiation therapy; neoplastic lesions; or over the heart, vagus nerve, or sympathetic innervation routes to the heart of cardiac patients [7,8]. Precautionary application should be considered when using LLLT over epiphyseal regions of long bones in children, gonads, infected areas, or areas with compromised somatosensation and when treating patients who display mental confusion, fever, or epilepsy [7,8]. Although there are few reports of adverse responses to LLLT, episodic tingling, burning sensations, mild erythema, numbness, increased pain, and skin rash associated with LLLT have been reported in individual cases [8].

The available literature shows a mixed picture of efficacy findings regarding the therapeutic effects of LLLT for various pain conditions. Proposed mechanisms have plausibility, yet they are incompletely understood. The use of LLLT is increasing in North America, and recent approval by the US Food and Drug Administration may accelerate its clinical implementation for the temporary reduction of pain. It is not in widespread use by physical therapists, and, although some clinics are providing this service, most do not have the apparatus or training to offer it.

Electrical current

Traditionally, the use of electrical currents to modulate pain is via transcutaneous electroneural stimulation (TENS). Unlike physical agents, whose primary site of action in pain control is the tissue level, TENS is thought to operate by facilitating interruption of the neural transmission of pain [9]. Using capacitance coupling, surface electrical current produced by the TENS unit generates action potentials in underlying peripheral nerves. Specific axons affected are determined by three interacting factors: fiber diameter, anatomic proximity of nerve fibers to the skin surface, and external current intensity [8]. There are choices for the placement of stimulating electrodes: around or near the lesion site, along the course of the peripheral nerve carrying the nociceptive message, on the back near spinal nerve root entry, or at related acupuncture points [8]. Four levels of stimulus intensity may be delivered by TENS units: subsensory, sensory, motor, and noxious.

Subsensory-level TENS uses a phasic charge of insufficient amplitude to depolarize peripheral nerve axons, reach sensory threshold, or depolarize muscle membranes [9]. This approach is sometimes referred to as subliminal stimulation [182], low-intensity direct current [5], or microcurrent electrical nerve stimulation (MENS) [8,9,183]. In the absence of neural stimulation, it is uncertain which mechanism microcurrents use to modulate pain. Postulated mechanisms include placebo effects, augmented tissue healing, and altering energy flow along acupuncture meridians [8]. Two authors have stated that there is no evidence for the use of subsensory-level electrical currents in pain management [8,9]. Several studies have found MENS to be no more effective than no treatment or placebos and significantly less effective than sensory-level TENS [183–189].

Although subsensory microcurrent does not operate by exciting peripheral nerves, it may enhance tissue healing [7]. Numerous studies have reported microcurrents being generated by the skin in areas around wounds [189–192]. These naturally occurring microcurrents, called "currents of injury" [189], have been observed in the skin of regenerating newt stumps [193,194]. It has been hypothesized that exogenous microcurrent may augment this endogenous activity and enhance or maintain skin healing [7]. Grade I investigations have found microcurrent efficacious in augmenting healing for epicondylitis [195], peritendinitis [196], and indolent and diabetic ulcers [197,198]. Two controlled studies found microcurrent to be of no benefit in the treatment of delayed-onset muscle soreness [199,200]. Mixed results have been reported in controlled studies for the treatment of pressure ulcers [201,202]. However, in reference to pressure ulcers, the United States Agency for Health Care Policy and Research concluded in 1994 that "At this time, electrical stimulation is the only adjunctive therapy with sufficient supporting evidence to warrant recommendation" [7]. From the perspective of pain management, microcurrent application may assist wound resolution but seems to be of no value in attenuating pain that is not associated with an active nociceptive lesion.

Operating at higher current amplitude than microcurrent, sensory-level (or "conventional") TENS is thought to attenuate the perception of pain via stimulation of large-diameter afferent peripheral nerve fibers and subsequent interruption of pain transmission at the dorsal horn due to the gate control mechanism [8,9,203]. Because it primarily operates neurally through the ascending analgesia pathway, sensory-level TENS produces a rapid onset of pain reduction, yet its effects typically cease quickly after stimulation has stopped [8]. Sensory-level TENS units are often worn for many hours during the day and use frequent random modulation of the stimulus wave to prevent neural habituation. Some studies have suggested that this level of stimulation may trigger limited endorphin release in instances where its effects seem to outlast the period of electrical stimulation [204,205].

Sensory-level TENS is primarily indicated for acute and subacute pain but also has utility in chronic pain conditions. One suggested chronic pain application is to reduce pain as early as possible in the development of the condition to fight dorsal horn remodeling of N-methyl-D-asparate (NMDA) receptors as a central pain generation site [11]. It may also be plausible to use sensory-level stimulation at a body site other than the painful region to provide a competing attentional counterirritant to fight long-term cortical remodeling.

To achieve a more prolonged analgesic response from TENS, current amplitudes may be increased to induce motor- or noxious-level stimulation, which activates the descending endogenous-opioid–based analgesic pathway [7–9,206,207]. Motor-level stimulation occurs when TENS amplitude is high enough to produce visible skeletal muscle contractions [8,9]. Rhythmic muscle contractions may be induced electrically without exciting nociceptive afferent fibers [9]. These contractions have been shown to stimulate therelease of enkephalins and dynorphins [208]. Analgesic responses to motor level TENS have a slower onset (15–60 minutes) but have longer duration after stimulation is discontinued (several hours) than sensory TENS [8].

Noxious-level TENS helps reduce pain perception by stimulating nociception at a site near or remote to the painful region. Current amplitudes are great enough to produce painful stimulation with or without skeletal muscle contraction [9]. Pain relief onset occurs within seconds or minutes after initiating the stimulus and may last for several hours [8]. Studies have demonstrated that noxious-level–induced decreases in pain last longer and are more pronounced than the relief generated from sensory- or motor-level TENS [206,207,209–211]. It is hypothesized that noxious-level stimulation may cause rapid pain modulation via "hyperstimulation analgesia," which interferes with central patterned-reverberation pain circuitry [9].

Although sensory-level TENS is the most widely used modality, due to patient intolerance for rhythmic muscle contractions and painful stimuli presented to a person already experiencing pain, motor- and noxious-level applications may be indicated if insufficient relief has been achieved with sensory-level stimulation [8]. Motor-level TENS is recommended for patients who have chronic pain and low endogenous endorphin levels (eg, from prolonged opiate use) [8]. Noxious-level TENS may be indicated for patients who have chronic pain and have not had a successful response to motor-level TENS [8].

Clinical efficacy literature related to chronic pain applications of TENS is extensive and has yielded relatively consistent findings. Six controlled studies have demonstrated significant clinical effectiveness for TENS in the management of pain associated with osteoarthritis [212–217]. Other conditions for which TENS has demonstrated effectiveness in grade I studies include trigeminal neuralgia [218], postamputation and phantom limb pain [219,220], neck pain [221], pain due to peripheral neuropathy [222,223], painful shoulder secondary to stroke [224], and migraine headache [225]. Mixed results have been reported for rheumatoid arthritis [226–228], low back pain [229–235], and myofascial pain [236,237]. Conditions for which the literature consistently shows TENS to be of no benefit over control subjects include a limited number of acute and post-surgical pain conditions [7].

In addition to TENS, electrical currents are used to enhance healing, resolve inflammation, and transdermally deliver topical medication [8,238]. Interferential current and iontophoresis are of potential utility in managing chronic pain.

Interferential current (IC) involves intersecting two alternating current sources of slightly different middle frequencies to create an interference pattern at a target tissue site. The resulting IC is in the form of a low-frequency "beat," whose frequency is the arithmetic difference between the two intersecting currents, typically in the 1 to 200 Hz range [8]. Suggested indications are for pain modulation via inhibitory gating at the dorsal horn and edema management.

Efficacy literature supporting the use of IC is lacking. Evidence for its use is largely based on clinical anecdotes and unsupported beliefs [239]. Regarding analgesia, one study reported that healthy subjects receiving IC showed significantly increased thresholds for "ice-pain" compared with control subjects not receiving IC [240]. Conversely, IC failed to show any effect on pain when using the RIII reflex as an experimental pain model [241]. Although there is a case report indicating successful treatment of a patient who had migraine headache using IC [242], grade I controlled studies applying IC to the treatment of acute low back pain [243] and jaw pain [244] have failed to demonstrate beneficial results. No benefit for low back pain was observed for IC in an investigation comparing it with motorized lumbar traction and massage [245]. In spite of the paucity of supporting evidence, IC is widely used in physical therapy clinics.

Similar in function to phonophoresis, iontophoresis uses direct current to assist the local transdermal delivery of ionizable medications, such as local anesthetics and antiinflammatories [238]. Positively charged ionic compounds are repelled from anode electrodes and attracted to cathodes, whereas negatively charged compounds manifest the opposite behavior [246]. For managing chronic pain conditions, several medications have been recommended that are capable of forming ionic compounds in solution: lidocaine for soft tissue pain and inflammation, dexamethasone and hydrocortisone for inflammation, magnesium sulfate for skeletal muscle spasms, and salicylates for acute and chronic muscle and joint pain [238]. Because iontophoresis relies upon direct current, it is important to note that a sodium hydroxide alkaline reaction naturally occurs beneath the cathode electrode and hydrochloric acid concentrates beneath the anode [238]. With excessive use, electrochemical skin burns may occur beneath the electrodes due to these pH changes. Although changes in tissue pH beneath the electrodes may affect drug ionization and stability, there is evidence that iontophoresis can effectively deliver some medications to the site of interest [247–249].

Few studies have investigated the use of iontophoresis for managing chronic pain. It has been found to be effective in a grade I study using dexamethasone to manage plantar fasciitis [247], beneficial using a combination of dexamethasone and lidocaine to treat shoulder myofascial syndrome in a grade II comparative study [248], and effective as an adjunct to managing post-herpetic neuralgia pain in an uncontrolled follow-up investigation [249].

There are other electrical current configurations with reported use in managing chronic pain whose application and availability in the United States is limited. Three of these are multiplexed anodal stimulation, high-voltage pulsed current [7,250,251], and diadynamic current [7,252,253].

Contraindications to the use of electrical stimulation include applying current over the anterior cervical region, carotid sinuses, heart, transthoracic area, insensate skin, and the abdomen of a pregnant woman; in conjunction with a cardiac pacemaker, implanted defibrillator, or any other implanted electrical device; during ECG testing or while operating diathermy devices; and for patients with venous or arterial thrombosis or thrombophlebitis [7,8].

Precautions should be taken delivering electrical stimulation over tissues susceptible to hemorrhage or hematoma; on craniofacial regions for patients with a history of cerebrovascular accidents or seizures; on patients who have movement control disorders, impaired cognition, malignancies, osteoporosis (motor-level TENS), or cardiopathies; and on patients while driving or operating heavy machinery [7,8]. Iontophoresis is specifically contraindicated for use over open skin lesions and for patients with known sensitivity to the therapeutic ions [7]. Precautions should be taken to prevent skin damage due to adhesive irritants and electrochemical pH changes under the electrodes.

Supporting evidence is strong for the use of TENS as adjunctive therapy for treating many pain conditions. Most physical therapy clinics are equipped to administer interferential current and iontophoresis (provided the patient brings to the clinic the ionic medication preparation prescribed by the referring physician), to conduct a TENS trial, and to arrange for the acquisition of a home TENS unit. A TENS trial frequently requires some time and experimentation to determine an effective electrode placement site.

Desensitization

In contrast to the normal hyperalgesic response of body tissue to acute injury, allodynia is a painful response to a non-noxious somatosensory stimulus such that the affected individual may guard the limb from even the most delicate tactile contact, even refraining from wearing clothing over the painful site [12,254,255]. It is one of the hallmark symptoms of CRPS, with 74% of patients reportedly experiencing allodynia [256]. For physical and occupational therapists, the treatment of allodynia via desensitization is an essential component in helping to restore functional use of the affected body part [257]. A number of authors cite desensitization training as one of the essential core therapeutic elements in the physical or occupational therapists' management of CRPS [4,257–260]. Using this technique, the therapist may directly treat pain symptoms that are restricting function [259].

Somatosensory desensitization therapy for allodynia generally involves having the patient rub the affected body region over time with a series of progressively coarser and more irritating tactile stimuli [257]. A complete treatment protocol may span 10 to 15 weeks, including home practice and at least weekly in-clinic rechecks and progressions [255,260].

Although the operating mechanism of desensitization has yet to be established or may be multidimensional, several plausible theories are offered. For a person experiencing allodynia, restricting or avoiding tactile contact to the painful area has become a way of life [4]. By reintroducing tactile stimulation, the person may rehabituate to formerly irritating somatosensory input [261]. Repeated exposure to progressively irritating materials may reset altered central processing of somatosensory input at the dorsal horn or cortically [257,261] or may prevent the development of permanent pain pathways in the central nervous system by manipulation of cortical centers responsible for pain perception [262]. Reintroducing normal tactile input may restore large-fiber–diameter afferent inhibition of pain, which had been eliminated through restricted normal tactile contact [257]. As a goal of desensitization, the patient may begin normalizing exposure of the effective body area to the distal environment [263]. This helps reestablish the benefits of ascending analgesia from large-diameter somatosensory fibers and, with guidance from the therapist, aids in reintroduction of the limb or body area into functional usage. Enhanced usage may create a positive spiral of analgesia and activity, thus turning normal activity into a continuation of the desensitization therapy [12,257].

Although clinical use of desensitization is common and considered part of standard care when working with patients manifesting allodynia [259] and individual patients are reported to manifest notable functional usage gains after its implementation [252–260], efficacy evidence supporting its use is sparse [264] and is predominantly limited to case studies of grade III with an absence of available controlled studies.

The earliest reports of using desensitization therapy come from prophylactic intervention against postamputation phantom limb pain [260,263, 264]. An early reported use of treating chronic allodynia used the chemical irritant capsaicin as the desensitizing agent in the treatment of CRPS [265]. Multiple reports have indicated that patients desensitized to light touch or never manifesting light touch allodynia may experience painful responses to non-noxious levels of thermal variation, pressure, or vibration [10,62,255, 257,266]. There are case reports of treatment success in managing thermal- [62] and pressure-related allodynia when the desensitizing agents were matched to the specific somatosensory modality producing the painful response, resulting in functional improvements along with reductions in pain intensity and pain medication usage [255,266]. This suggests that desensitization therapy may be somatosensory specific and that desensitizing agents should be chosen to represent the particular problematic sensory stimulus type that is triggering the allodynia [255,257,266].

Desensitization therapy may be indicated for conditions involving somatosensory allodynia. The clinician should consider the scarcity of supporting evidence and evaluate individual patient response. Its application is contraindicated when working with any painful skin field where there is an active lesion that may be physically harmed by exposure to somatosensory irritating agents.

Clinical implications: application of physical agents to prototypical cases

Physical therapy treatment approaches for the following prototypical cases may vary considerably, based on a therapist's treatment philosophy and the patient's functional goals. However, the following cases represent examples of how physical agents might be used in each case.

Case 1: Chronic right lower extremity pain secondary to closed head trauma

Because the patient's right lower extremity pain is not primarily nociceptive, a TENS trial is indicated. Placement of stimulating electrodes could be near the painful region, on the contralateral limb, or over the spinal nerve root. Given that the primary pain generator is most likely rostral to any possible stimulation site, TENS would serve as a potential counterirritant. With secondary pain aggravation due to spasticity, cryotherapy is indicated to ease the spasticity in the form of cold packs or vapocoolant sprays. A prolonged consequence of diminished movement and spasticity is contracture, which could create secondary structural pain-generation sites. This may be addressed with ultrasound, to facilitate collagen extensibility, combined with stretching. The patient's diminished cognitive status requires assessment to determine if comprehension and communication are adequate for the safe use of these agents and their potential for home implementation.

Case 2: Chronic bilateral distal lower extremity pain secondary to diabetic polyneuropathy

To treat bilateral distal lower extremity pain due to diabetic polyneuropathy, TENS is indicated for analgesia. Specific electrode placement sites need to be explored for effectiveness and convenience. If TENS analgesia is effective to help her increase activity, she decreases the possibility of developing new pain-generation sites secondary to inactivity. The patient's history of hypertension and myocardial infarction does not present elements that would contraindicate TENS.

Case 3: Chronic neck and back pain/possible fibromyalgia syndrome

It seems plausible that the spread of pain for this patient is due to diminished movement and muscle guarding after the initial episode of posterior neck pain. Myofascial release and treating the trigger points of the upper trapezius and levator scapulae muscles is beneficial in this case. This may be addressed in a variety of ways. One approach would be cryostretch of hypertonic, shortened muscles via vapocoolant sprays. The trigger points may also respond to superficial heat. Laser therapy may be helpful with trigger points, but the literature is divided over such treatment. A consideration with laser application is that LLLT penetrates 1 to 4 mm below the skin surface, which may not be deep enough to affect the trigger points in question. Patient response to each of these options should be assessed to determine the most effective option or combination of agents. TENS may also be applied to provide analgesia that might allow increased neck, back, and shoulder girdle mobility. Gradually increasing motion may break the exacerbation cycle spreading the pain and is consistent with therapeutic approaches for patients manifesting the tender points and restricted movements associated with fibromyalgia syndrome.

Case 4: Chronic low back pain without radicular symptoms

This patient may represent a case where physical agents are not indicated. With no specific pain generator identified, agents operating at the tissue level are not likely to be beneficial. A TENS trial might be useful, but careful attention should be paid to the psychobehavioral impact of a passive analgesia approach. Although the patient's interventional history includes extensive physical therapy, it may be appropriate to ascertain what specific treatment approaches were used. The development of deactivation pain is a concern, so the patient may be a likely candidate for reactivation therapy, with careful attention to physical activity dosing and pacing.

Summary

Evidence supporting the use of specific physical agents in the management of chronic pain conditions is not definitive; it is largely incomplete and sometimes contradictory. However, the use of agents in chronic pain management programs is common [78]. Within the broad use of physical agents, they are rarely the sole modality of treatment. A 1995 American Physical Therapy Association position statement asserts that "Without documentation which justifies the necessity of the exclusive use of physical agents/modalities, the use of physical agents/modalities, in the absence of other skilled therapeutic or educational intervention, should not be considered physical therapy" [13]. Physical agents may serve as useful adjunctive modalities of pain relief or to enhance the effectiveness of other elements in therapy geared toward resolution of movement impairments and restoration of physical function.

Given that a conclusive aggregate of findings is unlikely to exist for all permutations of patient conditions, combined with interacting therapeutic modalities, an evidence-based approach to pain management is not always possible or beneficial to the patient. In the face of inconclusive evidence, a theory-based approach may help determine if the therapeutic effect of a given physical agent has the possibility of being a useful clinical tool in the context of treating a particular patient's mechanism of pain generation. Until controlled efficacy findings are definitive, careful individual patient response monitoring of thoughtful theoretical application of adjunctive physical agents may be a prudent approach to the management of chronic pain.

References

[1] Loeser JD, Turk DC. Multidisciplinary pain management. In: Loeser JD, editor. Bonica's management of pain. Baltimore (MD): Williams & Wilkins; 2001. p. 2069–79.

[2] Witttink H, Michel TH. Chronic pain management for physical therapists. Boston: Butterworth Heinemann; 2002.

[3] Strong J, Unruh AM, Wright A, et al. Pain: a textbook for therapists. Edinburgh: Churchill Livingstone; 2002.

[4] Galer BS, Schwartz L, Allen RJ. The complex regional pain syndromes: type I / reflex sympathetic dystrophy & type II causalgia. In: Loeser JD, editor. Bonica's management of pain. Baltimore (MD): Williams & Wilkins; 2001. p. 388–411.

[5] American Physical Therapy Association. Guide to physical therapy practice. Fairfax (VA): American Physical Therapy Association; 2001.

[6] Wells PE, Frampton V, Bowsher D. Pain management in physical therapy. Norwalk (CT): Appleton & Lange; 1988.

[7] Belanger AY. Evidence based guide to therapeutic physical agents. Philadelphia: Lippincott Williams & Wilkins; 2002.

[8] Cameron MH. Physical agents in rehabilitation: from research to practice. Philadelphia: W.B. Saunders; 2003.

[9] Snyder-Mackler L. Electrical stimulation for pain modulation. In: Robinson AJ, Snyder-Mackler L, editors. Clinical electrophysiology: electrotherapy and electrophysiologic testing. 2nd ed. Baltimore (MD): Williams & Wilkins; 1995. p. 333–58.

[10] Berger JM, Katz RL. Sympathetically maintained pain. In: Ashburn MA, Rice LJ, editors. The management of pain. Philadelphia: Churchill Livingstone; 1998. p. 335–49.

[11] Foley R. Neuroplasticity of pain and the psychology of pain. Presented at the American Physical Therapy Association - Combined Sections Meeting. Tampa (FL), February 12, 2003.

[12] Allen RJ, Hulten JM. Effects of tactile desensitization on allodynia and somatosensation in a patient with quadralateral complex regional pain syndrome. Neuro Rep 2001;25:132–3.

[13] American Physical Therapy Association. Position on exclusive use of physical agents modalities. House of Delegates Reference Committee. Fairfax (VA): American Physical Therapy Association; 1995.

[14] Allen RJ. Deactivation pain: developmental sequelae of secondary pain generation sites resulting from reduced mobility. Presented at the Annual Conference & Exposition of the American Physical Therapy Association. Anaheim (CA), June 21, 2001.

[15] Allen RJ, Koshi LR. Development of chronic pain secondary to excessive limb immobilization following orthopaedic trauma. J Ortho Sports Phys Ther 2005;35:A63–4.

[16] Terman GW, Bonica JJ. Spinal mechanisms and their modulation. In: Loeser JD, editor. Bonica's management of pain. Baltimore (MD): Williams & Wilkins; 2001. p. 73–152.

[17] Chandler EH, Bonica JJ. Supraspinal mechanisms of pain & nociception. In: Loeser JD, editor. Bonica's management of pain. Baltimore (MD): Williams & Wilkins; 2001. p. 388–411.

[18] Butler SH, Galer BS, Bernirshka S. Disuse as a cause of signs and symptoms of CRPS-1. Presented at the International Association for the Study of Pain meeting. Vancouver (BC). August 20, 1996.

[19] Butler SH, Nyman M, Gordh T. Immobility in volunteers transiently produces signs and symptoms of complex regional pain syndrome. In: Devor M, Rowbotham MC, Wiesenfield-Hallin Z, editors. Proceedings of the 9th World Congress on Pain. Progress in pain research and management, vol. 16. Seattle: IASP Press; 2000. p. 657–60.

[20] Spitzer WO. The periodic health examination. Can Med Assoc J 1979;121:1–45.

[21] Spitzer WO, LeBlanc FE, Dupuis M, et al. Scientific approach to the assessment and management of activity-related spinal disorders. Spine 1987;12(Suppl):S1–59.

[22] Lehmann JF, DeLateur BJ. Therapeutic heat. In: Lehmann JF, editor. Therapeutic heat and cold. Baltimore (MD): Williams & Wilkins; 1990. p. 429–32.

[23] Mense S. Effects of temperature on the discharges of muscle spindles and tendon organs. Pflugers Arch 1978;374:159–66.

[24] Rennie GA, Michlovitz SL. Biophysical principles of heating and superficial heating agents. In: Michlovitz SL, editor. Thermal agents in rehabilitation. Philadelphia: FA Davis; 1996. p. 107–38.

[25] Fountain FP, Gersten JW, Senger O. Decrease in muscle spasm produced by ultrasound, hot packs and IR. Arch Phys Med Rehabil 1960;41:293–9.

[26] Newton RA. Contemporary views on pain and the role played by thermal agents in managing pain symptoms. In: Michlovitz SL, editor. Thermal agents in rehabilitation. Philadelphia: FA Davis; 1990. p. 18–42.

[27] Benson TB, Copp EP. The effects of therapeutic forms of heat and ice on the pain threshold of the normal shoulder. Rheumatol Rehabil 1974;13:101–4.

[28] Fox HH, Hilton SM. Bradykinin formation in human skin as a factor in heat vasodilation. J Physiol 1958;142:219–32.

[29] Kramer JF. Ultrasound: evaluation of its mechanical and thermal effects. Arch Phys Med Rehabil 1984;65:223–7.

[30] Ayling J, Marks R. Efficacy of paraffin wax baths for rheumatoid arthritic hands. Physiotherapy 2000;86:190–201.

[31] Mainardi CL, Walter JM, Spiegel PK, et al. Rheumatoid arthritis: failure of daily heat therapy to affect its progression. Arch Phys Med Rehabil 1979;60:390–3.

[32] Sukenick S, Buskila D, Neumann L, et al. Mud pack therapy in rheumatoid arthritis. Clin Rheumatol 1992;11:243–7.

[33] Sukenick S, Buskila D, Neumann L, et al. Sulfur bath and mud pack treatment for rheumatoid arthritis in the Dead Sea area. Ann Rheum Dis 1990;49:99–102.

[34] Sukenick S, Newmann L, Flusser D, et al. Balneotherapy for rheumatoid arthritis in the Dead Sea. Isr J Med Sci 1995;31:210–4.

[35] Dellhag B, Wollersjo I, Bjelle A. Effect of hand exercixe and wax bath treatment in rheumatoid arthritis patients. Arthritis Care Res 1992;5:87–92.

[36] Harris R, Millard JB. Paraffin-wax baths in treatment of rheumatoid arthritis. Ann Rheum Dis 1953;14:278–82.

[37] Harris ED, McCroskery PA. The influence of temperature and fibril stability on degradation of cartilage collagen by rheumatoid synovial collagenase. N Engl J Med 1974;290:1–6.

[38] Constant F, Collin JF, Guillemin F, et al. Effectiveness of spa therapy in chronic low back pain: a randomized clinical trial. J Rheumatol 1995;22:1315–20.

[39] Konrad K, Tatrai T, Hunka A, et al. Controlled trial of balneotherapy in treatment of low back pain. Ann Rheum Dis 1992;51:820–2.

[40] Guillemin F, Constant F, Collin JF, et al. Short and long term effect of spa therapy in chronic low back pain. Br J Rheumatol 1994;33:148–51.
[41] Landen BR. Hear or cold for the relief of low back pain? Phys Ther 1967;47:1126–8.
[42] Constant F, Guillemin F, Collin JF, et al. Use of spa therapy to improve the quality of life of chronic low back pain patients. Med Care 1998;35:1309–14.
[43] Cordray YM, Krusen EM. Use of hydrocollator packs in the treatment of neck and shoulder pains. Arch Phys Med Rehabil 1959;39:105–8.
[44] McCray RE, Patton NJ. Pain relief at trigger points: a comparison of moist heat and shortwave diathermy. J Othop Sports Phys Ther 1984;5:175–8.
[45] Douglas WW, Malcolm JL. The effect of localized cooling on cat nerves. J Physiol 1955;130: 53–4.
[46] Bassett FH, Kirkpatrick JS, Engelhardt DL. Cryotherapy induced nerve injury. Am J Sport Med 1992;22:516–28.
[47] Travell J. Ethyl chloride for painful muscle spasm. Arch Phys Med Rehabil 1952;32: 291–8.
[48] Travell J. Myofascial trigger points: clinical view. In: Bonica JJ, Able-Fessard DG, editors. Advances in pain research and therapy, vol. 1. New York: Raven Press; 1976. p. 919–26.
[49] Prentice WE. An electromyographic analysis of the effectiveness of heat or cold and stretching for inducing relaxation in injured muscle. J Orthop Sports Phys Ther 1982;3:133–7.
[50] Mennel J. Spray-stretch for the relief of pain from muscle spasm and myofascial trigger points. J Am Podiatr Assoc 1976;66:873–6.
[51] Nielson AJ. Spray and stretch for myofascial pain. Phys Ther 1978;58:567–9.
[52] Nielson AJ. Case study: myofascial pain of the posterior shoulder relieved by spray and stretch. J Orthop Sports Phys Ther 1981;3:21–6.
[53] Melzack R, Jeans ME, Stratford JG, et al. Ice massage and transcutaneous electrical stimulation: comparison of treatment for low-back pain. Pain 1980;9:209–17.
[54] Robbins LD. Cryotherapy for headache. Headache 1989;29:598–600.
[55] Diamond S, Freitag FG. Cold as an adjunctive therapy for headache. Postgrad Med 1986; 79:305–9.
[56] De Coster D, Bossuyt M, Fossion E. The value of cryotherapy in the management of trigeminal neuralgia. Acta Stomatol Belg 1993;90:87–93.
[57] Halliday Pegg SM, Littler TR, Littler MD. A trial of ice therapy and exercise in chronic arthritis. Physiotherapy 1969;55:51–6.
[58] Ziskin MC, McDiarmid T, Michlovitz SL. Therapeutic ultrasound. In: Micklovitz SL, editor. Thermal agents in rehabilitation. Philadelphia: FA Davis; 1990. p. 134–69.
[59] Reobroeck ME, Dekker J, Oostendorp RAB. The use of therapeutic ultrasound by physical therapists in Dutch primary health care. Phys Ther 1998;78:470–8.
[60] Robertson VJ, Spurritt D. Electrophysical agents: implications of EPA availability and use in private practices. Physiotherapy 1998;84:335–44.
[61] Currier DP, Kramer JF. Sensory nerve conduction: heating effects of ultrasound and infrared. Physiother Can 1982;34:241–6.
[62] Allen RJ, Stephenson KM, Sundahl BT, et al. Thermal desensitization for treatment of severe thermal sensitivity and associated functional deficits secondary to complex regional pain syndrome of the upper limb. Phys Ther Case Reports 2001;4:59–66.
[63] Michlovitz SL, Lynch PR, Tuma RJ. Therapeutic ultrasound: its effects on vascular permeability. Fed Proc 1982;41:1761.
[64] Hogan RD. The effect of ultrasound on microvascular hemodynamics in skeletal muscle: effect on arterioles. Ultrasound Med Biol 1982;8:45.
[65] Hogan RD, Burke KM, Franklin TD. The effect of ultrasound on microvascular hemodynamics in skeletal muscle: effects during ischemia. Microvasc Res 1982;23: 370–9.
[66] Baker KG, Robertson VJ, Duck FA. A review of therapeutic ultrasound: biophysical effects. Phys Ther 2001;81:1351–8.

[67] Van der Heijden GJMC, Leffers P, Wolters PH, et al. No effect of bipolar interferential electrotherapy and pulsed ultrasound for soft tissue shoulder disorders: a randomized controlled trial. Ann Rheum Dis 1999;58:530–40.

[68] Fountain FP, Gersten JW, Sengu O. Decrease in muscle spasm produced by ultrasound, hot packs and IR. Arch Phys Med Rehabil 1960;41:293–8.

[69] Ebenbichler GR, Erdogmus CB, Resh KL, et al. Ultrasound therapy for calcific tendonitis of the shoulder. N Engl J Med 1999;340:1533–8.

[70] Ebenbichler GR, Resch KL, Nicolakis P, et al. Ultrasound treatment for treating the carpal tunnel syndrome: randomized "sham" controlled trial. BMJ 1998;316:731–5.

[71] Nwuga VCB. Ultrasound in treatment of back pain resulting from prolapsed intervertebral disc. Arch Phys Med Rehabil 1983;64:88–9.

[72] Binder A, Hodge G, Greenwood AM, et al. Is therapeutic ultrasound effective in treating soft tissue lesions? BMJ 1985;290:512–4.

[73] Portwood MM, Lieberman JS, Taylor RG. Ultrasound treatment of reflex sympathetic dystrophy. Arch Phys Med Rehabil 1987;68:116–8.

[74] Tepperberg I, Marjey E. Ultrasound therapy of painful postoperative neurofibromas. Am J Phys Med 1953;32:27–30.

[75] Lehmann JF, Erickson DJ, Martin GM, et al. Comparison of ultrasonic and microwave diathermy in the physical treatment of periarthritis of the shoulder. Arch Phys Med Rehabil 1954;35:627–34.

[76] Cline PD. Radiographic follow-up of ultrasound therapy in calcific bursitis. Phys Ther 1963;43:16–8.

[77] Bommannan D, Okuyama H, Stauffer P. Sonophoresis, I: the use of high frequency ultrasound to enhance transdermal drug delivery. Pharm Res 1992;9:559–64.

[78] Loeser JD. Multidisciplinary pain programs. In: Loeser JD, editor. Bonica's management of pain. Baltimore (MD): Williams & Wilkins; 2001. p. 255–64.

[79] Munting E. Ultrasonic therapy for painful shoulders. Physiotherapy 1978;64:180–1.

[80] Roden D. Ultrasonic waves in the treatment of chronic adhesive subacromial bursitis. J Ir Med Assoc 1952;30:85–8.

[81] Falconer J, Hayes KW, Chang RW. Effect of ultrasound on mobility in osteoarthritis of the knee. Arthritis Car Res 1992;5:29–35.

[82] Svarcova J, Trnavsky K, Zvarova J. The influence of ultrasound, galvanic currents and shortwave diathermy on pain intensity with osteoarthritis. Scan J Rheumatol 1988; 67(Suppl):83–5.

[83] Ortas O, Turan B, Bora I, et al. Ultrasound therapy effect in carpal tunnel syndrome. Arch Phys Med Rehabil 1998;79:1540–4.

[84] Perron M, Malouin F. Acetic acid iontophoresis and ultrasound for the treatment of calcifying tendonitis of the shoulder: a randomized control trial. Arch Phys Med Rehabil 1997; 78:379–84.

[85] Hasish I, Hai H, Harvey W. Reproduction of postoperative pain and swelling by ultrasound treatment: a placebo effect. Pain 1988;33:303–11.

[86] Hasish I, Harvey W, Harris M. Anti-inflammatory effects of ultrasound therapy: evidence for a major placebo effect. Br J Rheumatol 1986;25:77–81.

[87] Flax HJ. Ultrasound treatment of peritendonitis calcerea of the shoulder. Am J Phys Med 1964;43:117–24.

[88] Creates V. Study of ultrasound treatment to the painful perineum after childbirth. Physiotherapy 1987;73:162–5.

[89] Everett T, McIntosh J, Grant A. Ultrasound therapy for persistent post-natal perineal pain and dyspareunia: a randomized placebo-controlled trial. Physiotherapy 1992;78:263–7.

[90] Downing DS, Weinstein A. Ultrasound therapy of subacromial bursitis: a double blind trial. Phys Ther 1986;66:194–9.

[91] ter Haar G, Dyson M, Oakley EM. The use of ultrasound by physiotherapists in Britian. Ultrasound Med Biol 1985;13:559–63.

[92] Young S. Ultrasound therapy. In: Kitchen S, Bazin S, editors. Clayton's electrotherapy. 10th ed. London: W.B. Saunders; 1996. p. 243–67.
[93] Hayne CR. Pulsed high frequency energy: its place in physiotherapy. Physiotherapy 1984; 70:459–66.
[94] Markov MS. Electric current electromagnetic field effects on soft tissue: implications for wound healing. Wounds 1995;7:94–110.
[95] Markov MS, Pilla AA. Electromagnetic field stimulation of soft tissues: pulsed radio frequency treatment of post-operative pain and edema. Wounds 1995;7:143–51.
[96] Pilla AA, Markov MS. Bioeffects of weak electromagnetic fields. Rev Environ Health 1994; 10:90–3.
[97] Canaday DJ, Lee RC. Scientific basis for clinical application of electric fields in soft tissue repair. In: Brighton CT, Pollack SR, editors. Electromagnetics in biological medicine. San Francisco (CA): San Francisco Press; 1991. p. 275–91.
[98] Mayrovitz HN, Larsen PB. A preliminary study to evaluate the effect of pulsed radio frequency field treatment on lower extremity peri-ulcer skin microcirculation of diabetic patients. Wounds 1995;7:90–3.
[99] Mayrovitz HN, Larsen PB. Effects of pulsed electromagnetic fields on skin microvascular blood perfusion. Wounds 1992;4:197–202.
[100] Bassett CA. Fundamental and practical aspects of therapeutic uses of pulsed electromagnetic fields (PEMFs). Crit Rev Biomed Eng 1989;17:451–529.
[101] Bassett CA, Mitchell SN, Schink MM. Treatment of therapeutically resistant nonunions with bone grafts and pulsing electromagnetic fields. J Bone Joint Surg 1982;24: 1214–20.
[102] Konrad K, Sevcic K, Foldes K, et al. Therapy with pulsed electromagnetic fields in aseptic loosening of total hip prostheses: a prospective study. Clin Rheumatol 1997;15:325–8.
[103] Ryaby JT. Clinical effects of electromagnetic and electric fields on fracture healing. Clin Orthop Relat Res 1998;355(Suppl):S205–15.
[104] Di Massa A, Misuriello I, Olivieri MC, et al. Pulsed magnetic fields: observations in 353 patients suffering from chronic pain. Ninerva Anesthesiol 1989;55:295–9.
[105] Trock DH, Bollet AJ, Markoll R. The effect of pulsed electromagnetic fields in the treatment of osteoarthritis of the knee and cervical spine: report of randomized, double-blind placebo-controlled trials. J Rheumatol 1994;21:1903–11.
[106] Vallbona C, Hazlewood CF, Juirda G. Response of pain to static and magnetic fields in postpolio patients: a double-blind pilot study. Arch Phys Med Rehabil 1997;78: 1200–3.
[107] Todd DJ, Heylings DJ, Allen GE, et al. Treatment of chronic varicose ulcers with pulsed electromagnetic fields: a controlled pilot study. Ir Med J 1991;84:54–5.
[108] Stiller MJ, Pak GH, Shupack JL, et al. A portable pulsed electromagnetic field (PEMF) device to enhance healing of recalcitrant venous ulcers: a double-blind, placebo-controlled clinical trial. Br J Dermatol 1992;127:147–54.
[109] Leclaire R, Bourgoin J. Electromagnetic treatment of shoulder periarthritis: a randomized controlled trial of the efficiency and tolerance of magnetotherapy. Arch Phys Med Rehabil 1991;72:284–7.
[110] Chard MD, Hazleman BL. Pulsed electromagnetic field treatment of chronic lateral humeral epicondylitis. Clin Exp Rheumatol 1988;6:330–2.
[111] Foley-Nolan D, Barry C, Coughlan RJ, et al. Pulsed high frequency (27MHz) electromagnetic therapy for persistent neck pain: a double-blind placebo-controlled study of 20 patients. Orthopedics 1990;13:445–51.
[112] Foley-Nolan D, Moore K, Codd M, et al. Low energy high frequency pulsed electromagnetic therapy for acute whiplash injuries. Scand J Rehabil Med 1992;24:51–9.
[113] Hamilton DE, Bywaters EG, Please NW. A controlled trial of various forms of physiotherapy in arthritis. BMJ 1959;2:542–5.
[114] Wright V. Treatment of osteoarthritis of the knees. Ann Rheum Dis 1964;23:389–91.

[115] Kabler-Moffett JA, Richardson PH, Frost H, et al. A placebo controlled double-blind trial to evaluate the effectiveness of pulsed shortwave therapy for osteoarthritic hip and knee pain. Pain 1996;67:121–7.
[116] Svarcova J, Trnavsky K, Zvarova J. The influence of ultrasound, galvanic currents and shortwave diathermy on pain intensity in patients with osteoarthritis. Scand J Rheumatol 1988;67(Suppl):83–5.
[117] Clarke GR, Willis LA, Stenners L, et al. Evaluation of physiotherapy in the treatment of osteoarthrosis of the knee. Rheum Rehabil 1974;13:190–7.
[118] McGill SN. The effect of pulsed shortwave therapy on lateral ligament sprain of the ankle. N Z J Physiother 1988;10:21–4.
[119] Pasila M, Visuri T, Sundholm A. Pulsating shortwave diathermy: value in the treatment of recent ankle and foot sprains. Arch Phys Med Rehabil 1978;59:383–6.
[120] Barker AT, Barlow PS, Porter J, et al. A double-blind clinical trial of low-power pulsed shortwave therapy in the treatment of a soft tissue injury. Physiotherapy 1985; 71:500–4.
[121] Comorosan S, Pana L, Pop L, et al. The influence of pulsed high peak power electromagnetic energy (Diapulse) treatment on posttraumatic algoneurodystrophies. Rev Roum Physiol 1991;28:77–81.
[122] Wagstaff P, Wagstaff S, Downey M. A pilot study to compare the efficacy of continuous and pulsed magnetic energy (shortwave diathermy) on the relief of low back pain. Physiotherapy 1986;72:563–6.
[123] Baxter GD, Bell AJ, Allen JM, et al. Low-level laser therapy current clinical practice in Northern Ireland. Physiotherapy 1991;71:171–8.
[124] Anderson RR, Parrish JA. The optics of the skin. J Invest Dermatol 1981;77:13–9.
[125] Baxter GD. Therapeutic lasers: theory and practice. New York: Churchill Livingstone; 1994.
[126] Schindl A, Schindl M, Pernerstorfer-Schon H, et al. Low intensity laser therapy: a review. J Invest Med 2000;48:312–26.
[127] Calderhead RG. Basics. In: Ohshiro T, Calderhead RG, editors. Low-level laser therapy: a practical introduction. New York: John Wiley & Sons; 1988. p. 1–18.
[128] Young S, Bolton P, Dyson M, et al. Macrophage responsiveness to light therapy. Lasers Surg Med 1989;9:497–505.
[129] Lam TS, Abergel RP, Castel JC, et al. Laser stimulation of collagen synthesis in human skin fibroblast cultures. Laser Life Sci 1986;1:61–77.
[130] Lyons RF, Abergel RP, White RA, et al. Biostimulation of wound healing in vivo by a helium-neon laser. Ann Plast Surg 1987;18:47–50.
[131] Kaupin IV, Pykov VS, Ivanov AV, et al. Potentiating effects of laser radiation on some immunologic traits. Neoplasma 1982;29:403–6.
[132] Passarella S, Casamassima E, Quangliariello E, et al. Quantitative analysis of lymphocyte-Salmonella interaction and effects of lymphocyte irradiation by Ne-He laser. Biochem Biophys Res Commun 1985;130:546–52.
[133] Snyder-Mackler L, Bork CE. Effect of helium-neon laser irradiation on peripheral sensory nerve latency. Phys Ther 1988;68:223–5.
[134] Basford JR, Hallman HO, Matsumoto JY, et al. Effects of 830 nm continuous laser diode irradiation on median nerve function in normal subjects. Lasers Surg Med 1993;13: 597–604.
[135] Baxter GD, Walsh DM, Allen JM, et al. Effects of low-intensity infrared laser irradiation upon conduction in the human median nerve in vivo. Exp Physiol 1994;79:227–34.
[136] Lowe AS, Baxter GD, Walsh DM, et al. The effect of low-intensity laser (830 nm) irradiation upon skin temperature and antidromic conduction latencies in the human median nerve: relevance of radiant exposure. Lasers Surg Med 1994;14:40–6.
[137] Greathouse DG, Currier DP, Gilmore RL. Effects of clinical infrared laser on superficial radial nerve conduction. Phys Ther 1985;65:1184–7.

[138] Basford JR, Daube JR, Hallman HO, et al. Does low-intensity helium-neon laser irradiation alter sensory nerve action potentials or distal latencies? Lasers Surg Med 1990;10:35–9.
[139] Santoianni P, Mofrecola G, Martellota D, et al. Inadequate effect of helium-neon laser on venous leg ulcers. Photodermatol 1984;1:245–9.
[140] Lundeberg TM. Low-power He-Ne laser treatment of venous leg ulcers. Ann Plast Surg 1991;27:537–9.
[141] Schindl M, Kerschan K, Schindl A, et al. Induction of complete wound healing in recalcitrant ulcers by low-intensity laser irradiation depends on ulcer cause and size. Photodermatol Photoimmunol Photomed 1999;15:18–21.
[142] Palmgren N, Jensen GF, Kaa K, et al. Low-power laser therapy in rheumatoid arthritis. Laser Med Sci 1989;4:193–6.
[143] Goldman JA, Chiapella J, Casey H, et al. Laser therapy in rheumatoid arthritis. Laser Surg Ther 1980;1:93–101.
[144] Walker JB, Akhanjee LK, Cooney MM, et al. Laser therapy for pain of rheumatoid arthritis. Clin J Pain 1987;3:54–9.
[145] Goats GC, Flett E, Hunter JA, et al. Low-intensity laser and phototherapy for rheumatoid arthritis. Physiotherapy 1996;82:311–20.
[146] Johannsen F, Hauschild B, Remvig L, et al. Low-energy laser therapy in rheumatoid arthritis. Scand J Rheumatol 1994;23:145–7.
[147] Hall J, Clarke AK, Elvins DM, et al. Low-level laser therapy is ineffective in the management of rheumatoid arthritic finger joints. Br J Rheumatol 1994;33:142–7.
[148] Bliddal H, Hellesen C, Ditlevsen P, et al. Soft-laser therapy of rheumatoid arthritis. Scand J Rheumatol 1987;16:225–8.
[149] Lonauer G. Controlled double-blind study on the efficacy of HeNe laser beams versus HeNe infrared laser beams in the therapy of activated osteoarthritis of finger joints. Lasers Surg Med 1986;6:172–5.
[150] Willner R, Abeles M, Myerson G. Low-power infrared laser biostimulation of chronic osteoarthritis in hand. Lasers Surg Med 1985;5:149–50.
[151] Jensen H, Herreby M, Kjer J. Infrared laser-effect in painful arthrosis of the knee? Ugeskr Laeger 1987;149:3104–6.
[152] Walker JB. Relief from chronic pain by low-power laser irradiation. Neurosci Lett 1983;43: 339–44.
[153] Stelian J, Gil I, Habot B. Improvement of pain and disability in elderly patients with degenerative osteoarthritis of the knee treated with narrow band light therapy. J Am Geriatr Soc 1992;S40:23–6.
[154] Basford JR, Sheffield CG, Mair SD, et al. Low energy helium-neon laser of thumb osteoarthritis. Arch Phys Med Rehabil 1987;68:794–7.
[155] Bulow PM, Jensen H, Danneskiold-Samsoe B. Low-power Ga-Al-As laser treatment of painful osteoarthritis of the knee. Scand J Rehabil Med 1994;26:155–9.
[156] Olavi A, Pekka R, Pertti K. Effects of the infrared laser therapy at treated and non-treated trigger points. Acupunct Electrother Res 1989;14:9–14.
[157] Snyder-Mackler L, Barry AJ, Perdns AI, et al. Effects of helium-neon laser irradiation on skin resistance and pain in patients with trigger points in the neck or back. Phys Ther 1989; 69:336–41.
[158] Waylonis GW, Wilke S, O'Toole D, et al. Chronic myofascial pain: management by low-output helium-neon laser therapy. Arch Phys Med Rehabil 1988;69:1017–20.
[159] Thorsen H, Gam AN, Jensen MK, et al. Low-energy laser treatment: effect in localized fibromyalgia in the neck and shoulder regions. Ugeskr Laeger 1991;153:1801–4.
[160] Thorsen H, Gam AN, Svensson BH, et al. Low-level laser therapy for myofascial pain in the neck and shoulder girdle: a double-blind, cross-over study. Scand J Rheumatol 1992;21: 139–41.
[161] Siebert W, Seichert N, Seibert B, et al. What is the efficacy of "soft" and "mild" lasers in therapy of tendinopathies? A double-blind study. Arch Orthop Trauma Surg 1987;106:358–63.

[162] Vecchio P, Cave M, King V, et al. A double-blind study of the effectiveness of low-level laser treatment of rotator cuff tendonitis. Br J Rheumatol 1993;32:740–2.

[163] Darre EM, Klokker M, Lund P, et al. Laser therapy of Achilles tendonitis. Ugeskr Laeger 1994;156:6680–3.

[164] England S, Farrell AJ, Coppock JS, et al. Low-power laser therapy of shoulder tendonitis. Scand J Rheumatol 1989;18:427–31.

[165] Vasseljen O, Hoeg N, Kjelstad B, et al. Low-level laser versus placebo in the treatment of tennis elbow. Scand J Rehabil Med 1992;24:37–42.

[166] Lundeberg T, Haker E, Thomas M. Effect of laser versus placebo in tennis elbow. Scand J Rehabil Med 1987;19:135–48.

[167] Krasheninnikoff M, Ellitsgaard N, Rogvi-Hansen B, et al. No effect of low-power laser in lateral epicondylitis. Scand J Rheumatol 1994;23:260–3.

[168] Haker E, Lunderberg TC. Laser treatment applied to acupuncture points in lateral humeral epicondylalgia: a double-blind study. Pain 1990;43:243–7.

[169] Haker E, Lunderberg TC. Lateral epicondylalgia: report of noneffective midlaser treatment. Arch Phys Med Rehabil 1991;72:984–8.

[170] Eckerdal A, Bastian HL. Can low reactive-level laser therapy be used in the treatment of neurogenic facial pain? A double-blind placebo-controlled investigation of patients with trigeminal neuralgia. Laser Ther 1996;8:247–52.

[171] Walker JB, Akhanjee LK, Cooney MM. Laser therapy for pain of trigeminal neuralgia. Clin J Pain 1987;3:183–7.

[172] Moore KC, Hira N, Kumar PS, et al. A double-blind crossover trial of low-level laser therapy in the treatment of post herpetic neuralgia. Laser Ther 1988;1:7–9.

[173] Schindl A, Neumann R. Low-intensity laser therapy is an effective treatment for recurrent herpes simplex infection: results from a randomized, double-blind, placebo-controlled trial. J Invest Med 1999;113:221–3.

[174] Moore KC, Hira N, Broome IJ, et al. The effect of infrared diode laser irradiation on the duration and severity of post-operative pain: a double-blind trial. Laser Ther 1992;4:145–50.

[175] De Bie RA, de Vet HC, Lenssen TF, et al. Low-level laser therapy in ankle sprains: a randomized clinical trial. Arch Phys Med Rehabil 1998;79:1415–20.

[176] Conti PC. Low-level laser therapy in the treatment of temporomandibular disorders (TMD): a double-blind pilot study. Cranio 1997;15:144–99.

[177] Craig JA, Barlas P, Baxter GD, et al. Delayed-onset of muscle soreness: lack of effect of combined phototherapy / low-intensity laser therapy at low pulse repetition rates. J Clin Laser Med Surg 1996;14:375–80.

[178] Craig JA, Barron J, Walsh DM, et al. Lack of effect of combined low-intensity laser therapy/phototherapy (CLILT) on delayed onset muscle soreness in humans. Lasers Surg Med 1999;24:223–30.

[179] Basford JR, Melanga GA, Krause DA, et al. A randomized controlled evaluation of low-intensity laser therapy: plantar fasciitis. Arch Phys Med Rehabil 1998;79:249–54.

[180] Rogvi-hansen B, Ellitsgaard N, Funch M, et al. Low-level laser treatment of chondromalacia patellae. Int Orthop 1991;15:359–61.

[181] Hansen HJ, Thoroe U. Low-power laser biostimulation of chronic oro-facial pain: a double-blind, placebo controlled cross-over study in 40 patients. Pain 1990;43:169–79.

[182] Rolle WC, Alon G, Nirschl RP. Comparison of subliminal and placebo stimulation in the management of elbow tendonitis. J Clin Electrophysiol 1994;6:4–9.

[183] Picker RI. Current trends: low-volt pulsed microamp stimulation, part I. Clin Manag Phys Ther 1989;9:10–4.

[184] Wolcot C, Dudek D, Kulig K. A comparison of the effects of high volt and microcurrent stimulation on delayed onset muscle soreness. Phys Ther 1991;71(Suppl):S116.

[185] Rapaski D, Isles S, Kulig K. Microcurrent electrical stimulation: comparison of two protocols in reducing delayed onset muscle soreness. Phys Ther 1991;71(Suppl):S116.

[186] Kulig K, Jarski R, Drewek E. The effects of microcurrent stimulation on CPK and delayed onset muscle soreness. Phys Ther 1991;71(Suppl):S115.
[187] Kulig K, DeYoung L, Maurer C. Comparison of the effects of high-velocity exercises and microcurrent neuromuscular stimulation on delayed onset muscle soreness. Phys Ther 1991;71(Suppl):S115.
[188] Picker RI. Current trends: low-volt pulsed microamp stimulation, part II. Clin Manag Phys Ther 1989;9:28–33.
[189] Becker RO, Selden G. The body electric: electromagnetism and the foundation of life. New York: William Morrow; 1987.
[190] Barker AT, Jaffe LF, Vanable JW. The glabrous epidermis of cavies contain a powerful battery. Am J Physiol 1982;242:358–66.
[191] Foulds IS, Barker AT. Human skin battery potentials and their possible role in wound healing. Br J Dermatol 1983;109:512–22.
[192] Becker RO, Murray DG. Method of producing cellular dedifferentiation by means of very small electrical current. Trans N Y Acad Sci 1967;29:606–15.
[193] Borgens RB, McGinnis ME, Vanable JW, et al. Stump currents in regenerating salamanders and newts. J Exp Zool 1984;23:249–56.
[194] Borgens RB, Vanable JW, Jaffe LF. Bioelectricity and regeneration: large current leaves the stumps of regenerating new limbs. Proc Natl Acad Sci USA 1977;74:4528–32.
[195] Johannsen F, Gam A, Haudschild B, et al. Rebox: an adjunct in physical medicine? Arch Phys Med Rehabil 1993;74:438–40.
[196] Hatten E, Hervik JB, Kalheim T, et al. Pain treatment with Rebox. Fysiotherapeuten 1990; 11:8–13.
[197] Baker LL, Chambers R, DeMuth SK, et al. Effects of electrical stimulation on wound healing in patients with diabetic ulcers. Diabetes Care 1997;20:405–12.
[198] Carley PJ, Wainapel SF. Electrotherapy for acceleration of wound healing: low-intensity direct current. Arch Phys Med Rehabil 1985;66:443–6.
[199] Allen JD, Mattacola CG, Perrin DH. Effect of microcurrent stimulation on delayed-onset muscle soreness: a double-blind comparison. J Athl Train 1999;34:334–7.
[200] Weber MD, Servedio FJ, Woodall WR. The effect of three modalities on delayed-onset muscle soreness. J Orthop Phys Ther 1994;20:236–42.
[201] Baker LL, Rubayi S, Villar F, et al. Effect of electrical stimulation waveform on healing of ulcers in human beings with spinal cord injury. Wound Repair Regen 1996;4:21–8.
[202] Wood JM, Evans PE, Shallreuter KU, et al. A multicenter study on the use of pulsed low intensity direct current for healing chronic stage II and III decubitus ulcers. Arch Dermatol 1993;129:999–1009.
[203] Melzack R, Wall PD. Pain mechanisms: a new theory. Science 1965;150:971–9.
[204] Almay BGL, Johansson F, von Knorring L. Long-term high frequency transcutaneous electrical nerve stimulation (hi-TNS) in chronic pain: clinical response and effects on CSF-endorphins, monoamine metabolites, substance P-like immunoreactivity (SPLI) and pain measures. J Psychosom Res 1985;29:247–57.
[205] Salar G, Job I, Mingrino S. Effect of transcutaneous electrotherapy on CSF β-endorphine content in patients without pain problems. Pain 1981;10:169–72.
[206] Chung JM, Fang ZR, Cargill CL. Prolonged Naloxone-reversible inhibition of the flexion reflex in the cat. Pain 1983;15:35–53.
[207] Chung JM, Fang ZR, Hori Y. Prolonged inhibition of primate spinothalamic tract cells by peripheral nerve stimulation. Pain 1984;19:259–75.
[208] Han JS, Chen XH, Sun SL. Effect of low- and high-frequency TENS on Met-enkephalin-Arg-Phe and dynorphin A immunoreactivity in human lumbar CSF. Pain 1991;47:295–8.
[209] Lee KH, Chung JM, Willis WD. Inhibition of primate spinothalamic tract cells by TENS. J Neurosurg 1985;62:276–87.
[210] Sjolund BH. Peripheral nerve stimulation suppression of C-fiber-evoked flexion reflex in rats. Part I: parameter of continuous stimulation. J Neurosurg 1985;63:612–6.

[211] Sweet JE, Law JD. Analgesia with peripheral nerve stimulation: absence of a peripheral mechanism. Pain 1983;15:55–70.
[212] Taylor P, Hallett M, Flaherty L. Treatment of osteoarthritis of the knee with transcutaneous electrical nerve stimulation. Pain 1981;11:233–40.
[213] Fargas-Babjak A, Rooney P, Gerecz E. Randomized trial of Codetron for pain control in osteoarthritis of the hip/knee. Clin J Pain 1989;5:137–41.
[214] Smith CR, Lewith GT, Machin D. TENS and osteoarthritis: preliminary study to establish a controlled method of assessing transcutaneous electrical nerve stimulation as a treatment for pain caused by osteoarthritis. Physiotherapy 1983;69:266–8.
[215] Grimmer K. A controlled double-blind study comparing the effects of strong burst mode TENS and high rate TENS on painful osteoarthritic knees. Austr J Physiother 1992;38: 49–56.
[216] Lewis D, Lewis B, Sturrock R. Transcutaneous electrical nerve stimulation in osteoarthritis: a therapeutic alternative? Ann Rheum Dis 1984;43:47–9.
[217] Zizic TM, Hoffman KC, Holt PA, et al. The treatment of osteoarthritis of the knee with pulsed electrical stimulation. J Rheumatol 1995;22:1737–61.
[218] Taylor DN, Katims JJ, Ng LK. Sine-wave auricular TENS produces frequency-dependent hypoesthesia in the trigeminal nerve. Clin J Pain 1993;9:216–9.
[219] Finsen V, Persen L, Lovlien M, et al. Transcutaneous electrical nerve stimulation after major amputation. J Bone Joint Surg 1988;70B:109–12.
[220] Katz J, Melzack R. Auricular transcutaneous electrical nerve stimulation (TENS) reduces phantom limb pain. J Pain Symptom Manage 1991;6:73–83.
[221] Nordemar R, Thorner C. Treatment of acute cervical pain: a comparative group study. Pain 1981;10:93–101.
[222] Kumar D, Marshall HJ. Diabetic peripheral neuropathy: amelioration of pain with transcutaneous electrical nerve stimulation. Diabetes Care 1997;20:1702–5.
[223] Thorsteinsson G, Stonnington HH, Stillwell GK, et al. Transcutaneous electrical stimulation: a double-blind trial of its efficacy for pain. Arch Phys Med Rehabil 1977;58:8–13.
[224] Leandri M, Parodi CI, Corrieri N, et al. Comparison of TENS treatments in hemiplegic shoulder pain. Scand J Rehabil Med 1990;22:69–72.
[225] Solomon S, Guglielmo KM. Treatment of headache by transcutaneous electrical stimulation. Headache 1985;25:12–5.
[226] Abelson K, Langley GB, Sheppeard H, et al. Transcutaneous electrical nerve stimulation in rheumatoid arthritis. N Z Med J 1983;96:156–8.
[227] Langley GB, Sheppeard H, Johnson M, et al. The analgesic effects of transcutaneous electrical nerve stimulation and placebo in chronic pain patients: a double-blind non-crossover comparison. Rheumatol Int 1984;4:119–23.
[228] Moystad A, Krogstard BS, Larheim TA. Transcutaneous electrical nerve stimulation in a group of patients with rheumatic disease involving the temporomandibular joint. J Prosthet Dent 1990;64:596–600.
[229] Melzack R, Vetere P, Finch L. Transcutaneous electrical nerve stimulation for low back pain: a comparison of TENS and massage for pain and range of motion. Phys Ther 1983;9:209–17.
[230] Cheing GL, Hui-Chan CW. Transcutaneous electrical nerve stimulation: nonparalleled antinociceptive effects on chronic pain and acute experimental pain. Arch Phys Med Rehabil 1999;80:305–12.
[231] Lehmann TR, Russel DW, Spratt KF, et al. Efficacy of electroacupuncture and TENS in the rehabilitation of chronic low back pain patients. Pain 1986;26:277–90.
[232] Deyo RA, Walsh NE, Martin DC, et al. A controlled trial of transcutaneous electrical nerve stimulation (TENS) and exercise for chronic low back pain. N Engl J Med 1990;322: 1627–34.
[233] Melzack R, Jeans ME, Stratford JG, et al. Ice massage and transcutaneous electrical stimulation: comparison of treatment for low-back pain. Pain 1981;9:209–17.

[234] Marchand S, Charest J, Li J, et al. Is TENS purely a placebo effect? A controlled study on chronic low back pain. Pain 1993;54:99–106.

[235] Herman E, Williams R, Stratford P, et al. A randomized controlled trial of transcutaneous electrical nerve stimulation (CODETRON) to determine its benefits in a rehabilitation program for acute occupational low back pain. Spine 1994;19:561–8.

[236] Graff-Radford SB, Reeves JL, Baker RL, et al. Effects of transcutaneous electrical nerve stimulation on myofascial pain and trigger point sensitivity. Pain 1989;37:1–5.

[237] Kruger LR, van der Linden WJ, Cleaton-Jones PE. Transcutaneous electrical nerve stimulation in the treatment of myofascial pain dysfunction. S Afr J Surg 1998;36:35–8.

[238] Ciccone CD. Iontophoresis. In: Robinson AJ, Snyder-Mackler L, editors. Clinical electrophysiology: electrotherapy and electrophysiologic testing. 2nd ed. Baltimore (MD): Williams & Wilkins; 1995. p. 277–310.

[239] Johnson MI. The mystique of interferential currents when used to manage pain. Physiotherapy 1999;85:294–6.

[240] Stephenson R, Johnson M. The analgesic effects of interferential therapy on cold induced pain in healthy subjects: a preliminary report. Physiother Theory Pract 1995;11:89–95.

[241] Cramp FL, Noble G, Lowe AS, et al. A controlled study on the effects of transcutaneous electrical nerve stimulation and interferential therapy upon the RIII nociceptive and H-reflexes in humans. Arch Phys Med Rehabil 2000;81:324–33.

[242] Truscott B. Interferential therapy as a treatment for classical migraine: case reports. Aust J Physiother 1984;30:33–5.

[243] Hurley DA, Minder PH, McDonough SM, et al. Interferential therapy electrode placement technique in acute low back pain: a preliminary investigation. Arch Phys Med Rehabil 2001;83:485–93.

[244] Taylor K, Newton R, Personius W, et al. Effect of interferential current stimulation for treatment of subjects with recurrent jaw pain. Phys Ther 1987;67:346–50.

[245] Werners R, Pynsent PB, Bulstrode CJ. Randomized trial comparing interferential therapy with motorized lumbar traction and massage in the management of low back pain in a primary care setting. Spine 1999;24:1579–84.

[246] Henley EJ. Transcutaneous drug delivery: iontophoresis and phonophoresis. Crit Rev Phys Rehabil Med 1991;2:139–51.

[247] Gudeman SD, Eisele SA, Heidt RS, et al. Treatment of plantar fascitis by iontophoresis of 0.4% dexamethasone: a randomized, double-blind, placebo-controlled study. Am J Sports Med 1997;25:312–6.

[248] Delacerda FG. A comparative study of three methods of treatment for shoulder girdle myofascial syndrome. J Orthop Sports Phys Ther 1982;4:51–4.

[249] Ozawa A, Haruki Y, Iwashita K, et al. Follow-up of clinical efficacy of iontophoresis therapy for postherpetic neuralgia (PHN). J Dermatol 1999;26:1–10.

[250] Oliver GC, Robin RJ, Salvati EP, et al. Electrogalvanic stimulation in the treatment of levator ani syndrome. Dis Col Rectum 1985;28:662–3.

[251] Quirion de Girardi CQ, Seaborne D, Savard-Goulet F, et al. The analgesic effect of high-voltage galvanic stimulation combined with ultrasound in the treatment of low back pain: a one-group pre-test. Physiother Can 1984;36:327–33.

[252] Bernard PA. La therapie diadynamique. Paris: Les Editions Naim; 1950.

[253] Hamalainen O, Kemppainen P. Experimentally induced ischemic pain and so-called diaphase fix current. Scand J Rehabil Med 1990;22:25–7.

[254] Turk DC, Okifuji A. Pain terms and taxonomies of pain. In: Loeser JD, editor. Bonica's management of pain. Baltimore (MD): Williams & Wilkins; 2001. p. 17–25.

[255] Allen RJ, Wu C, Horiuchi GM, et al. Pressure desensitization effects on pressure tolerance and function in patients with complex regional pain syndrome. Ortho Phys Ther Prac 2004; 16:13–6.

[256] Harden RN, Bruehl S, Galer B. Complex regional pain syndrome: are the IASP diagnostic criteria valid and sufficiently comprehensive? Pain 1999;83:211–9.

[257] Allen RJ, Wu C. Multimodal somatosensory desensitization therapy for patients with chronic pain. Presented at the Washington Occupational Therapy Association 2004 Annual Conference. Ocean Shores (WA), October 2, 2004.
[258] Robinson JL. Complex regional pain syndrome. Bulletin: State of Washington Department of Labor and Industries 1997;PB97-051:1–9.
[259] Walsh MT, Muntzer E. Therapist's management of complex regional pain syndrome (reflex sympathetic dystrophy). In: Macklin EJ, editor. Rehabilitation of the hand and upper extremity. 5th ed. St. Louis (MO): Mosby; 2002. p. 1707–24.
[260] Waylett-Rendall J. Desensitization of the hand. In: Hunter JM, Macklin EJ, Callahan AD, editors. Rehabilitation of the hand. 4th ed. St. Louis (MO): Mosby; 1995. p. 693–700.
[261] Harden RN. Complex regional pain syndrome. Br J Anaesth 2001;87:99–106.
[262] Fisher GT, Boswick JA. Neuroma formation following digital amputations. J Trauma 1983;23:136.
[263] Melzack R. From the gate to the neuromatrix. Pain 1999;(Suppl 6):S121–6.
[264] Loeser JD. Pain after amputation: phantom limb and stump pain. In: Loeser JD, editor. Bonica's management of pain. Baltimore (MD): Williams & Wilkins; 2001. p. 412–23.
[265] Cheshire WP, Snider CR. Treatment of reflex sympathetic dystrophy with topical capsaicin: case report. Pain 1990;42:307–11.
[266] Allen RJ, Wu C, Horiuchi G, et al. Somatosensory specific desensitization in the treatment of patients with complex regional pain syndrome: effects of pressure desensitization. J Ortho Sports Phys Ther 2005;35:A27.

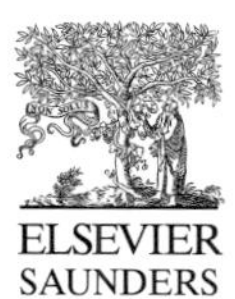
ELSEVIER
SAUNDERS

Phys Med Rehabil Clin N Am
17 (2006) 347–354

PHYSICAL MEDICINE
AND REHABILITATION
CLINICS OF
NORTH AMERICA

Nonsteroidal Anti-Inflammatory Drugs

Carin E. Dugowson, MD, MPH*,
Priya Gnanashanmugam, MD

Division of Rheumatology, University of Washington, Box 356428, Seattle, WA 98195-3414, USA

In Case 4, a 34-year-old male roofer fell off a roof 1 year ago and sustained an L1 vertebral body fracture. There was no neurologic compromise. An orthopedist recommended against surgical management. The patient was treated conservatively with bracing for several weeks and went through extensive physical therapy with only modest benefit. Radiographically, his condition stabilized, with no identifiable abnormality other than a 30% loss of height of the L1 vertebral body. He has undergone evaluation by an interventional pain physician. Diagnostic injections including medial branch blocks and discography at the thoracolumbar junction did not delineate any specific pain generator that might be a target for interventional therapy. The patient reports severe pain at the thoracolumbar junction. He has no symptoms in his lower extremities.

A patient like this one is almost certain to have undergone one or more trials of nonsteroidal anti-inflammatory drugs (NSAIDs). As a group, these medications are the most widely used medications in the world. Many are available over the counter. Although many of their adverse effects are well recognized, recent studies have identified new concerns. It is important to balance the benefits with the potential adverse effects of these drugs and to tailor therapy to the individual patient.

History

Derived from willow bark, salicin was used by MacIagan in 1874 to treat inflammation in rheumatic fever. Later, a more efficacious and better tolerated synthetic derivative, aspirin, was produced by Felix Hoffman of the Bayer company [1]. In 1963, indomethacin was introduced to treat

* Corresponding author.
E-mail address: carind@u.washington.edu (C.E. Dugowson).

doi:10.1016/j.pmr.2005.12.012

rheumatoid arthritis, and this was followed by the development of many other anti-inflammatory agents. The poor gastrointestinal (GI) tolerability of this class of drugs, coupled with their widespread use, led to the development of selective agents known as COX-2 inhibitors.

Mechanism of action

The mechanism of action of NSAIDs can be divided into their effects on inflammation, pain, and fever [1].

Anti-inflammatory effect

NSAIDs exert their anti-inflammatory effect through inhibition of prostaglandin G/H synthase, or cyclooxygenase, which is the enzyme catalyzing the transformation of arachidonic acid to prostaglandins and thromboxanes [1]. This enzyme has two recognized forms: cox-1 and cox-2. Selective inhibition of cox-2 leads to decreased GI side effects. Recent work suggests that activation of endothelial cells and expression of cell adhesion molecules play a role in targeting circulating cells to inflammatory sites. NSAIDs may inhibit expression of these cell adhesion molecules and may directly inhibit activation and function of neutrophils.

Analgesic effect

Although they are classified as mild analgesics, NSAIDs have a more significant effect on pain resulting from the increased peripheral sensitization that occurs during inflammation and leads nociceptors to respond to stimuli that are normally painless. In particular, it is believed that inflammation leads to a lowering of the response threshold of polymodal nociceptors [3].

Antipyretic effect

NSAIDs exert their antipyretic effect by inhibition of prostaglandin E2 (PGE2) synthesis, which is responsible for triggering the hypothalamus to increase body temperature during inflammation [3].

Pharmacokinetics

NSAIDS are metabolized primarily in the liver [1]. They vary in their half-lives and bioavailability. Given the multitude of available NSAIDs, the variability of their half-lives allows for different dosing regimens. Although decreased frequency of dosing improves compliance as a general rule, consideration must be given to the increase in renal dysfunction associated with longer-acting NSAIDs. It has also been speculated that use of daily dosed medications, by improving compliance, may increase the risk for GI bleeding. Variability in susceptibility to adverse effects of various NSAIDs does not seem to be due to difference in pharmacokinetics. Hepatic function, renal function, and age must be considered before prescribing and dosing.

Clinical uses

NSAIDs are classified as mild analgesics [4]. Although this designation says something about the potency of NSAIDs, it is misleading without the qualification that a major reason for the analgesic effect of NSAIDs is that they inhibit inflammation. Thus, pain mediated by inflammation is much more likely to be relieved by NSAIDs than pain that is unrelated to inflammation. Examples of the former include a variety of rheumatologic conditions, such as ankylosing spondylitis and rheumatoid arthritis. Osteoarthritis involves at least intermittent inflammation and can also respond to NSAIDs. Most importantly, local inflammation routinely occurs in response to acute injury of virtually any structure in the body [5]. Thus, NSAIDs are a logical choice for acute pain management after injury [6]. NSAIDs are widely used in the treatment of acute musculoskeletal injuries, and there is evidence for their ability to provide symptomatic relief of conditions such as acute low back pain [7,8].

NSAIDs are also commonly used in chronic musculoskeletal pain, although the rationale for their use in that setting is less clear because the degree to which inflammation plays a role in chronic musculoskeletal pain is not known. The literature on the efficacy of NSAIDs in chronic musculoskeletal pain is mixed. There is convincing evidence that NSAIDs are ineffective in treating fibromyalgia [9]. In contrast, there is evidence to support the use of NSAIDs in chronic spinal pain like that described in Case 4. However, this evidence comes from trials lasting no more than a few weeks [10–12], and other studies question the effectiveness of NSAIDs in spinal disorders [13].

Studies using large numbers of patients do not show a benefit of one type of NSAID over another, and their proven efficacy has not been shown to be superior to other agents, such as acetaminophen, narcotic analgesics, and muscle relaxants [2]. Variability in therapeutic response and susceptibility to toxicity is well recognized but poorly understood. Neither pharmacokinetics nor serum concentrations predict either of these outcomes. It is speculated that alteration of nonprostaglandin-mediated events may be important.

Adverse effects

In discussing adverse effects of anti-inflammatory medications, it is helpful to distinguish among aspirin, nonselective NSAIDs, and the newer selective cox-2 inhibitors. Although these three classes of drugs for the most part produce qualitatively similar adverse effects, they differ quantitatively in the risks that they pose.

Aspirin-induced asthma

NSAIDs should be avoided in patients who have established sensitivity to aspirin. All patients who are new to NSAIDs should be warned about this side effect. It is seen more commonly in patients who have asthma, nasal polyps, and history of rhinitis. The prevalence of aspirin-exacerbated respiratory tract disease is about 10% in the general population and about 21% in adults when determined by oral provocation testing. It is associated with rhinosinusitis and nasal polyps and presents most often as rhinitis and asthma. Although patients are described as having aspirin sensitivity or aspirin-induced asthma, they are at risk for adverse reactions from any NSAID that inhibits cox-1 [14,15]. There is recent evidence that suggests that selective cox-2 inhibitors are a safe alternative in this population, but this remains to be confirmed in large, well-controlled trials [16].

Aspirin should be used with caution in patients who have renal dysfunction or bleeding disorders and in elderly patients, in whom even baby aspirin can induce common side effects. Additionally, in elderly patients, tinnitus is commonly seen as therapeutic levels are reached. In practice, aspirin is uncommonly used for the management of musculoskeletal pain because the need for frequent dosing, the antiplatelet effect, and the risk of GI bleeding, and other issues make for a narrow therapeutic margin.

Effects on platelets

Aspirin and nonselective NSAIDs produce inhibition of platelet function via their inhibition of COX1. In the case of aspirin, the inhibition is irreversible, so the effect on platelet function continues for the life of the affected platelet (7–10 days). In contrast, nonselective NSAIDs cause a reversible inhibition of COX1, so that the effect on platelet function corresponds to the half-life of the specific drug, usually lasting from 2 to 12 hours [17]. Because COX-2 inhibitors have little effect on COX-1, they are less likely than nonselective NSAIDs to produce clinically significant effects on platelet function.

Gastrointestinal toxicity

Upper GI tract injury is a major side effect of NSAIDs and includes abdominal pain, dyspepsia, and gastroduodenal ulcers. Intolerance of GI side effects leads to withdrawal rates of about 10%. Also, nonselective NSAID users are four to eight times more likely to develop gastroduodenal ulcers during therapy. Although NSAID-induced ulcer complications are decreased with concomitant use of full-dose misoprostol, the usefulness of the latter drug is limited by the diarrhea it causes and by the need for multiple daily dosing [18]. Additionally, there is poor correlation between dyspeptic symptoms and the presence of ulcerations or erosions in the stomach or duodenum. Thus, symptoms may not be used as a guide regarding the risk of GI complications. A meta-analysis [19] of randomized controlled trials of comparing cox-2 inhibitors and nonselective NSAIDs showed that the cox-2 inhibitors were associated with a lower incidence of GI symptoms and symptomatic ulcers, but the studies did not provide data about the incidence of endoscopic ulcers.

In the CLASS study [20], fewer ulcers and ulcer complications were seen in the celecoxib group compared with ibuprofen or diclofenac in the initial 6 months. The effect was lost, but there is uncertainty about the cause. In particular, the use of low-dose aspirin in 20% of subjects and higher doses of celecoxib than used clinically complicate the analyses. There is also evidence that these agents do not decrease the risk of ulcers with complications in patients already at high risk for GI ulcers [21]. Also, of the COX-2 inhibitors, only rofecoxib was clearly shown to reduce the incidence of clinically significant GI bleeds and other ulcer complications. This has raised questions as to whether these drugs mask the presence of ulcers by decreasing dyspeptic symptoms [19].

Some studies suggest that double-dose H2-receptor blockers and proton pump inhibitors decrease the likelihood of gastroduodenal ulcers with long-term NSAID use, but this has not been borne out in randomized controlled trials; nor has there been clear evidence that one strategy is more effective than the other [22]. The preferred method of most physicians to avoid ulcer development is concomitant therapy with daily proton pump inhibitor or prescribing a selective COX-2 inhibitor.

GI side effects are more likely in elderly patients, patients who have a history of GI disease, patients who have concurrent *Helicobacter pylori* infection, patients using steroids or anticoagulants, and patients on higher doses of NSAIDs. The risk of GI ulcer is equal to that of nonselective NSAIDs in patients on cox-2 inhibitors who are also on aspirin [22]. GI bleeding in patients on warfarin is not less in patients using COX-2 drugs than nonselective NSAIDs [23].

Acute renal failure, nephrotic syndrome, and electrolyte complications

Due to constitutive expression of COX-2 in the kidneys, the effects of nonselective and COX-2 selective NSAIDs on renal function, electrolyte imbalance, and peripheral edema are similar [24]. There is an increase in renal toxicity when these agents are combined with antihypertensive agents and other potentially nephrotoxic drugs. There is a risk of peripheral edema and hyperkalemia, particularly in patients who have diabetes, elderly patients, and patients on other hyperkalemia-inducing agents such as potassium-sparing diuretics or angiotensin-converting enzyme (ACE) inhibitors.

Hypertension

In double-blind, randomized, controlled studies examining the effect of cox-2 inhibitors on blood pressure, the results are conflicting. Although rofecoxib seems to elevate blood pressure and interfere with antihypertensive effects of ACE inhibitors and beta blockers, the effect of celecoxib varies with the study design. Patients at particular risk of hypertension from the use of COX-2 inhibitors include those who have congestive heart failure, liver disease, and kidney disease and those taking ACE inhibitors or diuretics [25].

Cardiovascular effects

The selective COX-2 inhibitors do not inhibit platelet thromboxane A2, which is derived from COX-1. Animal studies show that the prostacyclin suppression mediated by COX-2 enhances responses to agonists that are thrombogenic and that increase blood pressure and atherosclerosis. As a result of these and other effects, COX-2 inhibitors, in comparison with nonselective NSAIDs, alter the balance antithrombotic and prothrombotic pathways in a way that promotes thrombogenesis [26]. This is the scientific basis behind the emerging evidence of risk of cardiovascular events with use of COX-2 inhibitors.

Cardiovascular toxicity was seen clinically in studies demonstrating that the use of rofecoxib (VIGOR) and valdecoxib (two studies of its use in post-CABG patients) led to an increase in atherosclerotic events and the withdrawal of rofecoxib from the market. The FDA's verdict regarding the cardiovascular hazard of the COX-2 inhibitors as a group remains to be seen. The evidence suggests that these drugs as a class increase the likelihood of a cardiovascular event, particularly in patients who are at increased risk. Many physicians have elected not to prescribe COX-2 inhibitors to patients who have a history of myocardial infarction or ischemic stroke. Consultation with a cardiologist is often appropriate for risk assessment and management of cardiovascular issues.

Addendum: case histories

Case 1

A 19-year-old man was involved in an accident while driving a motorcycle. He was not wearing a helmet. He hit his head into a telephone pole during the accident and sustained a skull fracture with intracerebral bleed. He was comatose for 10 days. He did not sustain any other significant injuries in the accident. After his coma resolved, he demonstrated significant cognitive difficulties, along with right-sided paresis and spasticity. He reports diffuse pain in his right lower extremity. There is no obvious orthopedic reason for this. His right lower extremity pain is thought to be a neuropathic type of pain secondary to his brain injury, with some aggravation caused by his spasticity.

Case 2

A 70-year-old woman has been treated for diabetes mellitus for the past 10 years. She complains of burning pain in both feet. The pain is severe enough that she reports substantial limitations in her physical activities and severe disruption of her sleep. She has undergone electrodiagnostic testing, which demonstrated abnormalities consistent with a diabetic polyneuropathy. The patient's general medical status is noteworthy in that she had a mild myocardial infarction 3 years ago, with subsequent angioplasty. Follow-up evaluations have shown normal left ventricular function and mild to moderate coronary artery stenosis. The patient has a history of hypertension adequately controlled with Lisinopril.

In cases of neuropathic pain (Cases 1 and 2), there is no clear long-term benefit of NSAIDs [27]. There may be a role in breakthrough pain when other long-term agents are in place. Combined use of NSAIDs with narcotic analgesics is thought to improve pain relief and to reduce opioid use [28]. Thus, in Case 1, NSAID use may decrease the patient's long-term need for opioids and may be a useful adjunctive therapy provided the bleeding from the acute traumatic episode is controlled. The decision to use an NSAID and the dose must be weighed against the individual patient's risk profile. In Case 2, the elderly hypertensive patient with coronary artery disease is on an ACE inhibitor, and aspirin use could put the patient at increased risk for adverse effects from NSAID use. Case 3 describes a pain syndrome (fibromyalgia) for which NSAIDs have been shown to be ineffective. NSAIDs are a commonly used and effective group of medications for many pain situations. However, the increased awareness of complications associated with their use mandates our increased caution when prescribing these drugs.

References

[1] Vane JR, Botting RM. The mechanism of action of aspirin. Thromb Res 2003;110:255–8.

[2] Brunton L, Lazo J, Parker K. Goodman & Gilman's the pharmacological basis of therapeutics. 11th ed. New York: McGraw-Hill Companies, Inc; 2006.

[3] Fitzgerald GA. COX-2 and beyond: approaches to prostaglandin inhibition in human disease. Nat Rev Drug Discov 2003;2:879–90.

[4] Burke A, Smyth EM, Fitzgerald GA. Analgesic-antipyretic agents; pharmacotherapy of gout. In: Brunton LL, Laxo JS, Parker KL, editors. Goodman & Gilman's the pharmacologic basis of therapeutics. 11th ed. New York: McGraw-Hill; 2006.

[5] Coltran RS, Kumar V, Robbins SL, editors. Robbins pathologic basis of disease. 5th ed. Philadelphia: Saunders; 1994.

[6] Ekman EF, Koman LA. Acute pain following musculoskeletal injuries and orthopaedic surgery: mechanisms and management. Instr Course Lect 2005;54:21–33.

[7] van Tulder MW, Scholten RJPM, Koes BW, Deyo RA. Non-steroidal anti-inflammatory drugs for low-back pain. Cochrane Database Syst Rev 2000;2:CD000396.
[8] Schnitzer TJ, Ferraro A, Hunsche E, et al. A comprehensive review of clinical trials on the efficacy and safety of drugs for the treatment of low back pain. J Pain Symptom Manage 2004;28:72–95.
[9] Goldenberg DL, Burckardt C, Crofford L. Management of fibromyalgia syndrome. JAMA 2004;292:2388–95.
[10] Hickey RF. Chronic low back pain: a comparison of diflunisal with paracetamol. NZ Med J 1982;95:312–4.
[11] Videman T, Osterman K. Double-blind parallel study of piroxicam versus indomethacin in the treatment of low back pain. Ann Clin Res 1984;16:156–60.
[12] Berry H, Bloom B, Hamilton EB, et al. Naproxen sodium, diflunisal, and placebo in the treatment of chronic back pain. Ann Rheum Dis 1982;41:129–32.
[13] Peloso P, Gross A, Haines T, et al. Medicinal and injection therapies for mechanical neck disorders. The Cervical Overview Group. Cochrane Database Syst Rev 2005;2:CD000319.
[14] Gollapudi RR, Teirstein PS, et al. Aspirin sensitivity: implications for patients with coronary artery disease. JAMA 2004;292:3017–23.
[15] Jenkins C, Costello J, Hodge L. Systematic review of prevalence of aspirin induced asthma and its implications for clinical practice. BMJ 2004;328:434–6.
[16] Woessner KM, Simon RA, Stevenson DD. Safety of high-dose rofecoxib in patients with aspirin-exacerbated respiratory disease. Ann Allergy Asthma Immunol 2004;93:339–44.
[17] Russell MW, Jobes D. What should we do with aspirin, NSAIDs, and glycoprotein-receptor inhibitors? Int Anesthesiol Clin 2002;40:63–76.
[18] Rostom A, Dube C, Wells G, et al. Prevention of NSAID-induced gastroduodenal ulcers. Cochrane Database Syst Rev 2002;4:CD002296.
[19] Wong VW, Chan FK. Review: misoprostol or COX-2-specific or selective NSAIDs reduce gastrointestinal complications and symptomatic ulcers. ACP J Club 2005;142:75.
[20] Silverstein FE, Faich G, Goldstein JL, et al. Gastrointestinal toxicity with celecoxib vs nonsteroidal anti-inflammatory drugs for osteoarthritis and rheumatoid arthritis. The CLASS study: a randomized controlled trial. JAMA 2000;284:1247–55.
[21] Chan FK, Hung LC, Suen BY, et al. Celecoxib versus diclofenac plus omeprazole in high-risk arthritis patients: results of a randomized double-blind trial. Gastroenterology 2004; 127:1038–43.
[22] Garner SE, Fridan DD, Frankish RR, et al. Celecoxib for rheumatoid arthritis. Cochrane Database Syst Rev 2002;4:CD003831.
[23] Battistella M, Mamdami MM, Juurlink DN, et al. Risk of upper gastrointestinal hemorrhage in warfarin users treated with nonselective NSAIDs or COX-2 inhibitors. Arch Intern Med 2005;165:189–92.
[24] Brater DC, Harris C, Redfern JS, et al. Renal effects of COX-2-selective inhibitors. Am J Nephrol 2001;21:1–15.
[25] Weir MR. Renal effects of nonselective NSAIDs and coxibs. Cleve Clin J Med 2002; 69(Suppl 1):SI53–8.
[26] Krotz F, Schiele TM, Klauss V, et al. Selective COX-2 inhibitors and risk of myocardial infarction. J Vasc Res 2005;42:312–24.
[27] Namaka M, Gramlich CR, Ruhlen D, et al. A treatment algorithm for neuropathic pain. Clin Ther 2004;26:951–79.
[28] Raffa RB, Clark-Vetri R, Tallarida RJ, et al. Combination strategies for pain management. Expert Opin Pharmacother 2003;4:1697–708.

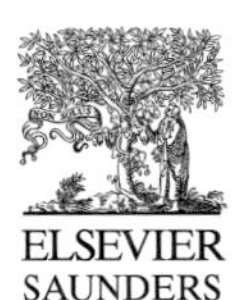
ELSEVIER
SAUNDERS

Phys Med Rehabil Clin N Am
17 (2006) 355–379

PHYSICAL MEDICINE
AND REHABILITATION
CLINICS OF
NORTH AMERICA

Opioids in the Treatment of Chronic Pain: Legal Framework and Therapeutic Indications and Limitations

Donna Bloodworth, MD[a,b,*]

[a]*Baylor College of Medicine, One Baylor Plaza, Houston, TX 77030, USA*
[b]*Outpatient Physical Medicine and Rehabilitation Clinics, Harris County Hospital District, 3601 N. MacGregor, Room 240B, Houston, TX 77004, USA*

Hill [1] writes that physicians have a threefold reluctance to prescribe opioids owing to: (1) the influence of disciplinary boards and state and federal drug enforcement agencies, (2) cultural and societal barriers to adequate and appropriate opioid use, and (3) knowledge deficits about the pharmacology of opioids. Thirty percent of physicians report no formal training in pain, and about half believe that prescribing strong opioids attracts medical review [2]. Physicians also endorse lower satisfaction and expectations when treating persons with chronic pain [2]. A high prevalence of personality disorder [3] and a 59% coincidence of depression, anxiety disorder, or substance abuse provide additional challenge [4]. This review will enable clinicians to develop informed therapeutic goals and limits for patients sustaining chronic pain by summarizing state and federal legislation regulating opioid prescription, the history and prevalence of opiophobia, and the efficacy, limitations, indications, and contraindications of opioids.

Federal regulation

Medical school curriculum rarely includes instruction about governmental regulation of medical practice. The government authorizes medical use of medications such as opioids through two distinct categories of laws: (1) controlled substance acts (CSAs) that regulate physiologically active chemicals, and (2) health care practice acts (HPAs) that set standards of medical practice [1]. Hierarchically, federal law takes precedence over state law, which

* Outpatient Physical Medicine and Rehabilitation Clinics, Harris County Hospital District, Houston, TX.
E-mail address: donna_bloodworth@hchd.tmc.edu

doi:10.1016/j.pmr.2005.12.001

can be more restrictive than federal legislation but not more permissive [5]. Any physician prescribing opioids should have working knowledge of the Federal CSA of 1970 and any CSA and HPA of the individual state in which he or she practices [5].

The Federal CSA of 1970 regulates the manufacture, distribution, prescription, and dispensing of opioids and other substances with the potential for diversion or abuse [5]. When registering for a number with the Drug Enforcement Administration (DEA), a branch of the US Department of Justice, the physician requests permission from the federal government to prescribe Schedule 2, 3, 4, and 5 substances. From Schedule 2 (most potential) to Schedule 5 (least potential), listed drugs and chemicals have descending abuse liability and risk of physical and psychologic dependence [6]. Examples of substances in Schedules 1 through 5 are as follows:

- Schedule 1: dihydromorphone (heroin); lysergic acid diethylamide (LSD); marijuana; various compounds of methamphetamine; phenylcyclohexyl piperidine (PCP)
- Schedule 2: cocaine, plain codeine and hydrocodone, hydromorphone, meperidine, fentanyl, methylphenidate, methadone, morphine, oxycodone
- Schedule 3: anabolic steroids and clostebol, butalbital, acetaminophen combinations of hydrocodone, ketamine, pentobarbital
- Schedule 4: alprazolam, butorphanol, clonazepam, diazepam, fenfluramine, meprobamate, modafinil, phentermine, temazepam, zolpidem
- Schedule 5: codeine in cough syrup preparations

Physicians may not prescribe Schedule 1 substances, which Congress has legislated have no legitimate medical purpose and extreme abuse potential [5].

A dynamic legislation, the CSA permits the addition of drugs as patterns of abuse emerge. The previous list of scheduled drugs is not complete and becomes dated. For example, anabolic steroids were added to Schedule 3 in 1991, and zolpidem, sold under the trade name Ambiens, is a relatively new drug added to Schedule 4. To keep abreast of the most current schedules of medications, physicians can access the DEA's website at www.usdoj.gov/dea [6].

Linked to the DEA's website is the Office of Diversion, accessible at www.deadiversion.usdoj.gov. This site contains practical information useful to the busy clinician, such as the following sample sections:

- FREQUENTLY ASKED QUESTIONS—provides DEA interpretation of opioid-related scenarios arising in clinical practice
- OFFICES & DIRECTORIES—lists DEA field offices by state
- PUBLICATIONS—links to the current downloadable version of the *CSA Manual* for physicians (currently being revised) or for pharmacists
- REGISTRANT ACTIONS—links to the Federal Register and actions against manufacturers, prescribers, and distributors of controlled substances

The link to the Federal Register reports that, in 2004, the DEA denied or revoked the registrations of 47 physicians, dentists, and veterinarians [7]. Because over 800,000 physicians practice in the United States, less than 0.006% of physicians lose their DEA registrations per annum. Nevertheless, the magnitude and notoriety of cases, such as that of Virginia physician William Hurwitz who was convicted in December 2004 on 50 counts of illegal drug distribution resulting in a 25-year prison term and 1 million dollar fine, offset the infrequency of prosecution [8].

The CSA does not prohibit prescribing scheduled substances to treat chronic pain. In fact, the DEA states [5], "Controlled substances, particularly narcotic analgesics, may be used in the treatment of pain experienced by a patient with a terminal illness or intractable pain. These drugs have legitimate uses...and may be issued for a legitimate medical purpose by a practitioner acting in the course of professional practice." Not an HPA, the CSA does not define "legitimate medical purpose" nor "set forth standards of professional practice" [5]. As regards physician practices, the CSA of 1970 limits or prohibits the refilling of certain medications, restricts the phone ordering of certain medications, and limits opioid prescription to treating pain only and not for treating physical dependence (Table 1) [5].

Federal legislation restricts prescribing opioids to treating pain [5]. With the exception of methadone and buprenorphine, opioid labeling on the package insert is strictly for pain treatment. Methadone (Methadose, Dolophine) is labeled to treat pain as well as for opioid detoxification and temporary maintenance treatment [9]. Physicians who prescribe methadone for opioid dependence in a narcotics maintenance treatment center require a special registration from the DEA [5]. Buprenorphine also has dual indications. As the brand name Buprenex, buprenorphine is labeled as an analgesic, whereas as the brand name Suboxone or SL Subutex, the labeling is for opioid dependence [10]. Physicians who prescribe Suboxone and Subutex for opioid dependence may do so only after attending mandated educational sessions and then applying for and receiving a special waiver from the DEA [11].

A practitioner not registered to practice in a narcotic treatment program or not waivered to prescribe buprenorphine for opioid dependence may administer narcotic substances to an addicted individual to relieve acute withdrawal symptoms for not more than 3 days while the practitioner refers the individual to a narcotic treatment program [5]. Only a 1-day supply of medication may be given per day, and the 3-day period may not be renewed [5]. All physicians need to understand the prohibition against treating addiction because any practice may encounter this condition.

The CSA of 1970 is federal legislation that regulates access to certain physiologically active chemicals. The CSA does not define "legitimate medical practice" but affects physician practice by prohibiting or limiting refills of controlled substances, requiring that all controlled substances be prescribed for an individual patient and not to "stock" use, and prohibiting the prescription of controlled narcotics for any indication but pain relief.

Table 1
The CSA of 1970 versus states' CSA laws: who restricts what?

Medications	Federal CSA	State CSA
Schedule 2 medications		
Requires a signed and dated prescription by the practitioner	Does require	Must require
Limits the time to fill a Schedule 2 prescription after being dated and signed by the practitioner	Does not limit	May limit
Limits quantity of pills prescribed at one time	Does not limit	May limit
Prohibits giving refills	Does prohibit	Must prohibit
Prohibits "calling medication in" to a pharmacy, except in an emergency (only a 3-day supply allowed; pharmacy must receive written script for these medications within 7 days)	Does prohibit	Must prohibit
Schedule 3 and 4 medications		
Prohibits more than five refills within 6 months of the date of prescription	Does prohibit	Must prohibit
Opioid medications in all schedules		
Prohibits prescribing for any purpose other than treating pain	Does prohibit	Must prohibit
Prohibits prescribing for "detoxification treatment" or "maintenance treatment"	Does prohibit	Must prohibit
Prohibits writing a prescription for office stock or "medical bag" use or general dispensing	Does prohibit	Must prohibit

Obviously, a patient treated for pain with narcotics but experiencing adverse effects from the medication, such as opioid-induced pain sensitivity, sedation, or constipation, may need the dosage tapered.

State regulations

The legislation of the state where a physician is licensed and practices may be more restrictive than federal law. The University of Wisconsin Medical School's Pain Policy website, www.medsch.wisc.edu/painpolicy, has compiled each state's legislation or medical board guidelines regarding chronic pain treatment or opioid prescription [12]. Policies regarding pain treatment (pt) or the use of controlled substances (cs) are as follows:

Medical Board Policy Statement (MBPS): CT (cs for pt); NY (cs for pt); NC (pt); WY

Medical Board Guideline (MBG): AZ (cs for pt); GA (cs); ID (cs for pt); KS (cs for pt); KY (cs); MD (cs); MA (pt; cs for pt); MT (cs for pt); SC (cs for pt); SD (cs for pt); UT (cs for pt); VT

Medical Board Regulation (MBR): AL (cs for pt); IA (cs for pt); LA (cs for pt); ME (cs for pt)

Intractable Pain Treatment Act (IPTA) only
Controlled Substance Act (CSA) only: ND; WI
Combination: AR (IPTA & MBR); CA (IPTA & MBG & MBPS); CO (CSA & IPTA & MBG); FL (IPTA & MBR); MN (IPTA & MBG); MS (MBR & MBPS); MO (IPTA & MBG); NE (MBG & public health statute); NV (MBR & Medical practice statute); NH (MBG and Statute); NJ (CSA and MBR); NM (MBG & MBR & Health Statute); OH (ITPA & MBR); OK (CSA & MBR & MBPS); OR (IPTA & MBR & MBPS); PA (MBR & MBG); RI (IPTA & MBG); TN (IPTA & MBR & MBPS); TX (IPTA & MBR & MBPS); VA (Medical Practice Statute & MBG); WA (CSA & MBR and Dept of Health Guideline); WV (IPTA & MBPS)
No Policy or other: AK; DE; DC; HI; IL; IN; MI (Public health statute)

Semantics, protections, and restrictions vary from state to state. Physicians practicing in several jurisdictions or moving should be familiar with each state's laws or medical board guidelines.

The Texas IPTA has served as an example for other states' legislatures. California's Medical Board Guidelines have served as an example for medical boards nationwide. In 1989, Texas became the first state to pass an IPTA, restricting opioid use but providing immunity to physicians compliant with the law. Although IPTAs "recognize in law…a legitimate place for opioids in the treatment of chronic pain," IPTAs are not a panacea for physicians prescribing opioids [13]. Experts admonish that IPTAs contain vague or undefined terms, deserving careful thought [1,14]. The federal language "legitimate medical practice" is not defined. In state regulations, the term *intractable pain* differs from the common medical parlance of *chronic pain*. Texas defines intractable pain as a state of pain in which "the cause of pain cannot be removed or otherwise treated and in the generally accepted course of medical practice no relief or cure of the cause of pain is possible or has been found after reasonable effort" [15]. Physicians in Texas and other states where the term intractable pain is used should verify that their patients with chronic pain on opioids fulfill the burden of this definition, and document the patient's condition as "intractable pain."

The Texas IPTA and Texas Medical Board regulations outline a management protocol to follow for persons with intractable pain on opioids [15,16]. Possible requirements of care while treating persons with opioids for intractable pain are as follows:

- Occurring in the usual course of professional practice
- The clinician is duly licensed where practicing
- Medication is ordered for legitimate medical practice (sometimes construed as "not to treat physical dependence or addiction")
- A recorded history and physical examination, including a review of pain, physical and psychologic function, the history and potential for substance abuse, coincident disease, and the presence of an indication for the use of a controlled substance

- A written treatment plan, including measurable objectives such as pain relief or improved physical functioning, as well as the need for other modalities, testing, or consultations
- A discussion of the risks and benefits of and alternative treatments to opioids; informed consent, required by some states for the prescription of opioids, may be indicated in this case
- Periodic review and documentation of the course and efficacy of treatment, and new information about the patient's condition.
- Complete and accurate records of care provided and substances, dosages, quantities, and refills prescribed

Some states' IPTAs, such as that of California, require consultation with a specialist in the organ system causing pain. Obtaining consultations even in jurisdictions where it is not explicit may benefit the patient and the clinician. Examination components that are not required but useful to assess opioid effects include pupillary constriction or dilation (which may indicate opioid use or withdrawal) and a sensory examination for allodynia and hyperalgesia (which may indicate neuropathic pain or opioid-induced pain hypersensitivity). Although not specifically named in the description of medical records, obtaining medical records from previous providers provides insight, details, and complications.

In addition to IPTAs and medical board regulations, some states pass controlled substance legislation more restrictive than the Federal CSA [5]. Common state restrictions include requiring that Schedule 2 prescriptions be filled within 7 days of being written [17], or limiting quantity amounts to 30-day supplies [18]. Neither are restrictions of the Federal CSA.

State controlled substance laws do alter physician behavior. Triplicate prescription bills in Texas, Rhode Island, New York, and Idaho decreased use of the targeted medications, including benzodiazepines in New York and Schedule 2 medications in Texas, by 50% or more [18,19]. Proponents of these laws interpreted decreased prescribing as evidence of antecedent overprescribing [18]. Critics of the laws noted that the laws resulted in the substitution of less effective and more dangerous nontargeted drugs [19,20].

The Federal CSA and states' HPAs, IPTAs, and CSAs impose various restrictions on physicians. Physicians should access available resources to familiarize themselves with the language, nuance, requirements, and controversies pertinent to these regulations.

Resources and tools

Various professional and patient organizations provide information and practice tools. The International Association for the Study of Pain (www.iasp-pain.org), its American chapter, the American Pain Society (www.ampainsoc.org), and its patient resource organization, the National Pain Foundation (www.painfoundation.org), provide links to pertinent sites and resources. The American Academy of Pain Medicine (www.painmed.org) provides links to an English language consent form for long-term opioids that discusses risks and benefits, as well as a "contract" for the use of long-term opioids that discusses physician and patient responsibilities. Physicians have ethical duties to patients that these forms subserve [21] as follows:

Autonomy—right of the individual to determine what will be done with his or her person, including confidentiality
Veracity—truthfulness and avoiding the withholding of information
Beneficence—doing or promoting good
Nonmalfeasance—avoiding doing harm
Fidelity—making and keeping promises
Right-to-know—principle of informed consent
Justice—fairness in distribution of scarce resources and treatments

The benefit to patients of informed consent should be evaluated scientifically. Forty percent of patients with a history of substance abuse who sign a long-term opioid contract and consent form do not fulfill its terms [22]. For the uncomplicated patient, these forms may achieve a different purpose of education. A simple survey of 12 opioid-naïve patients at the author's center found that 75% of patients who had requested opioids had questions about opioid therapy after discussing the risks and benefits. Examples of these issues are as follows:

Did not know Demerol is associated with seizures
Did not know opioids could cause death
Did not know the risks of acetaminophen independent of opioids
Did not know the signs of withdrawal
Did not know what constitutes delirium tremens (DTs)
Did not know Vicodin is a narcotic medication
Did not know that opioid and benzodiazepine cessation can be associated with withdrawal

Although alternative languages and illiteracy are common in the Unites States, alternative language consent forms and pain contracts are not available. The author's center is developing low-reading level and Spanish language forms. Partners Against Pain, an industry-sponsored, patient-oriented organization, offers Spanish language pain history intake packets.

Tools exist to educate patients, to help physicians conform to state and federal laws, and to promote a therapeutic relationship between physicians and persons with chronic pain. Electronic access facilitates this process.

Peer and patient attitudes

Although the World Health Organization has indicated that morphine and other opioids are "essential" drugs that should be available in all countries for medical treatment [18], even experts do not agree that opioids are appropriate treatment for persons with intractable pain [1]. Nonspecialists, patients, and regulators are uncertain about opioids' role. Turk and coworkers [23] surveyed clinicians nationwide and found that, although opioids were prescribed in all regions of the country by generalists and specialists, the frequency was uniformly low (1 to 1.5; range, 0 or never to 6). Moreover, physicians worried about the possibility of addiction and prosecution at a level of 3.5 and 4.5, respectively (range, 0 to 6) [23]. About one third of patients on opioids for intractable pain endorse concerns about addiction, but 86% percent report moderate pain-relieving benefit [24]. Physicians value improved function over pain relief as an outcome measure [23].

Only a decade ago, medical regulators may have had the most restrictive views about the use and benefit of opioids. Only 12% and 33% medical board members surveyed in 1991 and 1997, respectively, believed that extended opioid prescribing was "lawful and generally acceptable medical practice" for persons with chronic noncancer pain and no history of opioid abuse [25]. All others, except 6% to 7% in each year who were "not sure," believed the practice ranged from "not medically acceptable and should be discouraged" to "a violation of CSA and worthy of investigation" [25]. Educational interventions were offered and accepted by 12% of members. After education, the subgroup believing that long-term opioid prescription was "lawful and indicated" increased from 33% to 75% [25].

Related educational inroads led in 1998 to the Federation of State Medical Boards of the United States publishing model guidelines for the use of controlled substances for the treatment of pain [26]. These guidelines recognized that the use of opioids in the treatment of acute and chronic pain, including nonmalignant pain, might be essential [27]. The guidelines outlined expected essential components of care: patient evaluation, a treatment plan, informed consent and agreement for treatment, periodic review, consultation, maintenance of medical records, and compliance with state and federal controlled substance laws [27]. Nevertheless, in this recently negative regulatory climate, it is not surprising that the prescription of opioids for intractable pain remains a controversial and circumspect practice among the current generation of physicians.

Historical perspective

The soporific and medicinal use of opioids spans millennia. American suspicion regarding opioids spans more than a century. Arab traders propagated opium's medicinal use to Europe in the fifteenth century [28]. The bitter chemical could be smoked or ingested as a pill or an alcohol-opium mixture, laudanum [28]. Sertürner isolated morphine, the most active alkaloid in opium, in 1805 [29]. Historical uses of opiates included "intermittent fever" (malaria), wounds and fractures, burns, dysentery, cholera, colic and tetanus, dyspepsia, hysteria, asthma, rabies, seizures, and pain [30]. The hypodermic needle, invented in the 1850s, delivered smaller but more rapidly available doses of the drug [28,30]. When compared with blistering, purging, vomiting, and heavy metal–based medicines, opium pleasantly treated human suffering in the 1800s, when the use of opium quadrupled [30]. By the late 1890s when heroin was sold as the treatment for morphine addiction, cough, and diarrhea [28,31], 8% to 10% of all physicians used morphine with some frequency, and some authorities estimated that half of all opioid addicts had been made so at the hand of a physician [30].

Much like today, a subculture of substance abuse percolated into common consciousness and ultimately became legislative fodder. The word "yen," which entered the English language from Chinese around 1905, refers to the strong desire for opium [28]. Moving pictures about opium addiction condemned street dealers and unscrupulous prescribers in the 1910s and 1920s [28]. Dickens and O'Neill described the plight of the addicted in novels and plays [28,30]. Common citizens participated in antiopium movements [28].

Perhaps not causal links but comorbid at the time, physicians in America had variable training and few specific cures for disease, and government regulation of opioids did not exist [28,30,32]. Scientifically rigorous European medical training with laboratory and research opportunities contrasted with American medical schools that, through 1900, did not require a college degree for admission or even a high school diploma at one in five institutions [32]. The Carnegie Foundation, responding to the medical education crisis, commissioned Abraham Flexner to evaluate the quality of medical education in 1905 [30,32]. The Flexner report in 1910 effected the closing of 60% of all US medical schools in the ensuing years [32]. The US Congress responded to opioid abuse in 1914 and again in 1916 with two versions of the Harrison Narcotics Act, which restricted the availability, prescribing, and dispensing of opioids to specific physicians and pharmacies [28,30]. Thus began a 90-year struggle among patients, public perception, health care providers, and law enforcement in which [33], "Honest medical men have found dangers to themselves and their reputations in these laws... and they have simply decided to have as little to do as possible with drug addicts and their needs."

Considerations before and during opioid treatment: urine drug screens

Owing to federal regulation, physicians provide the only legal access to opioids in this country [34]. Because opioids not only treat pain, a medical prerogative, but also subserve addictive illness and black market commerce, physicians have become reluctant travelers on a convoluted course. Angarola and Joranson [18] argue that, "People suffering from pain...did not choose the disease that afflicts them. They should not have to suffer because a controlled substance is the appropriate treatment for their medical condition." Nevertheless, scheduled substances can be abused, which is why they are controlled [18]. Because physicians may treat pain with opioids but may not legally prescribe opioids for addiction, the first clinical divergence occurs separating patients with intractable pain from persons who have addictive illness and are drug seeking.

Addiction, abuse, dependence, and tolerance pertain to any opioid discussion. The literature often blurs these terms or simply does not define them. The DSM IV provides a consistent reference [35], providing the following definitions:

Dependence: maladaptive use with impairment of distress and three of the following concurrently: tolerance (the need to increase amount for effect, or diminished effect with use of the same amount); a characteristic withdrawal syndrome for the substance, or avoidance of withdrawal symptoms by use of the substance (presence indicates physiologic dependence); use of larger amounts of substance or for longer periods than planned; persistent desire to cut down on use; much time is spent obtaining substance; important social roles are given up because of substance use; substance use continues despite known harm

Substance abuse: maladaptive use with impairment of distress, manifested as one of the following: failure to fulfill a major obligation at work, school, or home; recurrent substance use in physically hazardous situations; recurrent substance-related legal problems; continued use despite recurrent interpersonal or social problems

Pain is a subjective complaint; its report cannot be challenged. Psychiatric comorbidity, including addiction, may exist. Drug diversion is criminal behavior and not a medical diagnosis; proving drug diversion burdens the legal system. Judging patients and jumping to conclusions on the physician's part clouds objectivity and may inadvertently cause malice. The physician's task becomes identifying subtle tissue damage and physical examination derangements consistent with a pain state, as well as behaviors suggestive of addiction, and then recommending a treatment plan in the patient's best interest.

Diagnosing addiction and abuse is difficult. As Fishman and coworkers [36] conclude, a "lack of accuracy in assessing abuse fosters conservative prescribing." IPTAs instruct physicians to inquire about past and current alcohol or substance abuse. The doctor–patient tradition is based on the physician accepting the veracity of the patient's report [37], but about 9% of chronic pain patients gave incorrect answers when asked if they use illicit substances [38]. Observation of behavior does not completely disclose substance abuse [37]. Forty-three percent of patients receiving treatment for chronic pain had inappropriate drug-taking behavior or positive urine drug screens (UDS) [37]. Behavior alone (unauthorized dose escalation, frequent phone calls, physician shopping, losing or reporting as stolen prescriptions, a drop in visits, and multiple allergies) identified one third of these patients; however, UDS alone identified another half of these persons whose behavior was normal. The small remainder had undesirable behavior and positive UDS [37]. In persons with a history of substance abuse seeking treatment for chronic pain, manifestation of the behaviors previously mentioned within 3 months correlated with the physician's subsequently diagnosing prescription abuse [39]. In this cohort, a history of alcohol abuse alone, stable family support, and active attendance of Alcoholics Anonymous predicted against concurrent substance abuse [39]. An audit of UDS from a clinic treating benign and malignant pain with long-term opioids found that half of all persons' tests were positive for alcohol, illicit substances, or unprescribed medications [40]. Risk factors for a positive result included having nonmalignant pain as opposed to malignant pain, and a positive HIV titer [40].

UDS and serum alcohol levels are initial and subsequent tools to identify persons with a primary or coincident diagnosis of substance abuse. Because many clinicians are not cognizant of the limitations of UDS, experts debate the generalized use of UDS. Nevertheless, some pain specialists require UDS before prescribing opioids [41]. Eight percent of family practitioners who treat pain order UDS [42]. The patient's full and informed consent should be obtained before drug testing. Standard language "pain contracts," such as that on the American Academy of Pain Medicine website, include permissions to obtain UDS [36]. Using positive UDS results in the context of other behavioral aberrances as a "three strikes" model to taper and discontinue opioid treatment has been proposed [36].

Initial UDS in clinical settings and even home test kits consist of an immunoassay. Immunoassay results are preliminary because cross-reactivity among similar compounds and false positives are possible (Box 1) [41,43]. Subsequent gas chromatography and mass spectrometry confirm the presence and concentration of a specific chemical [43]. Familiarity with the immunoassay specifications and limitations that a laboratory uses is recommended [36]. The physician can request this information from the laboratory. Screenings for marijuana, cocaine, opiate metabolites, PCP, and amphetamine are required tests for federal employment. Methadone, oxycodone, benzodiazepine, and barbiturate detection require distinct immunoassays.

Asking patients before UDS if they have taken any cold or flu preparations will prevent undesirable false positives. The immunoassay for amphetamines is nonspecific and often reacts with pseudoephedrine and other decongestants. If positive urine toxicology screens are identified, the physician must (1) be mindful that false positives occur and (2) have a plan of action to deal with a confirmed diagnosis of addiction, such as chemical dependency treatment. In 1915 Lewis and Woodruff argued that addiction was a medical problem and not a social affliction with "penological" remedies [33]. McLellen and coworkers [44] argued scientifically in 2000 that drug dependence is a chronic medical illness.

The goal of using UDS is to identify patient disease and comorbid addiction, and to permit appropriate patient referral to substance abuse counseling. As is true for all laboratory tests, UDS exist in a context of overall

Box 1. True and false positives in urine toxicology screens

True positives (detection period)

Opiates (1–2 days): morphine, codeine, heroin; unreliable for methadone, propoxyphene, oxycodone

Cocaine (2–4 days, 8 days high dose): only illicit cocaine or medical cocaine 2 to 3 days after a procedure

Amphetamines (1–2 days): medical or illicit amphetamines

Marijuana: active or recent marijuana use (2–8 days; up to 42 days in chronic users)

PCP (2–8 days)

Barbiturates (1–3 days, 10–14 days long acting)

Benzodiazepines

False positives

Technician/data entry error

Opiates: poppy seeds, quinolones

Cocaine: no cross-reactivity with other topical anesthetics

Amphetamines: diet agents (ephedrine, phentermine); decongestants (pseudoephedrine, phenylpropanolamine, phenylephrine); Parkinson medications (selegiline)

Marijuana: inhalation of secondary smoke and hemp seed ingestion are unlikely to cause a positive test; Marinol

patient behavior and compliance, as well as a context of testing limitations including sensitivity and specificity.

Opioid efficacy for intractable pain

One review article and two systematic reviews comment on the practice of prescribing opioids for the relief of chronic pain and summarize the available randomized controlled trials of the practice. Surveys and uncontrolled case series out to 6 years suggest that patients with chronic pain can achieve satisfactory analgesia on stable doses of narcotics with a minimal risk of addiction [34]. Except in the several days after opioid dose increases, psychomotor abilities such as driving are preserved [34]. Several randomized controlled trials exist, but practitioners should carefully consider the applicability of these results to unselected clinical populations [45,46]. What practitioners know about the use of opioids for the treatment of chronic pain is based on 15 to 16 randomized controlled studies involving fewer than 2000 subjects who were administered medication for less than 16 weeks [45,46]. Open label follow-up is available up to 2 years [45]. In clinical practice, persons on opioids for intractable pain may receive opioids for years or decades. The benefits, harms, and efficacy of long-term opioid therapy are not known but may include immunosuppressive and endocrinologic effects, such as suppressed libido [34].

Other limitations of the data, beyond small numbers and short follow-up, include adequate blinding, systemized identification of adverse events and standardized outcomes, as well as conservative patient selection [46]. Some studies excluded persons with psychiatric disease and histories of drug abuse, which does not reflect experience in general practice [45,46].

Patients and clinicians must understand the limited pain relief that opioids afford; otherwise, disappointment with the medication, the patient, or the physician will ensue. Satisfactory analgesia in most studies means a decrease in pain intensity of 30% [45]. Clinically, a 30% reduction means a patient rating pain at a score of 10 can hope for a 7, whereas persons starting at 7 might get to 5, still moderate levels of pain.

To avoid disappointment with the medication, the patient, or the physician, the high rate of side effects, namely, those expected with opioids, such as sedation, constipation, and stomach upset, should be disclosed to the patient [45,46]. Side effects are common with opioids, occurring in as many as 80% of patients [45]. The number needed to harm with opioids is 4.2. Kalso explains that for every four patients treated with opioids, one more would have experienced an adverse event than if they were treated with placebo [45]. Only about one third of available studies mention addiction, tolerance, or withdrawal; less than 20 subjects experienced these adverse events [45]. Inefficacy or side effects are the reasons why persons stop using opioids for pain over the long term, but details are not described [45]. Owing to side effects, costs, or other impediments to follow-up, less than half of patients started on opioids will continue beyond 7 to 24 months [45]. Physicians should inform patients that opioids have limitations not only in efficacy, with an average 30% relief, but also in side-effect profile and unknown long-term sequelae. For persons sustaining intractable pain, opioid limitations make alternative treatments such as paced exercise, stress management and coping skills, and restorative relaxation even more important.

Ballantyne and Mao [34] challenge "one of the fundamental principles of pain management…that the dose of an opioid should be increased until maximal analgesia is achieved with minimal side effects." The literature reports on moderate daily doses of opioids up to 200 mg morphine equivalents; high-dose opioid therapy has only been evaluated in two studies [34]. Increasing the opioids may not increase the pain relief. Ballantyne and Mao elegantly argue that, when opioids are not effectively treating pain, less opioid or a different opioid are possible clinical decisions.

Opioids become ineffective for the relief of pain owing to receptor alteration in two clinical scenarios—opioid tolerance and opioid-induced pain sensitivity [34]. In opioid tolerance, repeated opioid use causes the need to increase the dose to maintain the analgesic effect; downregulation or desensitization of opioid receptors by a variety of physiologic mechanisms is hypothesized [34]. Abnormal pain sensitivity, familiar in neuropathic pain states, manifests clinically as hyperalgesia and allodynia. Hyperalgesia occurs when a noxious stimulus evokes higher levels of pain in the affected area than the same stimulus applied to an intact area; allodynia describes when a nonnoxious stimulus evokes pain. The long-term use of opioids has been associated infrequently with the development of abnormal pain sensitivity, hypothetically owing to receptor sensitization [34]. Ballantyne and Mao contend that (1) doses above 180 mg of morphine daily have not been validated in the literature, and (2) the opioid itself may be inducing tolerance or pain sensitivity [34]. They present a reasonable and conservative management approach to the patient who may present to the office. The features of this approach include titrating up from a low dose of opioids as side effects allow to achieve analgesia (again, a 30% reduction from baseline), continuing as long as adverse drug reactions are not intolerable and follow-up is routine [34]. If dose escalation occurs, one should evaluate for the possibility of disease progression. Pain may worsen not because opioids are ineffective but because the disease process is advancing (eg, malignancy). Other strategies include rotating opioids, weaning the opioids, and restarting after a period of abstinence [34]. Treatment is a failure if evidence suggests addiction or noncompliance, or if pain relief is simply not forth coming [34].

Benefits of opioid treatment include improved sleep; however, depression scores did not change in six studies that assessed it, nor did overall activity or the pain disability index [45]. Physical function did not change in five of eight studies and improved in three; no studies have reported worsened function [45].

The systematic review by Chou and coworkers helps clinicians strategize [46]. They conclude that, based on the evidence, (1) no significant differences exist among long-acting opioids in regards to efficacy or safety profiles; (2) long-acting opioids as a class are not safer or more effective than short-acting opioids; and (3) no single long-acting opioid should be used first in the treatment of intractable pain. Practically, if a patient's pain is well controlled on three or four tablets daily of a short-acting acetaminophen and narcotic combination tablet, there may be no compelling reason to change the patient to a long-acting preparation. Additionally, the choice of a specific long-acting agent (eg, fentanyl patches versus long-acting morphine versus oxycodone products) has more to do with an individual patient's comorbidities than with the medication. For example, a patient with renal insufficiency or failure cannot excrete the metabolite of morphine, morphine-6-glucoronide; therefore, the physician should carefully weigh using morphine in a pain patient with renal disease [29]. In a patient with depression treated with Nardil or Parnate, monoamine oxidase (MAO) inhibitors, the use of meperidine to treat pain could precipitate malignant hyperthermia [47]. Because of inhibition of the cytochrome CYP3A4 system, a patient treated with erythromycin for infection or gastroparesis can experience prolonged respiratory depression with the intraoperative use of fentanyl [47]. In an HIV patient, rifampin or certain antivirals, inducers of the cytochrome CYP3A4, can precipitate withdrawal symptoms in a patient treated with methadone for pain or dependence [47].

Pharmacology of opioids

Acting on mu (μ) receptors in the periaqueductal gray, morphine and other opioids effect analgesia by inhibiting ascending pathway information about nociception. The affect of opioids could simplistically be said to be a function of the "descending pathways" that modulate the experience of pain. Morphine does not affect other sensory integration and, generally, more effectively decreases sharp intermittent pain than dull aching pain [29]. The analgesic and various other effects of opioids are mediated by at least three receptors with several subtypes (Table 2) [29]. The various chemicals that act on opioid receptors have different analgesic efficacies and different side-effect profiles because of unique affinities for the different opioid receptors. At each receptor, a chemical might be a full agonist, partial agonist, mixed agonist/antagonist, or antagonist, as follows [29]:

Full agonist: maximal physiologic response occurs with only a minimal percentage of receptors occupied
Partial agonist: requires maximal or full receptor occupancy for maximal physiologic response
Mixed agonist/antagonist: owing to different subtypes of receptors, an opioid may be an agonist at one receptor and a partial agonist or antagonist at another
Antagonist: binds to but does not activate the receptor

Table 2
Opioid receptors and the physiologic effects of opioids

Receptor subtype	Effect
μ_1	Supraspinal analgesia, dependence, withdrawal, and tolerance, euphoria, emesis, sedation, prolactin release, increased feeding behavior, immune suppression, possibly pruritus
μ_2	Spinal analgesia, respiratory depression, decreased gastrointestinal motility, decreased growth hormone
δ_1	Supraspinal analgesia, stimulates feeding, growth hormone release
δ_2	Supraspinal and spinal analgesia
κ_1	Dysphoric responses
κ_2	Decreased gastrointestinal transit, sedation, feeding behavior
κ_3	Supraspinal analgesia

Data from Maher TJ, Chaiyakul P. Opioids (Bench). In: Smith HS, editors. Drugs for pain. Philadelphia: Hanley and Belfus; 2003. p. 83–96.

Four families of chemicals are active at the opioid receptors as follows [29]:

Phenanthrenes: morphine, codeine, heroin, oxycodone, hydrocodone, hydromorphone
Phenylpiperidines: meperidine, loperamide, diphenoxylate, propoxyphene
Benzomorphan: pentazocine
Propionanilides: fentanyl, sufentanil, alfentanil

The medication and its metabolites may have physiologic activity. Of particular importance is morphine's conjugated form, morphine-6-glucuronide, which is a 100-times more potent analgesic than morphine [29]. Although it passes more slowly through the blood-brain barrier, it accumulates in tissues and, independent of morphine, causes respiratory depression, sedation, and vomiting [29]. Because glucuronide metabolites are renally excreted, renal insufficiency or renal failure may require conservative morphine dosing or a different agent entirely [48]. A minor metabolic pathway for opioids, N-demethylation, forms another problematic opioid metabolite, normeperidine, from meperidine (Demerol) [49]. This physiologically excitatory chemical may accumulate in renal insufficiency and failure and be epileptogenic [49].

The inability to metabolize a compound may also affect the analgesic efficacy of a drug. If not demethylated by the cytochrome P-450 CYP2D6 to morphine, codeine is a weak mu agonist [48]. As many as 10% of Caucasians lack CYP2D6 activity; therefore, reports of a lack of analgesic effect of codeine should be considered in the context of genetic predisposition and not only a context of possible drug-seeking behavior [48]. Other limitations of codeine include a tendency to cause nausea and vomiting in doses over 65 mg [48]. Because of its limited analgesic effect, variable metabolism, and notable side-effect liability at high doses, codeine's usefulness in the treatment of intractable pain may be limited.

Drug interactions also affect the analgesic efficacy of opioids [47,48]. Rifampin and retroviral drugs increase the metabolism of methadone and may precipitate withdrawal symptoms [47,48]. Quinidine inhibits CYP2D6 and may inhibit the analgesic effect of codeine [47,48]. Significantly, meperidine given in combination with MAO inhibitors or dextromethorphan can induce malignant hyperthermia [48]. Antidepressants, neuroleptics, and alpha-adrenoreceptor agonists, all sometimes used as adjuvant moieties in the treatment of intractable pain, enhance opioid analgesia and other effects. The use of tramadol and selective serotonin reuptake inhibitors (SSRIs) can produce serotonin syndrome involving mental status changes and agitation, hyperreflexia, incoordination, myoclonus, shivering, tremor, diaphoresis, diarrhea, fever, seizures, and coma [50]. Tramadol may be epileptogenic when used concomitantly with SSRIs, tricyclic antidepressants, opioids, and MAOIs [50]. The need to obtain a complete history and physical examination including laboratory studies, with full disclosure of medications prescribed by other physicians, is underscored by these potentially serious drug interactions.

Opioid rotation to treat tolerance

One strategy for restoring opioid efficacy when tolerance develops is opioid rotation [51,52]. Opioid rotation has also been employed to relieve opioid toxicity [53]. In the palliative care setting, subjects were rotated off one narcotic to another for signs of toxicity (cognitive failure, hallucinations, myoclonus, nausea and vomiting, local toxicity) or persistent pain [53]. Symptoms improved in a significant (73%) percentage of patients; also significant were a decrease in narcotic equivalents and an increase in pain control (from 4.4 to 3.6) [53]. Thomsen and Eriksen evaluated opioid rotation in subjects with nonmalignant pain [51]. Unlike in cancer subjects, the main reason for opioid rotation was insufficient pain relief [51]. Rotation resulted in 59% of patients experiencing better pain relief [51]. Opioid rotation from short-acting to long-acting opioids resulted in better pain relief but a doubling of opioid dose [51]. Quang-Cantagrel and coworkers evaluated opioid rotation in subjects with chronic noncancer pain as an initial management strategy to identify which narcotic best relieved pain and minimized side effects [52]. Subjects experienced significant pain relief with minimal side effects with the initial long-term opioid only one-third of the time [52]. Two thirds of patients required trials of other long-acting opioids [52]. If allowed a trial of up to five different long-acting opioids, an effective analgesic with minimal adverse effects could be identified for 90% of subjects [52]. Similar to Chou's meta-analysis, Quang-Cantagrel and colleagues showed that no initial long-acting opioid was superior in pain relief or side-effect profile when compared with other opioids.

Neuropathic pain and opioids

The occurrence and perpetuation of inflammatory pain, ischemic pain, and neuropathic pain involve the N-methyl-D-aspartate receptor, which is activated by glutamate and associated with a reduction in sensitivity to opioids [52]. In 1988, Arner and Meyerson [54] ignited a controversy regarding the efficacy of opioids for pain relief in neuropathic pain states. In a randomized, placebo-controlled trial of intravenous morphine, nociceptive pain was significantly relieved but neuropathic and idiopathic (chronic pain syndrome) pain were not [54]. They argued that the "therapeutic effect of [opioids] may be restricted to…suppression of nociceptive pain subserved by a functionally normal nervous system." They hypothesized that acute and chronic pain involve partly separate pathophysiologic mechanisms, with different susceptibility to analgesic drugs owing to different physiologic mechanisms [54]. Fundamental criticisms of the work include the variable experimental design among patient groups for pain rating and the number of doses and drugs administered [55]. Additionally, the nociceptive group was known to be opioid responsive and the neuropathic group was known to be resistant to all forms of previous treatment, including opioids [55].

Human scientific models for neuropathic pain include postherpetic neuralgia and diabetic peripheral neuralgia. In general, placebo or comparator trials of various opioids for the treatment of neuropathic pain reveal predictable findings (Table 3). Opioids partially relieve neuropathic pain, but the pain relief is not complete (Table 2) [56–61]. Depending on the diagnosis, opioids affect certain qualities of the pain experience differently [56,60,62]. For example, steady pain, paroxysmal pain, and allodynic pain, as well as disability, were significantly improved by oxycodone in the treatment of postherpetic neuralgia [56]. Side effects were common [57,59,61]. Cognitive adverse effects were more significant for certain comparators such as tricyclic antidepressants [57]. Clinicians need to be aware of the limitations of the trials. Generally, none of the studies exceeded 3 months [56–61]. Available follow-up to 2 years in open label trials suggests that about 80% of subjects discontinue opioids [62]. Another important difference between actual clinical practice and available clinical trials is that patients participating in studies undergo preselection processes and may not be representative of the responsiveness or comorbidities of the general population [61]. Adjuvant treatments such as tricylic antidepressants and gabapentin relieve pain more than placebo but less than opioid comparators [57,63]. Drug-sparing effects may be noted with opioid-adjuvant combinations [63].

Cases

Case 1

A 19-year-old man presents with motorcycle crash and traumatic brain injury and probably centrally mediated neuropathic pain. Tricylic antidepressants will probably compound compromised cognitive function. Opioids have not been shown to decrease central pain meaningfully, and, given their other liability, I would probably direct pain relief efforts at treatment of the spasticity.

Case 2

A 70-year-old woman presents with 10 years of diabetes mellitus, neuropathic type foot pain, and poor sleep. If the patient is not on SSRIs, tramadol should be considered for treatment of the patient's pain, as well as newer medications such as duloxetine (Cymbalta), which is labeled for the treatment of diabetic peripheral neuropathy, or pregabalin (Lyrica), which is also labeled for this purpose and has been shown to improve sleep. Another possibility is gabapentin. If the patient does not improve on these specifically labeled drugs, I would not hesitate to discuss with her the 30% pain relief possible with a low dose of long-acting opioid, or a twice daily to three times daily short-acting opioid. Side effects are likely and should be explained before treatment. Initial UDS and prior medical records should be obtained before starting opioid treatment.

Table 3
Neuropathic pain and trials of opioids

Author, year	Diagnosis	Medication	Design	Adverse effects	Pain relief	Comments
Watson, 1988 [56]	PHN for 2.5 years	10 mg LA oxycodone versus placebo	4-week crossover	1/4 drop out rate	Significant for oxycodone (decrease, 2.9) versus placebo (decrease, 1.8) and for all different types of pain	No effect of order; disability scores improved
Raja, 2002 [57]	PHN	Opioid versus TCA versus placebo	8-week crossover	Significantly more opioid (76%) ADR and drop out t han TCA (36%) arm	Sleep and pain relief significantly better with opioids (1.9 decrease) and TCA (1.4 decrease) than placebo	TCA worsened cognitive performance significantly more than opioids; no effect of order
Harati, 1998 [58]	DMPN	Tramadol versus placebo	42-day parallel, double blind		Significantly better pain relief with tramadol (2.5 decreased to 1.4) versus placebo (2.5 to 2.2)	Social and physical function also improved

Gimbel, 2003 [59]	DMPN	10 to 60 mg oxycodone versus placebo	42 day	96% ADR with oxycodone versus 68% with placebo	Average VNS with oxycodone 4.1 versus with placebo, 5.3	
Watson, 2003 [60]	DMPN	10 to 40 mg q12 oxycodone versus benzotropine	4-week crossover		Oxycontin experience significantly less total and daily pain and significantly less disability and all types of pain (brief, steady, and skin)	Number needed to treat for one person to experience 50% less pain was 2.6
Dellemijn 1998 [61]	Various neuropathic pain	Transdermal fentanyl, 25 to 100 µg, after administration of IV fentanyl	12 weeks	90% nausea, 70% other opioid effects	Marked pain relief in 13 of 48 and moderate in 5 of 48; at 2 years 1/5 of patients remained on fentanyl, with moderate-marked pain relief in 6	Depression scores did not change; quality of life increased 23%; maximal relief occurred at 9 weeks and was sustained in 40%

(*continued on next page*)

Table 3 (*continued*)

Author, year	Diagnosis	Medication	Design	Adverse effects	Pain relief	Comments
Attal, 2002 [62]	Central pain	IV morphine versus placebo, changed to sustained release morphine		Only 20% continued at 1 year	Only intensity of brush allodynia decreased; no effect on ongoing or evoked pains	
Gilron, 2005 [63]	PHN and DMPN	Morphine versus gabapentin versus (morphine plus gabapentin) versus placebo	5-week, crossover, 4 arms	1/4 drop out	Gabapentin with morphine provides better pain relief (average daily pain, 3.06) than either drug alone (morphine, 3.7; gabapentin, 4.15; placebo, 4.5; and baseline, 5.7)	More constipation with morphine-gabapentin combination

Abbreviations: ADR, adverse drug reactions; DMPN, diabetic peripheral neuropathy; IV, intravenous; PHN, postherpetic neuralgia; TCA, tricyclic antidepressant; VNS, verbal numerical (pain) score.

Case 3

A 35-year-old woman sustains a rear end motor vehicle accident with whiplash. MRI is negative, and there is no response to facet injections (keeping in mind that diagnostic injections have some false negativity). Examination suggests fibromyalgia and myofascial pain. If the patient has not had a course of physical therapy for stretch, strengthening, and myofascial interventions, she certainly should. Education about the benefit and importance of exercise, paced activity, focused relaxation, and time management should begin immediately. The patient should be asked about sleep and depressive symptoms, as well as employability. If there are psychosocial stressors, these should be anticipated, and the patient should be referred to social service workers. A tricyclic antidepressant with a more favorable anticholinergic profile and an anti-inflammatory medication can be considered if the patient has no contraindications. Several combinations can be tried. Tramadol may give the patient some relief and can be added or tried alone. If used with the tricyclic antidepressant, serotonin syndromes are theoretically possible. Opioids, either short or long acting, would be a last option. An extensive discussion about the limited efficacy of opioids (30% pain relief), the limitations owing to side effects, and the unknown long-term side effects, an initial UDS, and request of old medical records are all prerequisites to treatment.

Case 4

A 34-year-old male roofer falls and sustains an L1 compression fracture. No pain generator is identified subsequent to diagnostic injections. The considerations about diagnostic test sensitivity and specificity also apply to this patient. Education and psychosocial intervention need to begin immediately. One would have to question his employability in the construction field. Previous physical therapy interventions should be reviewed for the patient's compliance as well as the appropriateness of the interventions. If the patient did not meaningfully participate in an extension bias program and instruction in body mechanics, therapy should be reconsidered. The patient will likely have to concede some lifestyle, mobility, and activity considerations to his injury. Minimal bracing to block flexion may give the patient some symptomatic relief. Because this patient may be anticipating a four-decade use of pain medication, similar to Case 3, a frank discussion of medication limitations and unknown long-term side effects needs to be undertaken.

Summary

The most important message that physicians must communicate to persons with chronic pain is that, currently, no medication exists that will take away more than 30% of the pain they experience. Chronic pain is a chronic disease and, like diabetes or hypertension, requires chronic concessions and lifestyle modifications. In controlled trials of short duration and small sample size with highly selected patients, patients sustaining moderate-to-severe pain still experience moderate pain even on opioid medication. Adverse drug effects are predictable and common, and, in fact, long-term compliance with opioids is low owing to side effects. Screening for substance abuse by history taking, observing behavior, obtaining old medical records, and using UDS in patients before initiating opioid therapy is important to identify patients with comorbid addictive disease who require coincident or antecedent treatment. Familiarity with federal and state controlled substance legislation and state health care provider and pain treatment acts is a mundane but essential educational endeavor for all physicians prescribing opioids. If physicians educate their patients with chronic pain about the limited efficacy of the medications, patients' expectations for drug treatment can be more realistic.

References

[1] Hill CS. Government regulatory influences on opioid prescribing and their impact on the treatment of pain of nonmalignant origin. J Pain Symptom Manage 1996;11(5):287–98.

[2] Green CR, Wheeler JR, Marchant B, et al. Analysis of the physician variable in pain management. Pain Med 2001;2(4):317–27.

[3] Dersh J, Polatin PB, Gatchel RJ. Chronic pain and psychopathology: research findings and theoretical considerations. Psychosom Med 2002;64:773–86.

[4] Polatin PB, Kinney RK, Gatchel RJ, et al. Psychiatric illness and chronic low-back pain. Spine 1993;18(1):66–71.

[5] Drug Enforcement Administration. Pharmacist's manual: an informational outline of the Controlled Substance Act of 1970, p. 1–5, 32, 37–39, 53–55. Available at: http://www.deadiversion.usdoj.gov/pubs/manuals/pharm2/2pharm_manual.pdf. Accessed August 27, 2005.

[6] Drug scheduling. In: DEA briefs and background, drug policy, drug scheduling. Drug Enforcement Administration website. Available at: www.usdoj.gov/dea/pubs/scheduling.html. Accessed August 27, 2005.

[7] Registrant actions—2004. In: Federal Register Notices. Available at: www.deadiversion.usdoj.gov/fed_regs/actions/2004/index.html. Accessed August 27, 2005.

[8] News releases. In: News from DEA. Drug Enforcement Administration website. Available at: www.usdoj.gov/dea/pubs/pressrel/pr041505.html. Accessed August 27, 2005.

[9] Dolophine hydrochloride. In: Murray L, editor. Physician's desk reference. 56th edition. Montvale (NJ): Medical Economics Company; 2002. p. 3056–7.

[10] Buprenorphine hydrochloride (Buprenex and Suboxone and Subutex). In: Murray L, editor. Physician's desk reference. 59th edition. Montvale (NJ): Medical Economics Company; 2005. p. 2828–33.

[11] Intelligence bulletin: buprenorphine. Potential for abuse, September 2004, Product No. 2004–L0424–013, p. 1–4. Available at: http://www.usdoj.gov/ndic/pubs10/10123/10123t.htm. Accessed August 27, 2005.

[12] Database of statutes, regulations, and other policies. In: Pain and policies study group, University of Wisconsin, Comprehensive Cancer Center. Available at: http://www.medsch.wisc.edu/painpolicy/matrix.htm. Accessed August 27, 2005.

[13] Joranson DE, Gilson AM. State intractable pain policy—current status. APS Bulletin 1997; 7(2):7–9.

[14] Haddox JD. The AMA model intractable pain treatment act—a critique. Pain Medicine Network 1997;11(6):4.
[15] Texas Civil Statutes. Title 71: Health Public, Article 4495c. Intractable Pain Treatment Act. Amended September 1, 1997. Available at: http://www.medsch.wisc.edu/painpolicy/domestic/txipta.htm. Accessed August 27, 2005.
[16] Texas Administrative Code. Texas State Board of Medical Examiners, chapter 170. Authority of physician to prescribe for the treatment of pain. 22TAC∫∫170.1–170.3 Available at: http://www.medsch.wisc.edu/painpolicy/domestic/txmbreg.htm. Accessed August 27, 2005.
[17] Health and Safety Code, chapter 481.074. In: Texas Statutes in Texas Legislature website. Available at: http://www.capitol.state.tx.us/statutes/hs.toc.htm. Accessed August 27, 2005.
[18] Angarola RT, Joranson DE. State controlled substance laws and pain control. APS Bulletin 1992;2(3):10–1, 15.
[19] Sigler KA, Geurnsey BG, Ingrim NB, et al. Effect of a triplicate prescription law on prescribing of Schedule 2 drugs. Am J Hosp Pharm 1984;41:108–11.
[20] Weintraub M, Singh S, Byrne L, et al. Consequences of the 1989 New York State triplicate benzodiazepine prescription regulations. JAMA 1991;266(17):2393–7.
[21] Martin P. Medical ethics for physicians. CME Resource 2004;118(10):47–68.
[22] Dunbar SA, Katz NP. Chronic opioid treatment for nonmalignant pain in patients with a history of substance abuse. J Pain Symptom Manage 1996;11(3):163–71.
[23] Turk DC, Brody MC, Okifuji EA. Physicians' attitudes and practices regarding the long-term prescribing of opioids for noncancer pain. Pain 1994;59:201–8.
[24] Jamison RN, Anderson KO, Peeters-Asdourian C, et al. Survey of opioid use in chronic nonmalignant pain patients. Reg Anesth 1994;19(4):225–30.
[25] Gilson AM, Joranson DE. Controlled substances and pain management: changes in knowledge and attitudes of state medical regulators. J Pain Symptom Manage 2001;21(3):227–37.
[26] Joranson DE, Gilson AM, Dahl JL, et al. Pain management, controlled substances, and state board policy: a decade of change. J Pain Symptom Manage 2002;23(2):138–47.
[27] Model policy for the use of controlled substances for the treatment of pain. Federation of State Medical Boards of the United States. Available at: http://www.fsmb.org/Policy%20Documents%20and%20White%20Papers/2004_model_pain_policy.asp. Accessed August 27, 2005.
[28] Hodgson B. Opium portrait of the heavenly demon. San Francisco: Chronicle Books; 1999.
[29] Maher TJ, Chaiyakul P. Opioids (Bench). In: Smith HS, editor. Drugs for pain. Philadelphia: Hanley and Belfus; 2003. p. 83–96.
[30] Musto DF. Iatrogenic addiction: the problem, its definition and history. Bull N Y Acad Med 1985;61(5):694–705.
[31] Cohen S. Heroin. In: Encyclopedia Americana, vol. 14. Danbury (CT): Grolier; 1985. p. 149–50.
[32] Barry JM. The great influenza—the epic story of the deadliest plague in history. New York: Viking; 2004.
[33] Lewis HE, Woodruff CE. Editorial comment. American Medicine 1915;21(11):799–800.
[34] Ballantyne JC, Mao J. Opioid therapy for chronic pain. N Engl J Med 2003;349(20):1943–53.
[35] Substance-related disorders. In: First MB, Pincus HA, Frances A, et al, editors. Desk reference to the diagnostic criteria from DSM-IV-TR. Washington (DC): American Psychiatric Association; 2000. p. 105–51.
[36] Fishman SM, Wilsey B, Yang J, et al. Adherence monitoring and drug surveillance in chronic opioid therapy. J Pain Symptom Manage 2000;20(4):293–307.
[37] Katz NP, Sherburne S, Beach M, et al. Behavioral monitoring and urine toxicology testing in patients receiving long-term opioid therapy. Anesth Analg 2003;97(4):1097–102.
[38] Fishbain DA, Cutler RB, Rosomoff HL, et al. Validity of self-reported drug use in chronic pain patient. Clin J Pain 1999;15(3):184–91.
[39] Dunbar SA, Katz NP. Chronic opioid treatment for non-malignant pain in patients with a history of substance abuse. J Pain Symptom Manage 1996;11(3):163–71.

[40] Passik SD, Schreiber J, Kirsh KL, et al. A chart review of the ordering and documentation of urine toxicology studies in a cancer center: do they influence patient management. J Pain Symptom Manage 2000;19(1):40–4.
[41] Gourlay D, Heit HA, Caplan YH. Urine drug tests in primary care. San Francisco: California Academy of Family Physicians. 2002.
[42] Adams NJ, Plane MB, Fleming MF, et al. Opioids and the treatment of chronic pain in a primary care sample. J Pain Symptom Manage 2001;22:791–6.
[43] Eskridge KD, Guthrie SK. Clinical issues associated with urine testing of substances of abuse. Pharmacotherapy 1997;17(3):497–510.
[44] McLellen AT, Lewis DC, O'Brien CP, et al. Drug dependence, a chronic medical illness. JAMA 2000;284(13):1689–95.
[45] Kalso E, Edwards JE, Moore RA, et al. Opioids in chronic non-cancer pain: systematic review of efficacy and safety. Pain 2004;112(3):372–80.
[46] Chou R, Clark EC, Helfand M. Comparative efficacy and safety of long-acting oral opioids for chronic non-cancer pain: a systematic review. J Pain Symptom Manage 2003;26(5): 1026–48.
[47] Smith HS. Potential analgesic interactions. In: Smith HS, editor. Drugs for pain. Philadelphia: Hanley and Belfus; 2003. p. 453–63.
[48] Janicki PK, Parris WC. Clinical pharmacology of opioids. In: Smith HS, editor. Drugs for pain. Philadelphia: Hanley and Belfus; 2003. p. 97–118.
[49] Elliott JA, Opper SE. Opioids: adverse effects and their management. In: Smith HS, editor. Drugs for pain. Philadelphia: Hanley and Belfus; 2003. p. 133–51.
[50] Ripple MG, Psetaner JP, Levine BS, et al. Lethal combination of tramadol and multiple drugs affecting serotonin. Am J Forensic Med Pathol 2000;21(4):370–4.
[51] Thomsen AB, Eriksen J. Opioid rotation in chronic non-malignant pain patients: a retrospective study. Acta Anesthesiol Scand 1999;43:918–23.
[52] Quang-Cantagrel ND, Wallace MS, Magnuson SK. Opioid substitution to improve the effectiveness of chronic non-cancer pain control: a chart review. Anesth Analg 2000;90:933–7.
[53] DeStoutz ND, Bruera E, Suarez-Almazor M. Opioid rotation for toxicity reduction in terminal cancer patients. J Pain Symptom Manage 1995;10(5):378–84.
[54] Arner S, Meyerson BA. Lack of analgesic effect of opioids on neuropathic and idiopathic forms of pain. Pain 1988;33:11–23.
[55] Fields H. Can opiates relieve neuropathic pain? Pain 1988;35:365.
[56] Watson CPN, Babul N. Efficacy of oxycodone in neuropathic pain. Neurology 1998;50: 1837–41.
[57] Raja SN, Haythornewaite JA, Pappagallo M, et al. Opioids versus antidepressants in postherpetic neuralgia: A randomized placebo-controlled trial. Neurology 2002;59:1015–21.
[58] Harati Y, Gooch C, Swenson M, et al. Double-blind randomized trial of tramadol for the treatment of the pain of diabetic neuropathy. Neurology 1998;50:1842–6.
[59] Gimbel JS, Richards P, Portenoy RK. Continuous release oxycodone for pain in diabetic neuropathy: a randomized control trial. Neurology 2003;60(6):927–34.
[60] Watson CP, Moulin D, Watt-Watson J, et al. Controlled-release oxycodone relieves neuropathic pain: a randomized controlled trial in painful diabetic neuropathy. Pain 2003; 105(1–2):71–8.
[61] Dellemijn PLI, VanDuijn H, Vanneste JAL. Prolonged treatment with transdermal fentanyl in neuropathic pain. J Pain Symptom Manage 1998;16:220–9.
[62] Attal N, Guirimand F, Brasseur L, et al. Effects of IV morphine in central pain. Neurology 2002;58:554–63.
[63] Gilron I, Bailey JM, Tu D, et al. Morphine, gabapentin or their combination for neuropathic pain. N Engl J Med 2005;352(13):1324–34.

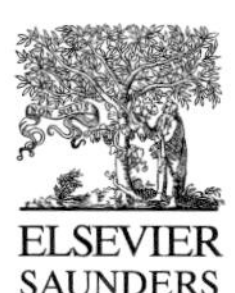

ELSEVIER
SAUNDERS

Phys Med Rehabil Clin N Am
17 (2006) 381–400

PHYSICAL MEDICINE
AND REHABILITATION
CLINICS OF
NORTH AMERICA

Antidepressant and Anticonvulsant Medication for Chronic Pain

Mark D. Sullivan, MD, PhD[a,*], James P. Robinson, MD, PhD[b]

[a]*Department of Psychiatry, University of Washington, 1959 Pacific Street, Box 356560, Seattle, WA 98195, USA*
[b]*Department of Rehabilitation Medicine, University of Washington, 1959 Pacific Street, Box 356044, Seattle, WA 98195, USA*

The evolution of contemporary clinical pain care dates back to the publication of Melzack and Wall's gate control theory in the journal *Science* in 1965 [1]. Around that time, most of the attention was given to the "gate" in this theory of pain, which referred to inhibitory interneurons within the substantia gelatinosa of the dorsal horn of the spinal cord. The gate closed when stimulation of large diameter fibers by touch or vibration activated these inhibitory interneurons, decreasing central neurotransmission from small diameter C fibers. At that time, little attention was paid to the role of descending control from the brain. Melzack and Wall did note this in their model, but little was known about descending pain modulation in 1965. Most of the pain research in the 40 years since that time has focused on the central control component of the gate control theory. Because central control is so important, antidepressants and anticonvulsants have a prominent role in the treatment of chronic pain problems.

Persons attending medical school in the 1970s and 1980s were still being taught that the neuroanatomy of pain essentially consisted of two ascending systems: the neospinothalamic and paleospinothalamic systems. It is now clear that this is only half of pain neuroanatomy. Equally important are the descending systems traveling from the central nervous system (CNS) to the periphery that continually modulate transmission in the ascending systems. The descending systems have opioid and nonopioid components. Activity in the opioid system can be blocked through use of the opioid

* Corresponding author.
E-mail address: sullimar@u.washington.edu (M.D. Sullivan).

1047-9651/06/$ - see front matter
doi:10.1016/j.pmr.2005.12.006 ***pmr.theclinics.com***

antagonist naloxone. The nonopioid component of the system uses many different neurotransmitters. Two of the important neurotransmitters active within the system are serotonin and norepinephrine. These substances are the same neurotransmitters altered by commonly used antidepressants. Norepinephrine-containing cell bodies are found in the dorsolateral pontine tegmentum. Serotonin-containing cell bodies are generally contained in the rostroventral medulla [2]. Currently, antidepressant medication is the primary means of augmenting transmission in these systems.

The old thinking about pain bequeathed to us from Descartes taught that pain was primarily a function of peripheral tissue damage. Many studies have documented that clinical pain is only loosely related to the amount of tissue damage in the periphery. The severity of clinical pain is best understood as a function of the overall threat to the organism rather than the amount of tissue damage in the part that hurts. The organism is continually adjusting the sensitivity of its pain system given its overall life situation. In situations of great threat to survival, such as those explored by stress-induced analgesia experiments, the pain system is adjusted to low sensitivity. In other situations of less life-threatening distress, the sensitivity of the system can be adjusted upward [3].

Reasons for using antidepressants

There are three basic reasons for considering antidepressant medications for patients with chronic pain. First, psychiatric disorders are common in patients with severe or disabling chronic pain. Second, sleep disturbance is common, even in patients who do not meet criteria for psychiatric disorders. Third, there is evidence that certain classes of antidepressants produce pain relief separate from relief of depression or other psychiatric disorders.

Psychiatric disorders

The DSM-IV defines major depression as 2 weeks or more of depressed mood or loss of pleasure. Patients with chronic pain may deny depressed mood and may attribute their lack of pleasure to the pain itself; however, according to the DSM-IV decision rules, these patients still qualify as meeting the symptoms of anhedonia. In addition to these core symptoms, it is required that a patient have four of the following symptoms to quality for the diagnosis of major depression: weight loss or gain, insomnia or hypersomnia, psychomotor agitation or retardation, fatigue or loss of energy, worthlessness or guilt, trouble concentrating or deciding, or thoughts of death or suicide. Two percent to 4% of the US general population meet the criteria for major depression at any time. Among ambulatory medical patients, this prevalence is doubled to 5% to 9% of patients. Among medical inpatients, the rate is doubled again to 15% to 20% who meet the criteria for major depression at any point in time. It has been difficult to obtain stable prevalence estimates of major depression from pain clinic populations, largely because these are such select groups. Prevalence rates have varied from 10% to 100%, with most estimates being greater than 50%. Certainly, major depression is common in patients with chronic pain and is often underdiagnosed owing to the stigma associated with psychiatric disorders and an often adversarial medical/legal environment focused on responsibility for the initial injury.

One of the most frequently asked questions by clinicians about depression and chronic pain is whether the depression causes the pain or the pain causes the depression. The appropriate answer to this question is yes. There are now 13 studies of the prevalence of pain complaints in depressed patients. The range of reported rates is between 15% and 100%, with a mean of 65% of depressed patients complaining of pain. Most of these studies were done in psychiatric settings, but similar rates have been evident in primary care studies. There have also been 41 studies of the prevalence of depression in patients with chronic pain. Rates reported include 38% in pain clinics, 35% in psychiatry clinics, 52% in rheumatology clinics, 78% in dental clinics, 23% in obstetric-gynecology clinics, and 27% in primary care clinics [4].

These studies demonstrate that depression and pain strongly reinforce each other. Multiple studies have shown that patients with pain have a depression risk two to five times that of the general population [5]. This risk is especially true for patients who have multiple pain complaints, multiple episodes of chronic pain, or especially severe pain. Patients with pain and depression have more pain complaints, more pain intensity, and more pain chronicity than those without depression [6].

Another psychiatric disorder with high prevalence in selected chronic pain populations is panic disorder. Panic disorder is defined as recurrent unexpected panic attacks in which at least one of the attacks has been followed by a month or more of persistent concern about additional attacks or worry about the implications of the attack or a significant change in behavior related to the attacks. Panic attacks themselves are defined as discrete periods of intense fear or discomfort in which four or more symptoms develop abruptly and reach a peak within 10 minutes. These symptoms include palpitations, sweating, trembling, shortness of breath, choking, chest pain, nausea, dizziness, derealization, paresthesias, and hot flashes, as well as fears of losing control, going crazy, or dying. In the general US population, 1% to 2% of adults meet the criteria for panic disorder at any given time. If patients presenting to an emergency room with chest pain are assessed for panic disorder, 16% to 25% will meet these criteria. If one goes a bit "further down the career" of a potential cardiac patient to patients who have had coronary angiography and are found to have normal coronary vessels, nearly half of these patients have panic disorder. Similarly, 28% of patients with irritable bowel syndrome have been found to have panic disorder, and 13% to 15% of patients with chronic headaches, particularly migraine headaches, have panic disorder [7].

A significantly underexplored problem among patients with chronic pain is posttraumatic stress disorder (PTSD). The prevalence of DSM-IV PTSD in the US general population is estimated to be approximately 8%, with 6% of men and 12% of women meeting the criteria. If one examines particular subsets of patients with chronic pain, high rates of PTSD are evident [8]. Motor vehicle accident patients who have persistent pain show a 30% to 50% rate of PTSD [9]. Injured workers referred for rehabilitative treatment have a 35% rate of PTSD [10]. Fibromyalgia patients have been reported to have a 20% current rate of PTSD and a 42% lifetime rate of PTSD [11].

As is true for pain and depression, many possible relationships are possible between chronic pain and PTSD. PTSD can give rise to pain as suggested by the high rates of chronic pain in patients with a history of severe childhood maltreatment. The physical trauma that gave rise to the pain complaint also can give rise to PTSD. Some evidence suggests that dissociation during the injury increases the risk of subsequent PTSD. The pain from the injury itself can produce PTSD, especially if the pain induces dissociation.

Although it may seem implausible that traumatic events such as childhood abuse could produce chronic pain problems many years after the abuse has ceased, data from animals and humans provide plausible mechanisms for this. Heim and coworkers [12] reported on 49 women aged 18 to 45 years separated into four groups: (1) one group with no childhood abuse or psychiatric disorder, (2) one group with current major depression and childhood abuse, (3) one group with no depression but having suffered abuse, and (4) one group with current major depression and no childhood abuse. They were able to show that the abused women showed a greater corticotropin (ACTH) response to a standardized speaking stress. The abused women who also had current major depression showed a six times greater rise in ACTH than those without depression or childhood abuse. This observation is consistent with animal research among rodents and primates suggesting that there are critical periods during development when the sensitivity of the hypothalamic pituitary adrenal axis is set. Young animals deprived of certain nurturing or subjected to particular stress during these critical periods have been demonstrated to show increased stress hormones in response to other stressors throughout their lives.

Antidepressant medication has been shown to treat these psychiatric disorders effectively. Cognitive-behavioral therapy also has been shown to work. These disorders are often missed or dismissed by clinicians who conceptualize the disorders as secondary to the injury or chronic pain problems. It is more appropriate to think of the disorders as comorbid illnesses that can benefit from treatment. There is clear evidence that treatment of concurrent psychiatric disorders improves the outcomes for patients with chronic pain [13].

Sleep disturbance

The second reason to use antidepressant medications in patients with chronic pain concerns the treatment of sleep disturbance. Fifty percent to

80% of patients with chronic pain have significant sleep disturbances [14]. Experimental disruption of slow-wave sleep has been shown to increase pain sensitivity in most studies. Clinical studies show a reciprocal relationship between sleep disturbance and pain. It is well known from depression treatment studies that persistence of insomnia strongly predicts persistence or relapse of depression.

Chronic pain patients are often prescribed benzodiazepines to address their sleep disturbance [15]; however, chronic benzodiazepine therapy does not correct the disturbed sleep architecture typical of many patients with chronic pain but may, in fact, further decrease slow-wave sleep. It is unclear whether the new "Z-drug" sleep agents, which are partial benzodiazepine receptor agonists, are any better. The most popular among these agents, zolpidem (Ambien) and the new eszopiclone (Lunesta), do seem to have some advantages when compared with the traditional benzodiazepines in terms of rebound after discontinuation and cognitive impairment, but it is not clear whether they affect sleep architecture more favorably [16].

Antidepressants almost all suppress rapid eye movement (REM) sleep, whereas they have variable effects on sleep continuity and slow-wave sleep. In general, the tricyclic antidepressants have a more predictably positive effect on sleep continuity and slow-wave sleep than do the popular selective serotonin reuptake inhibitors (SSRIs). This factor may be one important reason why the tricyclics have shown better effects in some chronic pain conditions. In some illnesses such as fibromyalgia, controlled trials suggest that the optimum treatment is the combination of a tricyclic with an SSRI [17]. The authors' interpretation of these data is that fibromyalgia patients frequently require full-dose antidepressant treatment, which is difficult to achieve with the tricyclic antidepressants owing to side-effect problems. Addition of an SSRI allows full antidepressant dosing, and the tricyclic portion of the regimen addresses problems with sleep continuity and slow-wave sleep. This theory has not been specifically tested.

Pain

The third principal reason to prescribe antidepressants to patients with chronic pain is that there is evidence of antidepressant analgesia independent of their effects on depression. Antidepressant analgesia has been well investigated over the past two decades. A 1992 review article documented that antidepressant analgesia could be found in over half of previous studies, although, on average, the pain relief was only 50% [18]. At that time, it appeared that the most responsive pain syndromes were neuropathic pain syndromes such as diabetes and postherpetic neuralgia. The next most responsive were headache, facial, and central pain syndromes. These findings have been largely confirmed in subsequent studies. Whether depression was present or an antidepressant effect noted appeared to make no difference in analgesia. The meta-analysis was unable to confirm the then popular presumption that serotonin was more important than norepinephrine. Instead, the investigators concluded that mixed agents affecting serotonin and norepinephrine were best.

The evidence suggesting that the tricyclics were better than the SSRIs for neuropathic pain began with the report by Max and coworkers [19] in 1992. His team at the National Institutes of Health performed two simultaneous crossover randomized controlled trials, with 38 subjects receiving amitriptyline or desipramine and 46 subjects receiving fluoxetine or placebo. Moderate or greater improvement in pain was noted by 74% of the amitriptyline group and 61% of the desipramine group. These differences were statistically equivalent. Moderate or greater improvement in pain was noted in 48% of the fluoxetine group and was not statistically significantly different from the 41% in the placebo group. Interestingly, it did not appear to make a difference in the response to tricyclics whether the patients were depressed; however, the SSRIs appeared to produce analgesia only if the patients were clinically depressed.

Subsequently, other mixed action antidepressants have been shown to be effective for neuropathic pain. Bupropion (Wellbutrin) has been shown in a trial of 41 patients with neuropathic pain to be superior to placebo over a period of 6 weeks [20]. Venlafaxine (Effexor) has also been shown to be superior to placebo for neuropathic pain. Rowbotham and coworkers [21] studied 244 patients with diabetic neuropathic pain and showed that the relief in the group receiving venlafaxine, 150 mg over a period of 6 weeks, was superior to that in the placebo group. An earlier study by Sindrup and coworkers [22] of 40 patients in a placebo-controlled crossover trial showed that venlafaxine, 225 mg, and imipramine, 150 mg, were superior to placebo for neuropathic pain [22].

Duloxetine (Cymbalta) is an antidepressant that has been approved by the Food and Drug Administration (FDA) for the treatment of diabetic neuropathic pain. Goldstein and coworkers [23] reported on a randomized trial of 457 patients treated for 12 weeks with 20, 60, or 120 mg a day of duloxetine. The 60 mg and 120 mg a day doses demonstrated greater improvement than placebo in the 24-hour average pain score beginning 1 week after randomization. Duloxetine has a similar pharmacology to venlafaxine in that it is a reuptake inhibitor for serotonin and norepinephrine. It differs from venlafaxine in that it is a norepinephrine reuptake inhibitor at lower doses. The clinical significance of this difference has yet to be demonstrated.

Mirtazapine is another atypical antidepressant with some norepinephrine reuptake action. It has been shown to be effective for chronic headache. Bendtsen and Jensen [24] showed that mirtazapine, 15 to 30 mg for 8 weeks, was superior to placebo for prophylaxis of chronic tension headache. An open label study by Samborski and coworkers [25] suggests its effectiveness in fibromyalgia. Mirtazapine is effective in improving sleep continuity. The same antihistaminic action that promotes sleep with mirtazapine unfortunately promotes weight gain, prompting many patients to discontinue mirtazapine.

St. John's wort, a popular naturopathic remedy that has been shown to treat depression successfully in European studies, was tested by Sindrup and coworkers [26] in a population with neuropathic pain, but it did not produce greater analgesia than placebo.

Multiple meta-analyses of antidepressant analgesia have been reported over the past few years. Tomkins and coworkers [27] analyzed 38 trials of antidepressants for chronic headache. The relative risk of improvement was 2.0 on antidepressants when compared with placebo, with 31% more antidepressant-treated patients improving. The number needed to treat (NNT) was 3.2, and the effect size was large on average. There did not seem to be a difference in response rates by drug class or headache type. Depression was not well monitored in these trials. In general, chronic headache is one disorder in which the SSRI medications seem to function just as well as the tricyclic or mixed reuptake inhibitor medications. There is a good database demonstrating efficacy for SSRIs in prophylaxis in patients who have chronic tension and recurrent migraine headaches. Holroyd and coworkers [28] reported that stress management added significantly to an antidepressant regimen for chronic tension headache. Rates of achieving at least a 50% reduction in the headache index were 64% for a combination of stress management and amitriptyline or nortriptyline versus 38% for tricyclics alone and 34% for stress management alone. The response rate was 29% for placebo alone.

O'Malley and coworkers [29] performed a meta-analysis of trials testing antidepressant treatment for fibromyalgia in 2000. They reviewed 13 adequate randomized trials and found that there was evidence for antidepressant treatment of fibromyalgia with an odds ratio for improvement of 4.2; the NNT was 4. They were able to show that antidepressants improved sleep, fatigue, pain, and well-being but not trigger points. Only one of these trials showed a significant correlation of analgesia with improvement in depression. There have been subsequent trials of antidepressants in fibromyalgia [30], including a recent trial with duloxetine demonstrating a superior efficacy to placebo [31]; however, it is important to remember that patients with fibromyalgia are heterogeneous psychiatrically. Some are relatively easy to treat and some are extremely difficult to treat, being resistant to psychopharmacologic regimens or intolerant of them. In general, the author (MDS) has found that fibromyalgia patients will improve if they can sleep and exercise.

Although the research literature concerning antidepressants and low back pain is large, many trials are poor in design. Two trials that are an exception to this rule were performed by Atkinson and coworkers. The first was a nortriptyline versus placebo trial reported in 1998 [32]. The second was a trial of maprotiline or paroxetine versus diphenhydramine reported in 1999 [33]. The 1998 trial was able to demonstrate clearly that among older males with chronic low back pain nortriptyline produced greater pain relief than placebo. This difference was not related to pretreatment depression severity or depression response with treatment.

They followed this trial with a second trial to explore mechanisms. Maprotiline, an older tricyclic drug that was the most potent norepinephrine reuptake inhibitor at the time, was compared with paroxetine, a relatively pure serotonin reuptake inhibitor. These agents were compared with an active placebo (diphenhydramine), which is an antihistamine that produces a dry mouth and some sedation. An 8-week trial was performed randomizing 103 subjects. Seventy-nine of the patients completed the trial. Each subject had to have 6 months of back pain, and no one with a diagnosable mood disorder was entered into the trial. Pain relief by the highly sensitive descriptor differential scale was 45% in the group that received maprotiline (up to 150 mg), 27% for those receiving placebo (up to 37.5 mg of diphenhydramine), and 26% for those receiving paroxetine (up to 30 mg). Pain intensity diminished more markedly than pain unpleasantness. Although this group had prolonged pain (median pain duration of 10 years), it was not a failed back syndrome group, because only 12% had had previous back surgery. This finding was not simply a replication of neuropathic pain studies, because only 14% had radicular pain. There was no change in self-reported or observer-rated depression in the active treatment groups. In addition, there was no significant correlation between the change in mood symptoms and the change in pain intensity. On the basis of the Atkinson trials, the author believes that the noradrenergic antidepressants may be preferable not just for neuropathic pain syndromes but also for common musculoskeletal pain syndromes such as neck and back pain.

Not all pain syndromes show increased responsiveness to noradrenergic antidepressants. Headaches, particularly chronic daily headache, respond to SSRI antidepressants as well as tricyclic and serotonin norepinephrine reuptake inhibitor (SNRI) medications. Nonischemic chest pain may be another area in which SSRIs do well. Cannon and coworkers [34] originally reported in 1994 that imipramine, 50 mg, was able to produce a 52% reduction in chest pain episodes in a noncoronary chest pain group compared with a 39% reduction in a group treated with 0.1 mg twice daily of clonidine and a 1% reduction in a placebo group. Varia and coworkers [35] reported in 2000 on a cohort of 30 patients treated for 8 weeks with sertraline, 50 to 200 mg/day, or placebo. Sixty-six percent of the sertraline-treated group met a criterion of greater than 50% pain relief versus 8% of the placebo group [35]. Somewhat oddly, they were unable to show an effect of sertraline treatment on quality of life or depression measures. These trials await replication.

Psychiatric disorders are common in patients with chronic pain, especially if the pain is associated with significant activity impairment. Antidepressants with norepinephrine reuptake are probably the psychotropic agents of choice for pain relief. These agents include nortriptyline, bupropion, venlafaxine, mirtazapine, and duloxetine. SSRI and SNRI antidepressants alone do not generally improve sleep continuity. This factor may be crucial in syndromes such as fibromyalgia and may mandate a combination of antidepressants with sedating agents such as the tricyclics trazodone or mirtazapine.

Anticonvulsants

Pain specialists typically discuss anticonvulsants primarily in relation to neuropathic pain, and the clearest evidence for their efficacy comes from studies of patients with this type of pain. As a first approximation, one could say that anticonvulsants should be used with enthusiasm in patients with neuropathic pain and with caution in patients with other types of pain; unfortunately, this simple rule is beguiling because the boundaries around neuropathic pain are far from clear.

Neuropathic pain

Neuropathic pain has been defined as "pain initiated or caused by a primary lesion, dysfunction, or transitory perturbation in the peripheral or central nervous system" [36]. Some experts have argued that the term should be limited to pain caused by abnormalities in the peripheral nervous system, or at least that neuropathic pain of peripheral origin should be distinguished from neuropathic pain of central origin [37].

A wide range of disorders of the peripheral nervous system can cause persistent pain, including peripheral polyneuropathies, entrapment neuropathies, radiculopathies, and traumatic injuries to nerves. Pain can also be associated with damage to the CNS. Examples include central poststroke pain and pain in spinal cord injury. The characteristic pain syndromes that occur in the context of these CNS lesions are sometimes called central pain syndromes. Some research supports the efficacy of treating central pain syndromes with anticonvulsants [38], although it is not as extensive or consistent as support for their use in painful disorders of the peripheral nervous system.

A much more difficult question is whether chronic pain syndromes associated with CNS hypersensitivity or dysfunction should be construed as neuropathic pain syndromes. To a large extent, the answer hinges on the interpretation given to the word "dysfunction" in the International Association of Pain definition of neuropathic pain [36]. As discussed in that text, nociception can lead to changes in the function of the CNS in the absence of any clear evidence of damage to the CNS. If pain associated with such functional changes is construed as neuropathic pain, the range of conditions falling under the rubric of neuropathic pain increases enormously. For example, complex regional pain syndrome [39,40] and fibromyalgia [41–43] have been construed by some as neuropathic pain disorders.

The issue of a narrow versus a broad conceptualization of neuropathic pain has been summarized by Rowbotham as follows [43], "An examination of how the term neuropathic pain is defined reveals a conceptual split into 2 partially overlapping groups of disorders: those with demonstrable pathology in the nervous system and those characterized primarily by enduring dysfunction of the nervous system. Requiring demonstrable pathology in the nervous system in the definition of neuropathic pain is the traditional approach. The expansion of the definition to require only enduring nervous system dysfunction is less palatable because it opens the classification to many disorders of uncertain etiology."

If fibromyalgia is construed as a neuropathic pain syndrome, only a short conceptual leap is needed to infer the presence of neuropathic pain in any chronic pain patient who demonstrates evidence of CNS hypersensitivity. It is beyond the scope of this article to discuss procedures for identifying CNS hypersensitivity in clinical populations, but one indicator of such hypersensitivity is widespread hyperalgesia in response to palpation over muscles. If this criterion is accepted, CNS hypersensitivity would probably be found to be the rule rather than the exception in chronic pain syndromes. For example, essentially all patients with myofascial pain would be construed as having CNS hypersensitivity [44].

Anticonvulsants in the treatment of neuropathic pain: research findings

Anticonvulsants are thought to inhibit seizures by multiple mechanisms, including functional blockade of voltage-gated sodium channels, functional blockade of voltage-gated calcium channels, direct or indirect enhancement of inhibitory GABAergic neurotransmission, and inhibition of glutamatergic neurotransmission [45,46]. The result is that they reduce the neuronal hyperexcitability that is fundamental to seizure disorders.

Because neuropathic pain is also characterized by neuronal hyperexcitability [47], clinicians and researchers have reasoned that anticonvulsants might alleviate it. This supposition is supported by a substantial amount of empirical data on the effectiveness of anticonvulsants in neuropathic pain. The multiple studies in this area have been the subject of recent systematic reviews and have been considered by expert panels devoted to developing guidelines for treating neuropathic pain. The discussion herein relies largely on guidelines developed by Dworkin and coworkers [48], three recent Cochrane systematic reviews [49–51], and a systematic review by Goodman and coworkers [52].

Goodman and coworkers searched for studies relevant to several anticonvulsants—phenytoin, valproic acid, carbamazepine, gabapentin, lamotrigine, oxcarbazepine, zonisamide, levetiracetam, tiagabine, and topiramate. The studies they included in their review dealt with the first five. As is typical of systematic reviews on therapies for chronic pain, Goodman and colleagues described significant methodologic flaws in the research on anticonvulsants in neuropathic pain and ended up with cautious conclusions. In combination with the guidelines developed by Dworkin and coworkers [48], the review permits the following conclusions to be reached with reasonable confidence:

- The effectiveness of anticonvulsants in the treatment of neuropathic pain has been studied extensively. For example, the review by Goodman and coworkers considered 37 studies.
- The preponderance of evidence supports the conclusion that, as a group, anticonvulsants are effective in the amelioration of neuropathic pain in comparison with placebos.
- This conclusion must be tempered by the fact that studies on anticonvulsants have been concentrated heavily on a few neuropathic pain conditions, especially diabetic neuropathy, postherpetic neuralgia, and trigeminal neuralgia. It is possible that some neuropathic pain conditions are responsive to anticonvulsants, whereas others are not. A related issue is that some observers have proposed that, for the purposes of treatment, neuropathic pain syndromes need to be classified according to the specific symptoms that patients experience (eg, spontaneous burning pain versus allodynia versus lancinating pain) or the pathophysiologic mechanisms underlying the neuropathic pain [37]. The general point is that research to date has not been broad enough to determine how robust anticonvulsants are in treating the broad scope of symptoms, pathophysiologic processes, and diagnostic entities that are subsumed under the broad definition of "neuropathic pain."
- There have been virtually no head-to-head comparisons between different anticonvulsants [52]. One indirect method for comparing the effectiveness of different drugs is to compare the NNT for them; however, comparisons with respect to NNTs must be interpreted cautiously (Table 1). The summary NNT data suggest that carbamazepine is more effective overall than gabapentin in the treatment of neuropathic pain, but the determination of NNT for carbamazepine was based primarily on studies of trigeminal neuralgia, whereas the NNT for gabapentin was based primarily on studies of diabetic neuropathy and postherpetic neuralgia. Given this difference, it may be meaningless to compare summary NNTs for the two drugs. Another problem is that data from some studies do not permit a reviewer to calculate the NNT. Summary NNTs are based on only a portion of the studies that have been done with a drug.
- Owing to the previously cited methodologic issues and several others, research to date does not permit any conclusive statements to be made about the relative efficacy of different anticonvulsants in the treatment of neuropathic pain. A few anticonvulsants (eg, carbamazepine, gabapentin, and lamotrigine) have been studied in several randomized controlled trials on neuropathic pain, whereas little or no systematic research has been done on the effectiveness of some of the newer anticonvulsants (eg, zonisamide, levetiracetam, tiagabine).

Table 1
NNT for CZP, gabapentin, and antidepressants in neuropathic pain: calculated from systemic reviews

	CZP	Gabapentin	Antidepressants
Trigeminal neuralgia	NNT = 1.9[a]	—	—
Postherpetic neuralgia	1 study – CZP group did better	NNT = 3.9[b]	NNT = 2.2[c]
Diabetic neuropathy	1 study – CZP group did better	NNT = 2.9[d]	NNT = 1.3[e]
Average for all neuropathic pain	NNT = 2.5[f]	NNT = 4.3[g]	NNT = 2.0[h]

The NNT is calculated by first dichotomizing subjects in a placebo controlled clinical trial into those who achieved a certain degree of pain relief (eg, moderate relief or more) and those who did not. The percentage of subjects who achieve moderate or better pain relief is calculated for those who received the drug under study and for those in the placebo control group. The difference between these two percentages is then determined, and this number is divided into 100 to determine the NNT for the drug. For example, if a study found that 60% of subjects receiving gabapentin achieved at least moderate pain relief versus 20% of subjects in the placebo control group, the NNT for gabapentin would be 100/40 = 2.5.

Abbreviations: CZP, carbamazepine; NNT, number needed to treat.

[a] Based on 2 studies, with total N = 47 [47].
[b] Based on 2 studies, with total N = 207. Dose ranged from 2400 to 3600 mg/d [48].
[c] Based on 4 studies, with total N = 77 [54].
[d] Based on 4 studies, with total N = 142. Dose ranged from 900 to 3600 mg/d [48].
[e] Based on 5 studies, with total N = 98 [54].
[f] Based on 4 studies, with total N = 91 [47].
[g] Based on 7 studies, with total N = 466 [48].
[h] For amitriptyline only; based on 7 studies, with total N = 112. Doses up to 150 mg/d [54].

- Assessing the relative effectiveness of different anticonvulsants is complicated by the fact that some of the newer ones have been investigated so recently that the relevant studies have not been considered in systematic reviews of anticonvulsants. For example, neither of the two most comprehensive reviews [51,52] considers several recent studies on topiramate [53–55].

Clinical use of anticonvulsants in neuropathic pain

A clinician who plans to use anticonvulsants in the treatment of neuropathic pain conditions will be heartened by evidence that as a class they are effective; however, he or she will immediately be confronted with a host of more specific questions that are not answered conclusively by research. This section discusses strategies for using anticonvulsants that are based on clinical experience rather than on research.

Diagnosis

The first step in using anticonvulsants to treat neuropathic pain is to establish that a patient has neuropathic pain. This step requires the identification of a disorder in the nervous system and reasonable clinical evidence that the patient's pain is a produced by the disorder. The latter determination is based on information about the distribution of symptoms, the quality of pain, and the settings under which the patient experiences pain [48].

With regard to distribution, neuropathic pain is suggested when the patient reports symptoms in a pattern that is consistent with the suspected neuropathy. The precise distribution, of course, depends on the neuropathy, for example, an L5 dermatome for an individual with an L5 radiculopathy and symptoms primarily in the feet in a patient with a diabetic neuropathy. With regard to quality, a combination of numbness and pain is suggestive of neuropathic pain. Also, the pain is frequently described as burning or lancinating. With respect to settings in which pain occurs, neuropathic pain is often distinctive in that it is worse when a patient is inactive. A patient with a diabetic neuropathy will often experience more symptoms when trying to sleep at night than when walking during the day. Another distinctive feature is that a patient with neuropathic pain will often describe discomfort from the light pressure of clothing on the body area that is symptomatic.

Anticonvulsants versus antidepressants

Antidepressants and anticonvulsants have demonstrable efficacy in the treatment of neuropathic pain [51,56], and both classes of medication have been recommended as first-line therapy for neuropathic pain [57].

Indirect comparisons based on NNTs suggest that antidepressants (especially amitriptyline) are more effective than anticonvulsants; however, this conclusion is challenged by three head-to-head comparisons between anticonvulsants and amitriptyline [58–60]. These studies failed to demonstrate any difference in effectiveness; therefore, the currently available research data do not provide a clear basis for choosing between an antidepressant and an anticonvulsant for initial therapy of neuropathic pain. The authors recommend that if a patient demonstrates significant depression, anxiety, or sleep disturbance, initial therapy should be with an antidepressant that affects the reuptake of norepinephrine and serotonin (eg, nortriptyline, duloxetine, or venlafaxine) at a dose that is effective for treating depression. In patients without significant emotional distress, anticonvulsants and antidepressants are equally appropriate as choices for initial therapy.

One recent consensus article [48] identified not only anticonvulsants (specifically gabapentin) and tricyclic antidepressants as first-line pharmacologic therapies for neuropathic pain but also three other agents: opiates, tramadol, and a 5% lidocaine patch (specifically for postherpetic neuralgia). No research permits a clinician to choose where to start in this list.

Which anticonvulsant

In the absence of head-to-head comparisons between different anticonvulsants, it is reasonable to start with the ones that have been studied the most—gabapentin and carbamazepine. In particular, gabapentin is attractive because it does not interact significantly with other drugs, and because its characteristic adverse effects are reversible with termination of the drug.

The authors recommend it for initial anticonvulsant therapy in most neuropathic pain. One exception to this general principle might be trigeminal neuralgia or any neuropathic pain condition in which lancinating pain dominates. The presence of significant lancinating pain should make one strongly consider carbamazepine. One might consider an anticonvulsant other than Gabapentin in a patient with cognitive impairment. In that setting, the authors have found lamotrigine to be a good choice, because it seems to cause less cognitive impairment than gabapentin.

Options for the patient who fails initial therapy with an anticonvulsant

If a patient fails to benefit from a maximally tolerated dose of gabapentin, one option would be to switch to another anticonvulsant. Although there are no scientific data to guide the clinician in choosing an alternative anticonvulsant, it seems logical to choose one (eg, carbamazepine or lamotrigine) that influences Na+ ion channels, because gabapentin is thought to stabilize neurons primarily by its effects on Ca++ ion channels or enhancement of GABAergic neurotransmission [45,61]. It would also be reasonable to consider valproate [62] or one of the less studied second-generation anticonvulsants, such as oxcarbazepine [63,64], topiramate [53–55], zonisamide [65], or levetiracetam [66]. Another possibility is pregabalin, which was released during the latter part of 2005. It has the disadvantage of being new but the advantage of having FDA approval for use in postherpetic neuralgia and painful diabetic neuropathy [67–71]. Although the effectiveness of phenytoin for neuropathic pain has been studied, the results have been equivocal [72,73], and the authors do not recommend its use [74].

An alternative strategy in the patient with a failed trial on gabapentin would be to switch an antidepressant, or to prescribe an opiate, tramadol, or a 5% lidocaine patch.

Combination therapy

Although monotherapy for neuropathic pain has been reported to produce significant benefit for approximately 70% of patients [57], the responses are often partial [48]. As a practical matter, one will commonly encounter patients who continue to complain of significant pain despite trials on anticonvulsants, antidepressants, and other first-line agents. In this setting, combination therapy is a reasonable strategy.

Unfortunately, combination therapy involving anticonvulsants has received only minimal attention in research. Simpson [75] found that among diabetic neuropathy patients who failed to respond to gabapentin, patients who subsequently received a combination of gabapentin and venlafaxine reported more pain relief than did controls who received gabapentin and a placebo. Gilron and coworkers [76] recently studied the effects of morphine, gabapentin, and a combination of morphine plus gabapentin in a crossover trial of patients with diabetic neuropathy and postherpetic neuralgia. Although both morphine and gabapentin led to pain reduction, the combination of the two agents was the most effective regimen. These studies suggest that combination therapy involving anticonvulsants may be effective, but more research is needed to determine what combinations are optimal.

The most logical drugs to combine would be an antidepressant and an anticonvulsant, because these two classes of drugs are thought to affect neuropathic pain by different mechanisms. The authors frequently see neuropathic pain patients who are receiving this type of combination therapy from their primary care providers. Typically, the anticonvulsant is prescribed for pain control, and the antidepressant is prescribed because of the patient's emotional dysfunction.

Anticonvulsants in other painful conditions

A considerable amount of research has been done on the efficacy of anticonvulsants in central pain syndromes, especially poststroke pain and pain in spinal cord injury [38]. Although the evidence for efficacy of anticonvulsants in these disorders is less impressive than it is in neuropathic pain from disorders of the peripheral nervous system, it is reasonable to give patients with any central pain syndrome a trial of anticonvulsants.

The role of anticonvulsants in migraine headache has been studied extensively, and the results are generally favorable, especially for valproate [63].

As discussed previously, some experts have proposed that fibromyalgia is a neuropathic pain syndrome. Regardless of the utility of this hypothesis, it is clear that fibromyalgia involves CNS hypersensitivity [42]. To the extent that this hypersensitivity is a reflection of hyperresponsiveness of neurons in nociceptive pathways, the use of anticonvulsants in patients with fibromyalgia could be rationalized in the same way that it is rationalized for the treatment of pain that is unequivocally neuropathic. Moreover, as discussed by Curatolo and colleagues elsewhere in this issue, CNS hypersensitivity is by no means restricted to fibromyalgia; in fact, it probably occurs in most chronic pain disorders. There is a conceptual rationale for considering anticonvulsants in the treatment of many patients with chronic pain.

Obviously, such an expansive use of anticonvulsants needs empirical support rather than just theoretical plausibility. Some data support the efficacy of anticonvulsants in musculoskeletal pain syndromes with CNS hypersensitivity. In particular, pregabalin, a new anticonvulsant, has been shown to reduce pain in fibromyalgia in a dose-dependent manner [77].

In contrast, studies of anticonvulsants in musculoskeletal conditions such as chronic low back pain have yielded inconsistent results [78,79]. These studies are difficult to evaluate in relation to the hypothesis that anticonvulsants are effective for disorders characterized by CNS hypersensitivity, because participants in the studies were not systematically assessed for the presence of indicators of CNS hypersensitivity. In an ideal study, patients with a common musculoskeletal condition such as axial low back pain would be divided into groups who did and did not show clinical evidence of CNS hypersensitivity, and both groups would be treated with an anticonvulsant. The expectation would be that only the patients demonstrating CNS hypersensitivity would benefit from the anticonvulsant therapy.

Clinicians in the authors' community frequently prescribe anticonvulsants (especially gabapentin) for patients with refractory musculoskeletal pain. In the absence of definitive research data, the authors' clinical experience suggests that a trial on an anticonvulsant is worth performing for a patient with chronic musculoskeletal pain and evidence of evidence of CNS hypersensitivity; however, these patients are often refractory to essentially all therapies, including anticonvulsants. If an anticonvulsant is prescribed, it is incumbent on the physician to monitor the patient's response carefully, and to discontinue the drug if it does not produce clear clinical improvement.

Prototypical cases

Case 1

The clinical information available on the patient in Case 1 in the introductory article suggests that his right lower extremity pain reflects a central pain syndrome. Although central pain syndromes represent a heterogeneous group of disorders with respect to the underlying CNS dysfunction, there is evidence that at least some of them respond to tricyclic antidepressants [80,81], lamotrigine [82], and possibly gabapentin [83]. It should be assumed that a patient with a history of prolonged coma from a traumatic brain injury would be sensitive to cognitive adverse effects from any centrally acting drug. This consideration implies that tricyclic antidepressants and gabapentin should be used with caution. Among the anticonvulsants, lamotrigine would probably be the best choice for this patient.

Case 2

Anticonvulsants and several antidepressants, including tricyclics, SSRIs, and dual reuptake inhibitors, have been shown to be effective in reducing pain associated with diabetic neuropathy; therefore, the patient in Case 2 provides the clinician with a plethora of pharmacologic options involving antidepressants or anticonvulsants. There is no obvious starting point for trials on these drugs, except that tricyclic antidepressants should be used with caution in an older individual with cardiovascular disease.

Case 3

Tricyclic antidepressants have repeatedly demonstrated effectiveness in the treatment of fibromyalgia, and one study has shown duloxetine to be effective. SSRIs and venlafaxine have demonstrated benefit in some studies. Among the anticonvulsants, only pregabalin has been shown to benefit patients with fibromyalgia [77]. Based on research to date, it would be reasonable for the clinician to have the patient in Case 2 undergo trials with several different sedating antidepressants and pregabalin.

Case 4

It is not obvious that antidepressants or anticonvulsants are likely to help the patient in Case 4 with persistent spinal pain in the absence of any evidence of radiculopathy; however, if this patient demonstrated widespread hyperalgesia, the clinician might conclude that CNS sensitization was contributing to his pain, and perhaps that the patient had a fibromyalgia-like condition. In that situation, it would be reasonable to consider medications that have been shown to help fibromyalgia (see Case 3), as long as the clinician is aware that there are no well-controlled studies validating the effectiveness of such medications for the type of patient described in Case 4.

References

[1] Melzack R, Wall PD. Pain mechanisms: a new theory. Science 1965;150:971–9.

[2] Fields HL. Pain modulation: expectation, opioid analgesia and virtual pain. Prog Brain Res 2000;122:245–53.

[3] Craig AD. A new view of pain as a homeostatic emotion. Trends Neurosci 2003;26(6):303–7.

[4] Bair MJ, Robinson RL, Katon W, et al. Depression and pain comorbidity: a literature review. Arch Intern Med 2003;163(20):2433–45.

[5] Gureje O, Von Korff M, Simon GE, et al. Persistent pain and well-being: a World Health Organization study in primary care. JAMA 1998;280(2):147–51.

[6] Gureje O, Simon GE, Von Korff M. A cross-national study of the course of persistent pain in primary care. Pain 2001;92(1–2):195–200.

[7] McWilliams LA, Cox BJ, Enns MW. Mood and anxiety disorders associated with chronic pain: an examination in a nationally representative sample. Pain 2003;106(1–2):127–33.

[8] Sharp TJ. The prevalence of post-traumatic stress disorder in chronic pain patients. Curr Pain Headache Rep 2004;8(2):111–5.

[9] Hickling EJ, Blanchard EB. Post-traumatic stress disorder and motor vehicle accidents. J Anxiety Disord 1992;6:285–91.

[10] Asmundson GJG, Norton G, Allerdings M, et al. Post-traumatic stress disorder and work-related injury. J Anxiety Disord 1998;12:57–69.

[11] Roy-Byrne P, Smith WR, Goldberg J, et al. Post-traumatic stress disorder among patients with chronic pain and chronic fatigue. Psychol Med 2004;34(2):363–8.

[12] Heim C, Newport DJ, Heit S, et al. Pituitary-adrenal and autonomic responses to stress in women after sexual and physical abuse in childhood. JAMA 2000;284(5):592–7.

[13] Guzman J, Esmail R, Karjalainen K, et al. Multidisciplinary biopsychosocial rehabilitation for chronic low back pain. Cochrane Database Syst Rev 2002;1:CD000963.

[14] Smith MT, Haythornthwaite JA. How do sleep disturbance and chronic pain interrelate? Sleep Med Rev 2004;8:119–32.

[15] Neutel CI. The epidemiology of long-term benzodiazepine use. Int Rev Psychiatry 2005;17(3):189–97.

[16] Stiefel F, Stagno D. Management of insomnia in patients with chronic pain conditions. CNS Drugs 2004;18(5):285–96.

[17] O'Malley PG, Balden E, Tomkins G, et al. Treatment of fibromyalgia with antidepressants: a meta-analysis. J Gen Intern Med 2000;15(9):659–66.

[18] Onghena P, Van Houdenhove B. Antidepressant-induced analgesia in chronic nonmalignant pain: a meta-analysis of 39 placebo-controlled studies. Pain 1992;49(2):205–19.
[19] Max MB, Lynch SA, Muir J, et al. Effects of desipramine, amitriptyline, and fluoxetine on pain in diabetic neuropathy. N Engl J Med 1992;326(19):1250–6.
[20] Semenchuk MR, Sherman S, Davis B. Double-blind, randomized trial of bupropion SR for the treatment of neuropathic pain. Neurology 2001;57(9):1583–8.
[21] Rowbotham MC, Goli V, Kunz NR, et al. Venlafaxine extended release in the treatment of painful diabetic neuropathy: a double-blind, placebo-controlled study. Pain 2004;110(3): 697–706.
[22] Sindrup SH, Bach FW, Madsen C, et al. Venlafaxine versus imipramine in painful polyneuropathy: a randomized, controlled trial. Neurology 2003;60(8):1284–9.
[23] Goldstein DJ, Lu Y, Detke MJ, et al. Duloxetine vs. placebo in patients with painful diabetic neuropathy. Pain 2005;116(1–2):109–18.
[24] Bendtsen L, Jensen R. Mirtazapine is effective in the prophylactic treatment of chronic tension-type headache. Neurology 2004;62(10):1706–11.
[25] Samborski W, Lezanska-Szpera M, Rybakowski JK. Open trial of mirtazapine in patients with fibromyalgia. Pharmacopsychiatry 2004;37(4):168–70.
[26] Sindrup SH, Madsen C, Bach FW, et al. St. John's wort has no effect on pain in polyneuropathy. Pain 2001;91(3):361–5.
[27] Tomkins GE, Jackson JL, O'Malley PG, et al. Treatment of chronic headache with antidepressants: a meta-analysis. Am J Med 2001;111(1):54–63.
[28] Holroyd KA, O'Donnell FJ, Stensland M, et al. Management of chronic tension-type headache with tricyclic antidepressant medication, stress management therapy, and their combination: a randomized controlled trial. JAMA 2001;285(17):2208–15.
[29] O'Malley PG, Balden E, Tomkins G, et al. Treatment of fibromyalgia with antidepressants: a meta-analysis. J Gen Intern Med 2000;15(9):659–66.
[30] Goldenberg DL, Burckhardt C, Crofford L. Management of fibromyalgia syndrome. JAMA 2004;292(19):2388–95.
[31] Arnold LM, Lu Y, Crofford IJ, et al. A double-blind multicenter trial comparing duloxetine to placebo in the treatment of fibromyalgia with or without major depressive disorder. Arthritis Rheum 2004;50:2974–84.
[32] Atkinson JH, Slater MA, Williams RA, et al. A placebo-controlled randomized clinical trial of nortriptyline for chronic low back pain. Pain 1998;76(3):287–96.
[33] Atkinson JH, Slater MA, Wahlgren DR, et al. Effects of noradrenergic and serotonergic antidepressants on chronic low back pain intensity. Pain 1999;83(2):137–45.
[34] Cannon RO 3rd, Quyyumi AA, Mincemoyer R, et al. Imipramine in patients with chest pain despite normal coronary angiograms. N Engl J Med 1994;330(20):1411–7.
[35] Varia I, Logue E, O'Connor C, et al. Randomized trial of sertraline in patients with unexplained chest pain of noncardiac origin. Am Heart J 2000;140(3):367–72.
[36] Merskey H, Bogduk N, editors. Classification of chronic pain. 2nd edition. Seattle (WA): IASP Press; 1994.
[37] Woolf CJ. Dissecting out mechanisms responsible for peripheral neuropathic pain: implications for diagnosis and therapy. Life Sci 2004;74:2605–10.
[38] Nicholson BD. Evaluation and treatment of central pain syndromes. Neurology 2004; 62(Suppl 2):S30–6.
[39] Ghai B, Dureja GP. Complex regional pain syndrome: a review. J Postgrad Med 2004;50(4): 300–7.
[40] Grabow TS, Christo PJ, Raja SN. Complex regional pain syndrome: diagnostic controversies, psychological dysfunction, and emerging concepts. Adv Psychosom Med 2004;25:89–101.
[41] Crofford LJ. The relationship of fibromyalgia to neuropathic pain syndromes. J Rheumatol 2005;32(Suppl 75):41–5.
[42] Price DD, Staud R. Neurobiology of fibromyalgia syndrome. J Rheumatol 2005;32(Suppl 75):22–8.

[43] Rowbotham MC. Is fibromyalgia a neuropathic pain syndrome? J Rheumatol 2005; 32(Suppl 75):38–40.
[44] Robinson JP, Arendt-Nielsen L. Muscle pain syndromes. In: Braddom R, editor. Physical medicine and rehabilitation. 3rd edition. In press.
[45] Czapinski P, Blaszczyk B, Czuczwar SJ. Mechanisms of action of antiepileptic drugs. Curr Top Med Chem 2005;5(1):3–14.
[46] Soderpalm B. Anticonvulsants: aspects of their mechanisms of action. Eur J Pain 2002; 6(Suppl A):3–9.
[47] Jensen TS. Anticonvulsants in neuropathic pain: rationale and clinical evidence. Eur J Pain 2002;6(Suppl A):61–8.
[48] Dworkin RH, Backonja M, Rowbotham MC, et al. Advances in neuropathic pain. Arch Neurol 2003;60:1524–34.
[49] Wiffen PF, McQuay HF, Moore RA. Carbamazepine for acute and chronic pain. Cochrane Database Syst Rev 2005;3:CD005451.
[50] Wiffen PF, McQuay HF, Edwards JE, et al. Gabapentin for acute and chronic pain. Cochrane Database Syst Rev 2005;3:CD005452.
[51] Wiffen P, Collins S, McQuay H, et al. Anticonvulsant drugs for acute and chronic pain. Cochrane Database Syst Rev 2005;3:CD001133.
[52] Goodman F, Glassman P, Qiufei M, et al. Drug class review on antiepileptic drugs in bipolar mood disorder and neuropathic pain. Santa Monica (CA): Rand; 2004.
[53] Dib JG. Focus on topiramate in neuropathic pain. Curr Med Res Opin 2004;20(12):1857–61.
[54] Raskin P, Donofrio PD, Rosenthal NR, et al. Topiramate vs. placebo in painful diabetic neuropathy: analgesic and metabolic effects. Neurology 2004;63:865–73.
[55] Thienel U, Neto W, Schwabe SK, et al. Topiramate in painful diabetic polyneuropathy: findings from three double-blind placebo-controlled trials. Acta Neurol Scand 2004;110(4): 221–31.
[56] Saarto T, Wiffen PF. Antidepressants for neuropathic pain. Cochrane Database Syst Rev 2005;3:CD005454.
[57] Namaka M, Gramlich CR, Ruhlen D, et al. A treatment algorithm for neuropathic pain. Clin Ther 2004;26(7):951–79.
[58] Dallochio C, Buffa C, Mazzarello P, et al. Gabapentin vs. amitriptyline in painful diabetic neuropathy: an open label pilot study. J Pain Symptom Manage 2000;20(4): 280–5.
[59] Leijon G, Boivie J. Central post-stroke pain—a controlled trial of amitriptyline and carbamazepine. Pain 1989;36(1):27–36.
[60] Morello CM, Leckband SG, Stoner CP, et al. Randomized double-blind study comparing the efficacy of gabapentin with amitriptyline on diabetic peripheral neuropathy pain. Arch Intern Med 1999;159(16):1931–7.
[61] Belliotti TR, Capiris T, Ekhato V, et al. Structure-activity relationships of pregabalin and analogues that target the alpha2-delta protein. J Med Chem 2005;48:2294–307.
[62] Kochar DK, Jain N, Agarwal RP, et al. Sodium valproate in the management of painful neuropathy in type 2 diabetes—a randomized placebo controlled study. Acta Neurol Scand 2002;106(5):248–52.
[63] Pappagallo M. Newer antiepileptic drugs: possible uses in the treatment of neuropathic pain and migraine. Clin Ther 2003;25(10):2506–38.
[64] Dogra S, Beydoun S, Mazzola J, et al. Oxcarbazepine in painful diabetic neuropathy: a randomized, placebo-controlled study. Eur J Pain 2005;9(5):543–54.
[65] Atli A, Dogra S. Zonisamide in the treatment of painful diabetic neuropathy: a randomized, double-blind, placebo-controlled pilot study. Pain Med 2005;6(3):225–34.
[66] Price MJ. Levetiracetam in the treatment of neuropathic pain: three case studies. Clin J Pain 2004;20(1):33–6.
[67] Hempenstall K, Nurmikko TJ, Johnson RW, et al. Analgesic therapy in postherpetic neuralgia: a quantitative systematic review. PLoS Med 2005;2(7):164.

[68] Freynhagen R, Strojek K, Griesing T, et al. Efficacy of pregabalin in neuropathic pain evaluated in a 12-week, randomised, double-blind, multicentre, placebo-controlled trial of flexible- and fixed-dose regimens. Pain 2005;115(3):254–63.
[69] Dworkin RH, Corbin AE, Young JP, et al. Pregabalin for the treatment of postherpetic neuralgia: a randomized, placebo-controlled trial. Neurology 2003;60:1274–83.
[70] Sabatowski R, Galvez R, Cherry DA, et al. Pregabalin reduces pain and improves sleep and mood disturbances in patients with post-herpetic neuralgia: results of a randomized, placebo-controlled clinical trial. Pain 2004;109:26–35.
[71] Richter RW, Portenoy R, Sharma U, et al. Relief of painful diabetic peripheral neuropathy with pregabalin: a randomized, placebo-controlled trial. J Pain 2005;6(4):253–60.
[72] Chadda VS, Mathur MS. Double-blind study of the effects of diphenylhydantoin sodium on diabetic neuropathy. J Assoc Physicians India 1978;32:403–6.
[73] Saudek CD, Werns S, Reidenberg MM. Phenytoin in the treatment of diabetic symmetrical polyneuropathy. Clin Pharmacol Ther 1977;22:196–9.
[74] Vinik A. Clinical review: use of antiepileptic drugs in the treatment of chronic painful diabetic neuropathy. J Clin Endocrinol Metab 2005;90:4936–45.
[75] Simpson DA. Gabapentin and venlafaxine for the treatment of painful diabetic neuropathy. J Clin Neuromusc Dis 2001;3:53–62.
[76] Gilron I, Bailey JM, Dongsheng T, et al. Morphine, gabapentin, or their combination for neuropathic pain. N Engl J Med 2005;352:1324–34.
[77] Crofford LJ, Rowbotham MC, Mease PJ, et al. Pregabalin 1008–105 Study Group. Pregabalin for the treatment of fibromyalgia syndrome: results of a randomized, double-blind, placebo-controlled trial. Arthritis Rheum 2005;52(4):1264–73.
[78] McCleane GJ. Does gabapentin have an analgesic effect on background, movement and referred pain? A randomized, double-blind, placebo-controlled study. Pain Clin 2001;13:103–7.
[79] McCleane GJ. Gabapentin reduces chronic benign nociceptive pain: a double-blind, placebo-controlled cross-over study. Pain Clin 2000;12:81–5.
[80] Leijon G, Boivie J. Central post-stroke pain—a controlled trial of amitriptyline and carbamazepine. Pain 1989;36(1):27–36.
[81] Panerai AE, Monza G, Molivia P, et al. A randomized, within-patient, cross-over, placebo-controlled trial on the efficacy and tolerability of the tricyclic antidepressants chlomipramine and nortriptyline in central pain. Acta Neurol Scand 1990;82(1):34–8.
[82] Vestergaard K, Andersen G, Gottrup H, et al. Lamotrigine for central poststroke pain: a randomized controlled trial. Neurology 2001;56:184–90.
[83] Tai Q, Kirshblum S, Chen B, et al. Gabapentin in the treatment of neuropathic pain after spinal cord injury: a prospective, randomized, double-blind, crossover trial. J Spinal Cord Med 2002;25:100–5.

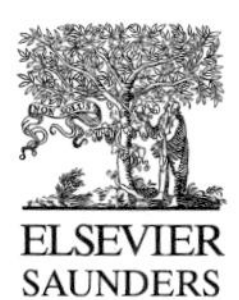
ELSEVIER
SAUNDERS

Phys Med Rehabil Clin N Am
17 (2006) 401–413

PHYSICAL MEDICINE
AND REHABILITATION
CLINICS OF
NORTH AMERICA

Muscle Relaxants and Antispasticity Agents

Alec L. Meleger, MD

Department of Physical Medicine and Rehabilitation, Spaulding Rehabilitation Hospital, 125 Nashua Street, Boston, MA 02114, USA

Pain of muscle origin or myogenic pain is commonly observed among patients experiencing chronic pain. A 30% prevalence of myofascial pain has been observed within the setting of general internal medicine practice [1]. The incidence of spasticity-related muscle pain in patients with stroke, multiple sclerosis, or after spinal cord injury can reach as high as 65%, 74%, and 67%, respectively [2–4]. A variety of pharmacologic agents is available for the treatment of myogenic pain. These agents are typically referred to as muscle relaxants, muscle relaxers, or antispastic medications. One study showed that up to 91% of physicians report using muscle relaxants, and that up to 35% of patients visiting a primary care physician with the complaints of low back pain have them prescribed [5,6]. This pharmacologic class is typically subdivided into central and peripheral depolarizing/nondepolarizing muscle relaxants. The former category is generally used for the treatment of myogenic pain and the latter for the induction of muscle paralysis as part of perioperative general anesthesia.

Pathophysiology of muscle pain

The pathophysiology of muscle pain is fairly complex and cannot be comprehensively addressed within the confines of this article. Nevertheless, a concise overview is attempted herein as it specifically pertains to the use of muscle relaxants and antispastic medications.

Local muscle pain is clinically elicited after the thinly myelinated Aδ and unmyelinated C nerve fibers become activated. This activation can be induced by thermal or mechanical stimuli, local inflammation, or muscle ischemia. Localized muscle ischemia can occur with vascular claudication,

E-mail address: ameleger@partners.org

doi:10.1016/j.pmr.2005.12.005 *pmr.theclinics.com*

and to some extent in clinical states such as increased muscular tension, muscle spasm, spasticity, and trigger point formation [7].

Various theoretical mechanisms have been proposed in an attempt to explain the chain of events leading up to the occurrence of chronic myogenic pain. One of the accepted explanations deals with the neuroplastic changes that occur at the level of the dorsal horn, where newly formed pathologic interneuronal synapses form. As a result, a previously nonpainful stimulus is interpreted as algesic or hyperalgesic owing to abnormal sensitization of the nociceptive neurons and the secondary neurons involved. Another explanation is pathologic functioning of the descending inhibitory pathways that, in the normal healthy state, serve as strong inhibitors of afferent stimulation. A third possibility is that constant peripheral sensitization of nociceptive intramuscular nerve endings occurs owing to the recurrent trauma or chronic local ischemic conditions. The local tissue ischemia is thought to occur as a result of vaso-occlusive events, as might be seen within trigger points, or owing to local neurogenic edema producing the same pathologic effect in the vascular supply. Perpetuating factors of a mechanical or systemic nature causing abnormal firing of the involved muscle groups can also lead to chronic muscle pain. Another theoretical mechanism is the well-documented mind-body connection in the context of chronic pain. Chronic pain patients with untreated depression or anxiety who are under significant stress tend to perceive pain at higher intensity. This effect can be explained by well-documented central nervous system connections involving ascending and descending nociceptive pathways and pathways relaying an emotional state of affairs [7].

Clinically, chronic muscle pain can be observed in individuals who sustain entities such as recurrent muscle spasms, spasticity, fibromyalgia, trigger points, and increased muscle tension. Typical complaints are a diffuse, aching, cramping pain of mild-to-severe intensity, which can be intermittent (ie, when induced by postural changes) or constant (ie, in fibromyalgia).

The pain of muscle spasms can be encountered as part of acute, subacute, or chronic pain states. It is defined as an involuntary muscular contraction that can be observed during electromyographic examination. A painful muscle spasm is typically referred to as a muscle cramp.

Spasticity, which is commonly seen in patients with previous stroke, multiple sclerosis, or spinal cord injury, is defined as a muscle tone disorder characterized by hyperactive tonic stretch reflexes. The exaggerated muscle tone is velocity dependent, producing progressive resistance to stretch with increased speed of applied passive movement. Other clinical findings in spasticity include hyperreflexia, clonus, the Babinski sign, and flexor spasms. Spasticity is thought to arise from an imbalance of excitatory and inhibitory inputs at the level of the spinal cord seen after injury to descending motor pathways.

Physiologic contracture, which is defined as a state of muscle contractile activity without the presence of electrical activity, can be found in disorders with abnormal regulation of calcium at the level of sarcoplasmic reticulum as well as in commonly seen taut muscle bands that surround myofascial trigger points [8]. The physiologic contracture should be differentiated from structural contracture involving the surrounding fascia, connective tissue, and ligaments commonly seen in chronically shortened muscles.

Myofascial trigger points are frequently observed and contribute to the overall level of pain in individuals sustaining chronic musculoskeletal conditions. It has been proposed that sustained muscle fiber shortening, induced by an abnormal increase in the release of acetylcholine, produces localized ischemia and subsequent sensitization of nociceptive nerve fibers [8].

The pain of fibromyalgia, which some physicians still believe is a controversial clinical diagnosis, is described as diffuse and constant muscle pain with pathognomonic tactile allodynia on physical examination. This often incapacitating pain is thought to be due to the pathologic sensitization of central nociceptive pathways.

Muscle relaxants

Muscle relaxants make up a heterogeneous group of drugs that mainly exert their pharmacologic effect centrally at the level of the spinal cord, the brainstem, or the cerebrum, and that have an insignificant, if any effect, at the muscle fiber level. Their centrally mediated mechanism of action can exert a clinically significant peripheral therapeutic effect.

Cyclobenzaprine

Cyclobenzaprine is probably the most commonly used muscle relaxant for nonspasticity-related muscle pain. Structurally, it resembles tricyclic antidepressants and differs from amitriptyline by only one double bond. Its therapeutic effect is centrally mediated and carries no direct peripheral action on the affected muscles. Its main pharmacologic action occurs at the brainstem and spinal cord levels and is partially explained by a depressant effect on the descending serotonergic neurons [9]. It is extensively metabolized in the liver and excreted as a glucuronated metabolite through the kidneys. It possesses a fairly long half-life of approximately 18 hours and can continue to accumulate for up to 4 days when administered at a frequency of three times per day. Given its structural similarity to tricyclic antidepressants as well as potent anticholinergic properties, caution should be exercised when considering its use in the elderly or in patients with heart disease. Likewise, concomitant use with monoamine oxidase inhibitors is absolutely contraindicated because this combination can cause a hyperpyretic crisis or even death. The initial starting dose should be 5 mg three times per day on as needed basis and can be titrated up to 10 mg three times per day per therapeutic effect or side effect. In patients with hepatic or renal insufficiency, it should initially be administered once per day given its relatively long half-life. Of note, one recent study showed equal efficacy of 5 and 10 mg doses, with the smaller dose showing a lower level of sedation [10]. The most common side effects are drowsiness, dry mouth, fatigue, and headache, followed by less often occurring adverse effects of diarrhea, dizziness, abdominal pain, nausea, nervousness, blurred vision, and confusion [11].

Methocarbamol

Methocarbamol is structurally related to the expectorant guaifenesin and the muscle relaxants chlorphenesin and mephenesin. It is a centrally acting muscle relaxant that suppresses spinal polysynaptic reflexes and has no direct effect on skeletal muscle. It is extensively metabolized in the liver and is excreted through the kidneys, with a small amount excreted with feces. Acutely, methocarbamol can be administered four times a day at a dose of 1500 mg. For maintenance therapy, 1500 mg can be given three times per day. This medication can also be administered via intravenous and intramuscular routes. Frequent side effects include drowsiness and dizziness, followed by nausea, anorexia, headache, blurred vision, muscular discoordination, and, in some instances, urine discoloration. Seizures have been reported with intravenous administration, especially with a history of epilepsy [11].

Orphenadrine

Orphenadrine is structurally related to diphenhydramine and carries relatively stronger anticholinergic and weaker sedative properties. It does not produce any direct effect on skeletal muscle, and its exact mechanism of action is unknown. Orphenadrine is mostly excreted through the kidneys. The typical adult oral dose is 100 mg administered at the frequency of twice per day owing to its relatively long half-life. The drug can also be administered intravenously as well as intramuscularly. Common side effects include drowsiness and dizziness, followed by other central nervous system effects such as agitation, hallucinations, and euphoria. The following adverse effects have been reported owing to orphenadrine's anticholinergic properties: dry mouth, nausea, constipation, urinary retention, tachycardia, blurred vision, and mental confusion, especially in the elderly. Rare reports of aplastic anemia have been documented [11].

Metaxalone

Metaxalone is a centrally acting muscle relaxant with an unknown mechanism of action. It is metabolized in the liver and excreted through the kidneys in the form of metabolites. Typical adult dosing consists of 800 mg three to four times per day. It is recommended to monitor liver function tests after initiation of this agent. Common side effects include drowsiness, dizziness, nervousness, nausea, and headache. The following rare but serious adverse reactions have been reported: leukopenia, hemolytic anemia, jaundice, and hypersensitivity reactions [11].

Tizanidine

Tizanidine is a centrally acting muscle relaxant that, through its alpha-2 adrenergic agonist properties, is thought to prevent the release of excitatory amino acids by suppressing polysynaptic excitation of spinal cord interneurons. Metabolism is through the liver, and excretion is 60% through the kidneys and 20% through the feces. Tizanidine should be administered through a gradual upward titration from an initial dose of 2 to 4 mg at bedtime up to the maximum of 8 mg three times per day. The bedtime dose can provide an analgesic effect as well as improve quality of sleep owing to the commonly occurring sedating side effect. Other common side effects are daytime drowsiness, hypotension, weakness, and dry mouth. Even though tizanidine's pharmacologic effect is similar to another alpha-2 agonist, clonidine, it possesses only a fraction of its blood pressure–lowering effect. Less commonly reported side effects of tizanidine are palpitations, bradycardia, dizziness, headache, nausea, elevated liver enzymes, and several rare cases of fulminant liver failure that led to death. Serial monitoring of liver enzymes is strongly recommended [11].

Quinine

In the not so distant past, quinine was extensively prescribed for the treatment of nocturnal leg muscle cramps; however, it lost this Food and Drug Administration indication owing to the seriousness of potential side effects, with increased morbidity in the older population. Structurally, quinine is a stereoisomer of a class IA antiarrhythmic quinidine and possesses some of its cardiac effects. Quinine's other pharmacologic properties include antimalarial, antipyretic, analgesic, and muscle relaxant effects. The last effect is achieved owing to its ability to increase the refractoriness of muscle and to decrease the excitability of the neuromuscular endplate. Quinine is extensively metabolized in the liver and is mainly excreted in the urine. The typical adult dosing for nocturnal leg cramps is 260 mg at bedtime. The more serious adverse effects include myelosuppression, thrombocytopenia, hemolysis, disseminated intravascular coagulation, torsades de pointes, angina, vasculitis, hypoglycemia, renal toxicity, hemolytic uremic syndrome, urine discoloration, liver toxicity, asthma, toxic epidermal necrolysis, and hearing loss. Less serious reported side effects are headache, confusion, dizziness, nausea, and blurred vision. If prescribed, regular checks of liver and kidney function tests, a compete blood count, and a performance of a 12-lead electrocardiogram are strongly recommended [11].

Carisoprodol

Carisoprodol is still a commonly prescribed muscle relaxant that should be dispensed with caution owing to the potentially addictive properties of its main metabolite, meprobamate. Carisoprodol produces its muscle relaxant effect by depressing the interneuronal activity at the spinal cord level as well as in the descending tracts of the reticular formation. It is not recommended for use in the pediatric age population. This drug is metabolized in the liver with meprobamate as its main metabolite. It is mainly excreted through the kidneys. The usual adult dosage is 350 mg four times per day. The most common side effect is drowsiness. Other central nervous system adverse effects that have been reported include ataxia, agitation, insomnia, and others. Adverse effects such as tachycardia, postural hypotension, nausea, erythema multiforme, and eosinophilia have also been seen [11].

Botulinum toxin type A, B

Clostridium botulinum is a spore-forming anaerobic bacillus that produces seven distinct antigenic types of botulinum toxin named from A to G. Toxins type A, B, and F are the only neurotoxins that have been used in the clinical arena. These neurotoxins exert their pharmacologic effect at the neuromuscular junction, where they prevent the calcium-dependent release of acetylcholine, producing a state of temporary drug-induced denervation. The therapeutic effect can take up to 1 week to take place fully and can last up to 3 months, at which point repeat injections can be considered. Injectable botulinum preparations are unstable and need to be stored and reconstituted with caution per the manufacturers' recommendations. Each unit of the respective clinically available neurotoxin carries a different level of biologic potency and cannot be reliably interconverted. Relative muscle weakness of the injected musculature as well as of adjacent muscle groups is to some degree expected from local spread of the neurotoxin. Caution should be exercised in using appropriate botulinum dosing to avoid functionally limiting muscle weakness. Headache, dizziness, fever, flulike symptoms, nausea, biliary colic, injection site pain, edema, and erythema are some of the adverse effects encountered. Dysphagia, dry mouth, and dysphonia can be observed with injections in the cervical area. Rare instances of arrhythmia, myocardial infarction, hypertension, and botulismlike syndrome have been reported. Patients who receive repeated botulinum injections can develop antibodies and become resistant to the neurotoxin's therapeutic effect. Trials of the other available antigenic types of the neurotoxin can be entertained in such cases [11].

Benzodiazepines (diazepam, lorazepam, clonazepam, etc)

Diazepam has commonly been used in the treatment of muscle spasm, especially in the acute setting. It belongs to a group of compounds called benzodiazepines, known for their potent anxiolytic, sedative, as well as muscle relaxant effects. Their main mechanism of action is through central potentiation of the inhibitory γ-aminobutyric acid (GABA) effect through presynaptic facilitation of GABA release. Benzodiazepines are extensively metabolized in the liver into inactive and in some cases active metabolites. Compounds that lack active metabolites should be used as first-line agents in the elderly and in patients with liver or kidney insufficiency. Such compounds are lorazepam, clonazepam, temazepam, and oxazepam. Excretion principally occurs through the kidneys. Some of the common side effects are drowsiness, confusion, ataxia, cognitive impairment, memory loss, agitation, and disinhibition. Of note, withdrawal symptoms may occur after only 4 to 6 weeks of use, and their potential for abuse should be taken into consideration [11].

Antispastic agents

Antispastic drugs are principally used for the treatment of spasticity observed in disease states with upper motor neuron pathology, such as stroke, spinal cord injury, traumatic brain injury, and multiple sclerosis. All but two of these agents exert their clinical effect through centrally mediated mechanisms.

Baclofen

Structurally, baclofen is related to the centrally occurring inhibitory neurotransmitter GABA. Clinically, it has commonly been used for its muscle relaxant effects in the treatment of spasticity, as well as for its neuropathic analgesic properties in the treatment of trigeminal neuralgia pain. Baclofen is a GABA-B receptor agonist with presynaptic and postsynaptic effects leading to a decrease in the excitatory neurotransmitter release as well as in substance P, which is involved in transmission of nociceptive impulses [12]. It is metabolized in the liver and excreted in the urine. Baclofen can be administered orally as well as intrathecally via an implanted pump mechanism when significant adverse effects preclude further dose escalation to achieve therapeutic effect. Initial dosing of baclofen should be gradual, starting with 5 to 10 mg three times per day. The maximum recommended dose is 80 mg per day in divided doses; however, higher therapeutic doses in cases of refractory spasticity have been used without any significant untoward side effects. Common side effects are weakness, sedation, and dizziness. At higher doses, baclofen can cause seizures, ataxia, and hallucinations. Abrupt withdrawal should be avoided because it can precipitate seizures and hallucinations [11].

Dantrolene

Dantrolene reduces muscle spasms by inhibiting the release of calcium from the sarcoplasmic reticulum and does not directly affect the central nervous system. It is metabolized in the liver and excreted through the kidneys. Because dantrolene tends to produce greater muscle weakness than baclofen, it should not be the first-line agent for patients who are capable of ambulation. Typically, this medication should be started at a relatively low dose of 25 mg per day and slowly titrated on a weekly basis per effect or side effect up to the maximum of 100 mg three times per day. Such slow titration can obviate the development of some of the common side effects: drowsiness, weakness, dizziness, and diarrhea. Less frequently observed side effects are constipation, nausea, insomnia, diplopia, tachycardia, depressed mood, anxiety, muscle pain, difficult urination/frequency, erectile dysfunction, and respiratory depression. More serious but relatively rare adverse effects are hepatitis, seizure, heart failure, aplastic anemia, leukopenia, thrombocytopenia, respiratory depression, pleural effusion, and pericarditis. Dantrolene should be used with caution in patients with heart failure, chronic obstructive pulmonary disease, and liver disease [11].

Tizanidine

For information on this agent, the reader is referred to the section on muscle relaxants.

Benzodiazepines (diazepam, lorazepam, clonazepam, etc)

For more information on the benzodiazepines, the reader is referred to the section on muscle relaxants. In the treatment of spasticity, the maximum daily doses of 40 to 60 mg and 10 to 20 mg of diazepam and clonazepam, respectively, can be gradually achieved as tolerated per therapeutic effect.

Botulinum toxin type A, B

For more information on botulinum toxin, the reader is referred to the section on muscle relaxants.

Clonidine

Clonidine is an antihypertensive agent available in an oral form as well as a transdermal preparation. It is an alpha-2 agonist that exerts its pharmacologic effect on the brainstem, leading to a reduced central sympathetic outflow. This effect in turn causes a reduction in the peripheral resistance, blood pressure, and heart rate. The oral preparation of clonidine is administered twice per day with a starting dose of 0.1 mg up to the maximum of 1.2 mg BID as tolerated. Transdermal clonidine patch, which is changed every 7 days, can be prescribed if compliance is an issue. It is metabolized in the liver with majority excretion through the kidneys. A small portion is eliminated through the biliary/fecal route. The most common side effects are drowsiness, dizziness, dry mouth, and constipation. Other adverse side effects include fatigue, headache, orthostatic hypotension, palpitations, syncope, Raynaud's phenomenon, congestive heart failure, conduction blocks, anxiety, insomnia, nausea, hepatitis, constipation, impotence, loss of libido, thrombocytopenia, muscle pain, and blurred vision [11].

Clinical implications

Available evidence

A large number of studies of varying quality and methodology have been conducted on the efficacy of muscle relaxants and antispastic agents in the treatment of muscle-related pain. Several systematic reviews and at least one meta-analysis have been performed, with three of these available through the Cochrane collaborative database.

The Cochrane review on the use of muscle relaxants for nonspecific low back pain was recently updated in May of 2005 and consists of 30 randomized, controlled and randomized, double-blinded, controlled clinical trials. The review concluded that there is strong evidence for statistically significant symptomatic relief within 1 week of therapy for non-benzodiazepine muscle relaxants in the treatment of acute low back pain; however, the evidence for benzodiazepines, specifically diazepam and tetrazepam, was less convincing. The various muscle relaxants were found to be equally effective (ie, tizanidine, cyclobenzaprine, orphenadrine, methocarbamol, metaxalone, carisoprodol), and there was a significantly higher prevalence of adverse effects in the muscle relaxant group than in the placebo group. Interestingly, antispasticity muscle relaxants (ie, baclofen, dantrolene) also showed clinical efficacy in the setting of acute low back pain. Likewise, muscle relaxants were found to be effective when used as adjunctive therapy in treating acute back pain. In regards to chronic low back pain, tetrazepam, flupirtine, and tolperisone, none of which are available in United States, showed short-term efficacy over placebo [13].

A meta-analysis by Browning and coworkers [14] evaluated the efficacy of cyclobenzaprine in the context of back pain. Fourteen randomized, placebo-controlled studies were included, three of which dealt with nonacute pain of spinal origin. The overall observation was that cyclobenzaprine was modestly more effective than placebo, with the greatest efficacy seen in the first 4 days of treatment, and that the agent showed a trend of declining effectiveness over time. Adverse effects were observed in more than 50% of patients, with drowsiness being the most common [14]. Three of the studies examined the muscle relaxant effects of cyclobenzaprine in patients with more of a chronic presentation. They included subjects with cervical as well as lumbosacral complaints. Basmajian [15] compared the effects of cyclobenzaprine, diazepam, and placebo in individuals with greater than a 30-day duration over the course of 18 days. Both treatment groups showed a statistically significant effect, more so in the cyclobenzaprine arm [15]. In a study by Bercel [16], cyclobenzaprine was compared with placebo in a population with greater than a 30-day symptom duration over 14 days, again showing superiority of the treatment arm. The study by Brown and Womble [17] was the only study of a true chronic pain population with a minimum symptom duration of 12 months comparing cyclobenzaprine and diazepam versus placebo. Unfortunately, this study was of relatively poor quality with a short treatment period of 14 days. Both treatment arms showed a significantly positive therapeutic effect [17].

The most recent update of the Cochrane review on the treatment of spasticity after spinal cord injury was conducted in March of 2005 and included 55 studies that met the inclusion criteria. This review reported the clinical efficacy of intrathecal baclofen in reducing spasticity and improving performance of activities of daily living in a comparison with placebo, as well as a significant effect of tizanidine in improving the Ashworth score but not activities of daily living [18].

Another Cochrane review update (February, 2004) also dealt with the efficacy of antispasticity agents and was inconclusive in regards to their use in the setting of multiple sclerosis. Less than half of the placebo-controlled trials, which used the Ashworth score as one of its outcome measures, showed a statistically clinical significance over placebo. None of the comparative trials showed a significant difference of one antispastic agent over another [19].

Clinical pearls

Before initiating the prescription of muscle relaxants to patients with chronic pain, a comprehensive assessment should be performed to determine whether these agents are indicated or contraindicated for the clinical scenario at hand. The first question that should be addressed is whether the pain of muscle origin is one of the main contributors. Is there evidence of muscle spasm, trigger points with a referral pattern, spasticity, increased muscle tension, decreased range of motion, muscle tightness, cramping, or other factors?

Unfortunately, exact pathophysiologic factors of chronic pain are not always easily teased out owing to its multifactorial nature and the significant overlap of causative mechanisms. When one is uncertain about the putative mechanisms and when other pharmacologic options have been exhausted, an empiric trial of muscle relaxants should be considered.

Has the patient already tried a muscle relaxant, and what was the response? Was the dose therapeutic and was an adequately long trial attempted? Sometimes one needs to titrate the specific agent gradually up to the maximum daily allowable therapeutic dose and perform a trial for at least 4 to 7 days before concluding that it is ineffective. Failure or poor tolerance of one muscle relaxant should not preclude the use of others because the mechanisms of action and side-effect profiles are different. Clinically, some of the side effects dissipate over time with longer use of a specific muscle relaxant. Because all of the muscle relaxants produce sedation to some degree, their introduction to the patient should begin at bedtime, especially if the patient is already suffering from insomnia.

What is the age of the patient? Are there any medical contraindications? In general, elderly patients do not tolerate muscle relaxants well, especially if they have anticholinergic properties, such as cyclobenzaprine, which can cause significant mental confusion. Initial doses should be minimal and titration gradual in this patient population.

Caution should be exercised in patients who have liver as well as kidney insufficiency, because all of the muscle relaxants undergo liver metabolism and principally are renally excreted. Patients with heart disease or conduction abnormalities should avoid using cyclobenzaprine and dantrolene owing to the proarrhythmic properties of the former and the cardiac muscle depressant effect of the latter.

Is the medication ineffective at the maximal oral dose, requiring an intrathecal route of administration? Do the adverse effects preclude ongoing use or prevent further dose escalation? Intrathecal infusion of the antispasticity drug baclofen allows administration of potent doses with a significantly improved side-effect profile [20].

Clinical scenarios

In Case 1 in the introductory article of this issue, that is, a 19-year-old male patient with a traumatic brain injury status post a motorcycle accident who presents with right-sided paresis, spasticity, and neuropathic pain involving his right lower extremity, the use of an agent with antispastic and neuropathic properties would be most advantageous. These agents include baclofen, which is one of the first-line agents used in the treatment of trigeminal neuralgia pain, as well as tizanidine and clonidine, which also possess antineuropathic pain properties [21,22]. Clonazepam could also be considered, because it might possess some analgesic properties for neuropathic pain [23]. Because all of these agents can affect the level of alertness and mentation, caution should be exercised in patients with a history of traumatic brain injury. Clonidine should not be used as the first-line agent owing to the possible hypotensive effects, especially if posttraumatic autonomic dysregulation is present.

A trial of bedtime cyclobenzaprine should be considered in Case 3, that is, the 35-year-old female patient with a diagnosis of posttraumatic fibromyalgia [24]. Initial dosing should start with 5 mg and be gradually titrated up to 30 to 40 mg at bedtime based on the therapeutic effects or side effects. Orphenadrine could also be tried, because it exhibited some therapeutic efficacy in at least one clinical study [25].

In Case 4, a 34-year-old roofer with an L1 vertebral fracture, an empiric trial of a muscle relaxant could be considered if a component of myogenic pain is present or if the other pharmacologic or nonpharmacologic therapies have failed. Local trigger points might have formed as a result of the initial injury, or the patient might be experiencing intermittent muscle spasms owing to altered vertebral biomechanics. If the patient does not have any history of liver abnormalities, a trial of tizanidine can be undertaken because it is relatively well tolerated.

Summary

Muscle relaxants make up a heterogeneous group of agents and can have a clinically significant role in the treatment of chronic muscle pain. These medications are not without possible serious side effects; hence, care should be taken in deciding on their appropriateness and ongoing monitoring performed, if prescribed.

References

[1] Skootsky SA, Jaeger B, Oye RK. Prevalence of myofascial pain in general internal medicine practice. West J Med 1989;151:157–60.
[2] McGuire JR, Harvey KL. The prevention and management of complications after stroke. Phys Med Rehabil Clin North Am 1999;10:857–74.
[3] MS Society. MS symptom management survey. London: MS Society; 1997.
[4] Maynard FM, Karunas RS, Waring WP. Epidemiology of spasticity following traumatic spinal cord injury. Arch Phys Med Rehabil 1990;71:566–9.
[5] Di Iorio D, Henley E, Doughty A. A survey of primary care physician practice patterns and adherence to acute low back problem guidelines. Arch Fam Med 2000;9(10):1015–21.
[6] Cherkin DC, Wheeler KJ, Barlow W, et al. Medication use for low back pain in primary care. Spine 1998;23(5):607–14.
[7] Bruckle W, Suckfull M, Fleckenstein W, et al. Gewebe-pO_2-Messung in der verspannten Ruckenmuskulatur (m. erector spinae). Z Rheumatol 1990;49:208–16.
[8] Mense S, Simons DG, Russell IJ. Muscle pain: understanding its nature, diagnosis, and treatment. Baltimore: Lippincott Williams & Wilkins; 2001. p. 7–15, 255.
[9] Kobayashi H, Hasegawa Y, Ono H. Cyclobenzaprine, a centrally acting muscle relaxant, acts on descending serotonergic systems. Eur J Pharmacol 1996;311(1):29–35.
[10] Borenstein DG, Korn S. Efficacy of a low-dose regimen of cyclobenzaprine hydrochloride in acute skeletal muscle spasm: results of two placebo-controlled trials. Clin Ther 2003;25(4): 1056–73.
[11] Thomson Micromedex. 1974–2005. Available at: http://www.micromedex.com. Accessed February 5, 2006.
[12] Hwang AS, Wilcox GL. Baclofen, gamma-aminobutyric acid B receptors and substance P in the mouse spinal cord. J Pharmacol Exp Ther 1989;248:1026–33.
[13] Tulder MW, Touray T, Furlan AD, et al. Muscle relaxants for non-specific low-back pain. Cochrane Database Syst Rev 2005;3.
[14] Browning R, Jackson JL, O'Malley PG. Cyclobenzaprine and back pain: a meta-analysis. Arch Intern Med 2001;161(13):1613–20.
[15] Basmajian JV. Cyclobenzaprine hydrochloride effect on skeletal muscle spasm in the lumbar region and neck: two double-blind controlled clinical and laboratory studies. Arch Phys Med Rehabil 1978;59:58–63.
[16] Bercel NA. Cyclobenzaprine in the treatment of skeletal muscle spasm in osteoarthritis of the cervical and lumbar spine. Curr Ther Res 1977;22:462–8.

[17] Brown BR Jr, Womble J. Cyclobenzaprine in intractable pain syndromes with muscle spasm. JAMA 1978;240:1151–2.

[18] Taricco M, Adone R, Pagliacci C, et al. Pharmacological interventions for spasticity following spinal cord injury. Cochrane Database Syst Rev 2000;2:CD001131.

[19] Shakespeare DT, Boggild M, Young C. Anti-spasticity agents for multiple sclerosis. Cochrane Database Syst Rev 2003;4:CD001332.

[20] Coffey RJ, Cahill D, Steers W, et al. Intrathecal baclofen for intractable spasticity of spinal origin: results of a long term multicenter study. J Neurosurg 1993;78:226–32.

[21] Semenchuk MR, Sherman S. Effectiveness of tizanidine in neuropathic pain: an open-label study. J Pain 2000;1(4):285–92.

[22] Kawamata T, Omote K, Yamamoto H, et al. Antihyperalgesic and side effects of intrathecal clonidine and tizanidine in a rat model of neuropathic pain. Anesthesiology 2003;98(6): 1480–3.

[23] Bartusch SL, Sanders BJ, D'Alessio JG, et al. Clonazepam for the treatment of lancinating phantom limb pain. Clin J Pain 1996;12(1):59–62.

[24] Bennett A. Comparison of cyclobenzaprine and placebo in the management of fibrositis. Arthritis Rheum 1988;31(12):1535–42.

[25] Abeles M. Long-term effectiveness of orphenadrine citrate in the treatment of fibromyalgia. In: American College of Rheumatology Scientific Abstracts. 113–A270.

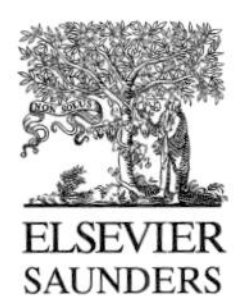

ELSEVIER
SAUNDERS

Phys Med Rehabil Clin N Am
17 (2006) 415–433

PHYSICAL MEDICINE
AND REHABILITATION
CLINICS OF
NORTH AMERICA

Psychologic Interventions for Chronic Pain

Travis L. Osborne, PhD[a,*], Katherine A. Raichle, PhD[a], Mark P. Jensen, PhD[a,b]

[a]*Department of Rehabilitation Medicine, Box 356490, University of Washington School of Medicine, Seattle, WA 98195-6490, USA*
[b]*Multidisciplinary Pain Center, University of Washington Medical Center–Roosevelt, 4245 Roosevelt Way Northeast, Seattle, WA 98105-6920, USA*

In recent decades it has becoming increasingly evident that restrictive biomedical models are not sufficient to explain the development and maintenance of chronic pain problems [1]. For many persons with chronic pain, a single pathophysiologic mechanism that underlies all of their pain and suffering cannot be identified, and medical/pharmacologic treatments rarely, if ever, provide adequate pain control [2]. To address the limitations of biomedical models of chronic pain, more comprehensive biopsychosocial conceptualizations were developed to take into account a variety of factors (eg, physical, social, cognitive, affective, behavioral, and sociocultural) that can contribute to chronic pain problems [3]. Since the development of these models, research on the psychologic factors associated with chronic pain has flourished, and several psychologically based treatments for pain management have been developed [4]. Most of these treatments have sound empirical support [5] and are routinely integrated into multidisciplinary chronic pain treatment programs [6]. This article provides an overview of four of the primary psychologic treatment approaches that are now used to help persons with chronic pain: operant behavioral therapy, cognitive-behavioral therapy, hypnotic analgesia, and motivational interviewing. In each case, methods of incorporating the principles of these interventions into a medical

Work for this article was supported by grant H133B980017 from the Department of Education's National Institute of Disability and Rehabilitation Research and by Management of Chronic Pain in Rehabilitation grant PO1 HD33988 from the National Institute of Child Health and Human Development, National Center for Medical Rehabilitation Research, National Institutes of Health.

* Corresponding author.
E-mail address: osbornet@u.washington.edu (T.L. Osborne).

doi:10.1016/j.pmr.2005.12.002 **pmr.theclinics.com**

practice and for considering when to refer patients for more specialized psychologically based pain treatment are discussed.

Operant behavioral therapy

Operant behavioral therapy was perhaps the first psychologic intervention that gained wide acceptance for treating chronic pain problems. According to the theory of operant conditioning, overt behaviors that might initially be biologic responses to stimuli eventually come under the control of environmental contingencies. Specifically, behaviors that are reinforced tend to increase in frequency and be maintained over time, whereas behaviors that are not reinforced or that are punished are likely to decrease in frequency or be extinguished. Reinforcement can include the application of a desired consequence (positive reinforcement) as well as the removal of a negative consequence (negative reinforcement), whereas punishment involves administering an undesired consequence. Operant theory also posits that when a neutral stimulus is repeatedly paired with a target behavior and the consequence for this behavior (ie, reinforcement or punishment), the stimulus can eventually become a discriminative cue that can influence the target behavior. The key to understanding what maintains specific behaviors often involves understanding the discriminative stimuli that actively maintain these behaviors [7].

Operant conditioning was first applied to the conceptualization and treatment of chronic pain by Fordyce and colleagues [7,8]. Fordyce's approach focused on overt pain behaviors (eg, limping, guarding, rubbing, pain medication use, inactivity) and well behaviors (ie, adaptive behaviors, such as working and engaging in activities) exhibited by persons with pain. He theorized that pain behaviors are natural responses to acute pain that can persist after healing if they are reinforced and if competing well behaviors are not sufficiently reinforced. Over time, this can lead to pain behaviors occurring, at least in part, in response to environmental contingencies and discriminative stimuli (eg, spouses, other family members, or health care providers who might reinforce pain behaviors) instead of only in response to nociception. The operant model of chronic pain hypothesizes that the perpetuation of pain behaviors after healing contributes to chronic pain problems and that these behaviors can contribute to suffering and disability. For the most part, such behaviors involve limiting one's activity and functioning.

Based on the operant conditioning model of chronic pain problems, Fordyce developed an operant treatment designed to eliminate pain behaviors and promote well behaviors in persons with chronic pain. The goal of this treatment is not to reduce an individual's subjective experience of pain but to restore functioning by modifying overt pain behaviors that can interfere with functioning and quality of life. Key components of operant treatment for chronic pain include identifying: (1) target pain behaviors or lack of well behaviors, (2) the discriminative stimuli that precede and influence these behaviors, and (3) the reinforcers and punishments for these behaviors [9]. Information about these factors is obtained by direct observation of the patient, behavioral assessment questionnaires, and self-monitoring by the patient and is used to develop a functional behavioral analysis (a conceptualization of the antecedents that lead to specific behaviors) of the behaviors that will be targeted during treatment [10]. These data are integrated with information about the patient's pathophysiology to set realistic expectations for physical functioning [9].

Following a thorough behavioral analysis, operant conditioning strategies can be used to decrease pain behaviors and increase well behaviors to work toward functional goals that have been set within the parameters of the patient's upper limits of functioning. For instance, maladaptive pain behaviors can be reduced or extinguished by removing the environmental contingencies (positive and negative reinforcers) associated with these behaviors. To accomplish this goal, a high degree of control is generally needed over the patient's environment. Consequently, treatment is typically most effective when it includes spouses or family members, because these individuals are often the ones providing various forms of reinforcement for patients' pain behaviors. Early stages of treatment frequently involve educating patients and significant people in their lives about pain behaviors and asking these significant others to ignore pain behaviors and reinforce competing well behaviors (such as activity, exercise, and expressions of confidence). Patients and their spouses/family members may also be asked to keep logs of pain behaviors and responses to these behaviors to track progress and raise awareness of the connection between patients' behaviors and the responses they receive from the environment [11].

Another way to weaken the association between pain behaviors and environmental contingencies is to work toward making behaviors time contingent rather than reinforcement contingent. For instance, a common problem among persons with chronic pain is taking pain medications in response to pain sensations rather than at regularly spaced intervals (which can provide greater overall pain control). From an operant conditioning perspective, it is easy to understand how this pattern of behaviors develops; the relief provided by the medication becomes a negative reinforcer for medication-taking behavior, thereby increasing the likelihood that an individual will engage in this behavior in the future. One way to modify this pattern is to establish a schedule whereby patients take pain medication at predetermined times during the day, as opposed to in response to pain sensations or experience, so that taking the medication becomes independent of current pain intensity. A time-contingent approach can also be used to reduce potentially maladaptive resting behaviors in response to pain. Patients can be encouraged to rest at regular intervals of time to pace their activity level appropriately, instead of resting primarily in response to pain. A time-contingent resting schedule can weaken the contingency-based association between pain and resting and can facilitate the replacement of a maladaptive strategy (pain-contingent resting) with a more adaptive behavior (activity pacing).

Operant conditioning can also be used in several ways to increase the frequency of well behaviors. Patients can be provided with positive reinforcement for engaging in well behaviors, and these behaviors can be shaped toward specific goals. Shaping involves graded tasks that successively approximate a target behavioral goal, coupled with positive reinforcement for meeting incremental goals. For example, if a treatment goal is to increase a patient's tolerance for exercise from 10 minutes to 30 minutes, the patient might initially be asked to exercise for 10 minutes a day and be given positive reinforcement for engaging in this behavior. At specific intervals (eg, a specific number of days), the length of time spent exercising is increased by predetermined increments (eg, a specific number of minutes) and is accompanied by additional positive reinforcement. This graded activity schedule, accompanied by positive reinforcement, is continued until the patient reaches the established goal. During the early stages of treatment, reinforcement is typically given in response to well behaviors on a consistent and regular basis. As well behaviors increase over time, reinforcement can be given on a more intermittent schedule (eg, 50% of the time) [10].

In general, operant behavioral therapy for chronic pain typically is most appropriate when a number of conditions are satisfied [9,10]. First, the patient should exhibit overt pain behaviors. Because the operant approach focuses on altering contingencies for specific maladaptive behaviors that are observable and measurable, if such behaviors are not clearly evident, the treatment may be difficult to implement. Second, meaningful positive and negative reinforcers must be identified, otherwise it will be difficult to create a behavioral contingency program. Third, there must be sufficient control over the patient's environment to modify effectively salient behavioral contingencies. It can be challenging to alter behavioral contingencies if significant persons in the patient's life are not involved in treatment. Any efforts made to change behavioral contingencies on the part of the clinician may be undermined if prior contingencies that perpetuate maladaptive behaviors continue in the home or other settings. Fourth, patients who have severe nonmedication-related cognitive-learning impairments may not be suitable for this treatment approach. Fifth, patients must be actively willing to engage in this treatment approach, because behavior change is unlikely to occur unless patients are motivated to participate in and adhere to the treatment protocol. Finally, high levels of ongoing identifiable nociception are a contraindication for this approach and should be treated with the appropriate medical intervention [9]. An operant approach is most appropriate when pain behaviors are judged to be in excess of what would be expected given the findings from physical/medical evaluation [10].

Empirical research provides support for operant behavioral treatments for chronic pain. A recent meta-analysis of randomized controlled trials of behavioral therapies for chronic pain found that treatments based on an operant approach had a significant effect when compared with wait list control conditions in reducing overt pain behaviors, subjective experiences of pain, interference with social role functioning, and difficulties with mood/affect other than depression (eg, anxiety) [5]. Operant-based treatments were also found to have a significant effect on reducing overt pain behaviors and interference with social role functioning when compared with active treatment control conditions [5]. Although the number of behavioral studies that met inclusion criteria for the meta-analysis was small, the results provide support for the operant model of chronic pain by demonstrating that operant behavioral treatments for chronic pain have a significant impact on the display of overt pain behaviors.

The operant model and operant treatment approaches for pain have the potential to be appropriate for all four of the clinical cases described in the introductory article to this issue. Although patients with neuropathic pain (Cases 1 and 2) often tend to respond better to biomedically based interventions, an assessment of the potential role that operant issues are playing in each patient's pain problem is indicated. To what extent are the pain complaints linked to the presence or absence of specific individuals? If pain intensity ratings are systematically higher in the presence of a spouse or family member, this particular individual may be inadvertently reinforcing the patient's pain complaints and perhaps even the patient's actual experience of pain. Additionally, in the absence of ongoing injury, the natural course of most pain problems is to improve rather than worsen. Evidence for increases in pain intensity and behaviors over time, as was reported in Case 3, is consistent with the presence of ongoing reinforcers for pain and illness behaviors, suggesting that this patient might benefit from an operant approach.

Operant principles can be incorporated into work in a rehabilitation setting with patients who experience chronic pain and exhibit pain behaviors that interfere with functioning in several ways. Physiatrists and members of the rehabilitation team can avoid reinforcing pain behaviors (eg, guarding, wincing) during medical appointments or treatment sessions. In contrast, reinforcement, often in the form of praise, should be provided in response to displays of well behaviors (eg, efforts to increase activity levels or to return to prior levels of functioning). These objectives can be reinforced by not focusing on pain intensity when interviewing patients but instead focusing on activity levels and attempts or plans to get reactivated. Physical and occupational therapy treatment protocols can be planned using a graded task approach so that pain-related well behaviors can be shaped toward target functional goals over time. Whenever possible, spouses, family members, or significant persons in patients' lives should be included in treatment and encouraged to reinforce any attempts by patients to become more active and functional. Medical providers can also establish and recommend time-contingent pain medication dosing schedules to help avoid the development of pain-contingent medication use patterns.

Clearly, the rehabilitation team will have greater control over pain-related behavioral contingencies in inpatient settings. In such cases, it may be most helpful for team members to work together when implementing a pain management intervention so that all members of the team apply behavioral contingencies consistently. When working with patients in an outpatient setting, it may be helpful to coordinate with other treatment providers around pain management issues to help ensure consistency across providers. Referral to a structured multidisciplinary pain treatment program that includes operant behavioral therapy may be indicated in some cases where such consistency cannot be established. A more detailed account of the use of an operant approach to treating chronic pain has been described by Sanders [10].

Cognitive-behavioral therapy

The cognitive-behavioral model of chronic pain takes into account the complex interactions among the cognitive, behavioral, affective, social, and sensory-physical aspects of the pain experience [9]. This model acknowledges the important roles that learning and behavior (eg, environmental responses to pain behaviors) play in patient functioning but also argues that cognitions (eg, attributions, beliefs) can enhance or interfere with effective behavioral coping. For example, patients who believe that there is nothing they can do to help manage their pain are thought to be unlikely to engage in adaptive pain management strategies or to make efforts to learn such strategies. The findings from numerous studies of persons with chronic pain indicate that individuals' beliefs about pain are associated with various indices of functioning [12]. Research also supports the hypothesis that changes in patients' beliefs about pain are associated with changes in functioning [13,14], consistent with the hypothesis that patient cognitions play a key role in adjustment to chronic pain.

Cognitive-behavioral treatments for chronic pain aim to assist individuals in addressing beliefs about pain that may interfere with functioning or adjustment, as well as learning effective strategies for managing stress and pain. A hallmark of this approach is that individuals are taught new coping skills so that, over time, they become able to manage pain-related difficulties on their own. Although reductions in pain intensity may occur in response to treatment, the primary objective of cognitive-behavioral treatments for pain is to enhance patients' abilities to self-manage pain-related difficulties and to increase functioning and well-being. Patients are frequently given exercises or assignments to work on between treatment sessions to reinforce skill development, to provide "real world" practice of the skills learned, and to enhance self-efficacy related to using the skills they have learned. Early stages of treatment typically focus on education about the treatment approach and skill acquisition, whereas later stages of treatment tend to focus on skill rehearsal, generalization, and maintenance [9].

Cognitive-behavioral treatments for chronic pain can include a wide range of cognitive and behaviorally focused interventions. Cognitively focused interventions typically involve teaching patients how to identify their thoughts and beliefs about pain, how to evaluate whether these cognitions are accurate or helpful, and how to change inaccurate or unhelpful cognitions into ones that are more accurate and balanced [15,16]. This process, often referred to as cognitive restructuring, also involves educating patients about the various ways that thoughts and beliefs about pain can influence the experience of pain as well as the adjustment to pain (eg, pain-related distress, pain-related interference with functioning). Patients are often asked to monitor their thoughts about pain to observe any patterns or themes in their thinking and then to look for evidence from their lives regarding the accuracy of their pain-related cognitions. Patients are taught to develop more adaptive balanced cognitions about pain, taking into account the evidence that supports and does not support a particular belief. Behaviorally focused interventions emphasize teaching patients adaptive coping skills that can be used to manage pain, as well as stress and distress that can exacerbate pain problems [17]. Depending on the patient's unique needs, skills training can include, but is not limited to, problem-solving skills, relaxation skills (breathing techniques and muscle relaxation training), assertiveness training, communication skills training, and exercise and activity pacing. Cognitive-behavioral treatments for chronic pain can include any combination of cognitive and behavioral interventions; therefore, this type of treatment may look somewhat different between treatment programs and providers. Nevertheless, all cognitive-behavioral treatments share a similar underlying theoretical conceptualization.

Randomized controlled trials have repeatedly shown that cognitive-behavioral treatments are effective for treating chronic pain. A recent meta-analysis of such trials found that cognitive-behavioral treatments were more efficacious than wait list control conditions for decreasing subjective experiences of pain, difficulties with mood/affect, negative cognitive coping, and interference with social role functioning, as well as for increasing positive cognitive coping and activity levels [5]. Cognitive-behavioral treatments were also found to have a significant effect on reducing subjective pain experience and overt pain behaviors and increasing positive cognitive coping when compared with active treatment control conditions [5].

The case descriptions presented in the first article in this issue do not indicate whether maladaptive patient appraisals about pain are having a negative impact on these patients' functioning or contributing to their experiences of pain and suffering over and above any effects from the injury (Cases 1, 3, and 4) or illness (Case 2) itself. Nevertheless, base rates of the occurrence of such maladaptive appraisals suggest the strong possibility that at least one of these patients, and likely more than one, have beliefs that will interfere with pain rehabilitation. To minimize the impact of such beliefs and to provide the patients with an opportunity to replace these with more adaptive ones, an assessment of the pain-related beliefs held by each of the patients described is warranted. Such assessment can be informal, such as asking the patient, "Tell me, what is your sense of what is causing your pain, and how do you see it changing over the next few months?" One should listen for responses indicating catastrophic thoughts about pain, beliefs that pain necessarily indicates physical harm, beliefs that one is disabled owing to pain, or beliefs that one cannot do anything to influence one's pain. Formal standardized measures of pain-related appraisals can also be used [18].

For patients who verbalize maladaptive thoughts/beliefs about pain, it is important to first empathize with their concerns and only then to challenge these cognitions gently. If patients' experiences are not validated before attempts are made to help them restructure unhelpful or inaccurate pain-related cognitions, this approach will likely be ineffective. Once a trusting clinical relationship is established, several strategies can be used to help patients challenge and change unhelpful or inaccurate beliefs about pain. First, patients can be asked to identify experiences from their own lives that contradict their maladaptive pain beliefs. For instance, if a patient states, "I can't do anything anymore because of this pain," he or she can be encouraged to keep a log of his or her activities for a designated period of time to determine whether this belief is accurate. Second, patients can be encouraged to change absolute statements about their pain (eg, "My pain is *always* the same." "Nothing *ever* helps to reduce my pain.") to statements that are more balanced and accurate and that take into account the fact that pain tends to fluctuate and change, even in subtle ways, over time. Patients who express these types of beliefs can be encouraged to track their pain to ascertain whether there are minor fluctuations in their pain sensations and to identify any factors that might be related to these changes. Third, patients can be encouraged to evaluate the helpfulness of their thoughts/beliefs about pain and to replace unhelpful cognitions (ie, thoughts that lead to increased distress or interfere with effective coping) with ones that are realistic but more reassuring or motivating. For example, the thought "This pain controls my life" could be changed to "I am going to continue to live my life despite this pain."

Assisting patients to restructure their unhelpful or inaccurate cognitions about pain is not simply asking them to engage in positive thinking. Patients are unlikely to believe overly positive statements or affirmations about their pain because such statements do not take into account the real challenges that patients face. Instead, patients should be encouraged to evaluate whether their thoughts and beliefs about pain are helpful and completely accurate and, if not, to work on replacing them with cognitions that are more balanced.

Regarding more behaviorally focused interventions, patients can be encouraged to use any number of coping strategies to help manage their pain, as well as any stress or distress related to the pain. These strategies can include engaging in relaxation exercises (eg, progressive muscle relaxation, breathing techniques, relaxing imagery), distracting themselves from focusing on pain by participating in enjoyable activities, scheduling activities to help promote social interaction and overall activity level, and, if medically appropriate, engaging in various forms of movement or exercise. When encouraging patients to use various behavioral coping strategies, it is important to set goals that are easily attainable so that patients can experience a sense of accomplishment and increased self-efficacy. This approach will not only increase the likelihood that patients will continue to use such strategies but will also help to challenge inaccurate or unhelpful cognitions that patients may hold about pain or themselves as persons who experience pain.

Although some patients may respond to the cognitive-behavioral interventions described herein, when implemented in the clinician's office, others may require a referral to a more structured cognitive-behavioral pain treatment program. The latter may be more appropriate for individuals whose maladaptive beliefs about pain are more strongly held, or who need more in-depth coping skills training. Readers are referred to the books by Turk [17], Thorn [15], and Winterowd and coworkers [16] for detailed descriptions of prototypical cognitive-behavioral interventions for chronic pain.

Hypnotic analgesia

There has recently been increased interest in hypnotic analgesia, or the use of hypnosis and hypnotic suggestions to reduce or alter pain sensations. This increased interest may be due in part to emergent evidence for the specific effects of hypnotic analgesia on neurophysiologic measures of pain processing from recent brain imaging studies. Using positron-emission tomography (PET) scans, Rainville and colleagues [19] found that changes in the affective dimension of pain in response to suggestions for decreased "pain unpleasantness" were associated with changes in cortical limbic regional activity (anterior cingulate cortical area 24). The results of another study, also using PET scans, indicated that reductions in activity in the somatosensory cortex were evident following suggestions for decreased pain [20]. These studies provide evidence that hypnotic analgesia does not merely alter self-reported pain but produces measurable changes in brain activity linked to pain experience, making the effects of hypnotic analgesia seem more "real" to skeptics. At the same time, recent controlled trials indicate that hypnotic analgesia interventions can significantly reduce health care costs (eg, reduced hospital time) associated with various medical procedures [21].

Hypnosis has a lengthy history within the medical field, particularly with regard to the treatment of pain. Although definitions of hypnosis vary, Barber [22] describes hypnosis as "an altered condition or state of consciousness characterized by marked increased receptivity to suggestion, the capacity for modification of perception and memory, and the potential for systematic control of a variety of usually involuntary physiologic functions (such as glandular activity, vasomotor activity, etc)." Hypnotic analgesia interventions seek to capitalize on this increased receptivity to suggestion and capacity for modifying perception by providing individuals with suggestions for decreased pain sensations and increased feelings of comfort to alter an individual's perceptions and experiences of pain.

In general, hypnotic analgesia sessions include three primary stages: (1) hypnotic induction, (2) suggestions for analgesia, and (3) arousal. The hypnotic induction serves as a transition from a normal waking state to a hypnotic state. For theorists who do not view hypnosis as involving a change in state of consciousness, the induction can be thought of as a situation in which the patient becomes more willing and able to respond to suggestions. To bring this about, the clinician usually engages the patient's attention and interest and encourages the individual to focus his or her range of attention on a particular stimuli (eg, the sound of the clinician's voice or a particular mental image). A common hypnotic induction technique involves the clinician counting from 1 to 10 while having the patient imagine that he or she is walking down a flight of stairs and becoming more relaxed and comfortable with each step downward [23].

After the induction, the clinician offers a variety of hypnotic suggestions directed at changing or eliminating the patient's painful sensations or altering how these sensations are perceived. Hypnotic analgesia suggestions can include the following [24]:

Reduction of pain intensity—having the patient imagine that the intensity of the sensory component of his or her pain is decreasing

Decreased unpleasantness—suggesting that the affective component of pain is separate from the sensory component of pain and that painful sensations do not have to be interpreted as unpleasant or bothersome

Sensory substitution—asking the patient to imagine that a painful or uncomfortable sensation is replaced by a sensation that is more tolerable and less distressing (eg, replacing a hot burning sensation with a sensation of cold)

Displacement of pain—suggesting that a localized painful sensation move from an area of the body where the patient perceives the pain as intolerable to a location in the body where the individual can better tolerate feelings of pain (eg, from the central part of the body to an extremity)

Posthypnotic suggestions can also be given with the intent of extending any changes or reductions in pain sensations (eg, suggestions for pain relief to continue for longer and longer periods of time or that it will become easier and easier for the patient to use hypnotic analgesia strategies).

The final component of hypnotic analgesia treatment involves assisting the patient to transition back into a normal waking state. Often, this is achieved by the use of phrases and images that are the reverse of those used during hypnotic induction, such as having an individual imagine that he or she is becoming increasingly alert as the clinician counts backward from 10 to 1.

Several randomized controlled trials have been conducted to evaluate the efficacy of hypnotic analgesia in treating a wide range of acute and chronic pain problems (for a comprehensive review of these studies, see the article by Patterson and Jensen [25]). Acute pain studies, which comprise the majority of such clinical trials, have focused primarily on pain secondary to a variety of invasive medical procedures (eg, surgery, burn care, bone marrow aspirations) as well as childbirth. Overall, the findings from these studies indicate that hypnotic analgesia is typically superior to control conditions (ie, no treatment, standard care, attention control) and often superior to other psychologic interventions (eg, cognitive-behavioral therapy, relaxation training, and emotional support) for treating acute pain [25].

Considerably fewer randomized controlled trials have examined the use of hypnotic analgesia for treating persons with chronic pain problems. Of those that have, most have examined chronic headache pain, although a few have focused on other chronic pain conditions (eg, cancer pain, fibromyalgia, back pain). The findings from these studies indicate that hypnotic analgesia is generally superior to a variety of control conditions. When compared with other viable treatment conditions, hypnotic analgesia has frequently been found to be comparably effective in treating chronic pain, particularly when compared with treatments with shared characteristics (ie, relaxation and autogenic training) [25]. None of the chronic pain controlled trials has found hypnotic analgesia to be less effective than other treatment conditions. One possible explanation for the fact that few studies have found hypnotic analgesia to be superior to other psychologic interventions for chronic pain is that such studies may not take into consideration the complex nature of chronic pain and its treatment [25]. Suggestions for how to address this issue have included: (1) incorporating hypnotic analgesia into multidisciplinary chronic pain treatment programs; (2) including hypnotic suggestions that target the sensory (ie, painful sensations) and affective (ie, pain-related suffering) components of chronic pain; and (3) teaching self-hypnotic skills that can be used over the long term [25].

Although no randomized controlled trials have been published regarding the use of hypnotic analgesia to treat chronic pain in persons with disabilities, data from a recent case series suggest that the intervention may be effective for this purpose. Jensen and coworkers [26] reported findings from 33 individuals with chronic pain secondary to a disability (ie, spinal cord injury, multiple sclerosis, amputation, cerebral palsy, post polio syndrome, or Charcot-Marie-Tooth disease) who received 10 sessions of hypnotic analgesia training. The results indicated a significant pre- to posttreatment reduction in average pain intensity and ratings of pain unpleasantness (both assessed on a 0 to 10 numeric rating scale) that was maintained at 3-month follow-up. Although a randomized controlled trial is needed to replicate the findings, these results suggest that hypnotic analgesia may hold promise for treating chronic pain secondary to a variety of physical disabilities.

Clinical lore suggests that hypnotic analgesia is more effective for focal pain problems, such as many neuropathic pain conditions, than for diffuse musculoskeletal pain. Based on this observation alone, one might expect the patients described in the clinical case vignettes with neuropathic pain (Cases 1 and 2) to benefit more from a trial of hypnotic analgesia than would the patients with musculoskeletal pain or fibromyalgia (Cases 3 and 4). Nevertheless, strong empirical evidence for the differential effect of hypnotic analgesia on different pain conditions has not been presented. Until then, and to the extent that a reduction in perceived pain intensity or an increase in the patient's sense of control over pain is the treatment goal, each of the four cases would deserve a trial of self-hypnosis training. Although hypnosis has traditionally been viewed as an "intervention" as opposed to a self-management approach, in fact, the successful application of hypnotic analgesia requires significant patient cooperation and usually involves practice for patients to learn to apply self-hypnosis to their particular pain problem.

Conducting hypnotic analgesia interventions requires specialized training in hypnosis and related techniques. As a result, persons with pain secondary to a disability who might benefit from, and are open to, this form of treatment should be referred to a qualified provider. Whenever possible, this individual should have experience working with rehabilitation populations and should be knowledgeable about the kinds of pain problems that can develop secondary to physical and neurologic conditions. After a referral for hypnotic analgesia treatment has been made, it is recommended that the referring provider remain in regular contact with the hypnotherapist to ensure continuity of care and to address any medical or functional concerns that might have an important bearing on the treatment.

Although in many instances the hypnotherapist will be someone outside the rehabilitation team, treating physiatrists and members of the rehabilitation team can have an important role in preparing patients for hypnotic analgesia treatment. In particular, it may be helpful for a member of the rehabilitation team to talk with patients about their attitudes and beliefs about hypnosis before making a referral for hypnotic analgesia treatment. Many individuals have inaccurate perceptions of hypnosis based on information from the media or experiences of witnessing hypnosis conducted as entertainment (eg, that hypnosis involves being under someone else's control, produces complete amnesia for the period of time one is hypnotized, or can be done against one's will). As a result, it may be necessary to debunk any inaccurate perceptions about hypnosis and to assess any other potential obstacles to patients engaging in the treatment (eg, some individuals may have spiritual or religious beliefs that would preclude them from participating in treatments involving hypnosis). Of course, doing this necessitates that team members themselves become familiar with the data regarding hypnotic analgesia and evaluate their own beliefs and attitudes about hypnosis.

Interested individuals are referred to the book by Barber [22] for an introduction to hypnotic analgesia and overview of its specific applications to a range of pain problems, as well as the article by Patterson and Jensen [25] for a review of the empirical research in this area.

Motivational interviewing

Although numerous studies have documented the efficacy of a variety of treatments for chronic pain, including those described previously, not everyone who receives these treatments improves or maintains treatment gains over the long term [27,28]. Motivation may have an important role in whether people benefit from chronic pain treatments [29,30]. Interventions for chronic pain typically require patients to learn and implement a set of pain-related coping and self-management skills, the acquisition of which involves making numerous behavioral changes. Given that motivation plays a key role in whether people make and follow through with behavioral changes, the pain management field has become increasingly focused on methods for increasing patient motivation and readiness to change to maximize the effects of existing treatments [29–31].

Motivational interviewing [32,33] is a therapeutic approach designed to increase motivation, or "the probability that a person will enter into, continue, and adhere to a specific change strategy" [32]. An underlying assumption of this approach is that people typically have the skills needed to engage in adaptive behaviors but may lack motivation to do so. The role of the clinician is to provide a therapeutic environment that increases patient motivation to make behavioral changes. This environment is accomplished via a set of therapeutic responses geared toward helping patients address and resolve feelings of ambivalence about making positive behavioral changes. Although the ultimate responsibility for making changes lies with the patient, from a motivational interviewing perspective, the clinician's behaviors play an integral role in developing and maintaining patient motivation [29].

There are five basic principles of motivational interviewing that guide clinician behaviors when working with patients [29,32]. First, expressing empathy involves conveying respect and acceptance of the patient by seeking to understand the patient's perspective and reflecting this understanding back to the patient. In this way, the clinician adopts a nonjudgmental stance that often frees patients to make behavioral changes. Second, the clinician seeks to develop a discrepancy between the patient's current behaviors and his or her important life goals. Instead of confronting the patient, the clinician seeks to raise the patient's awareness of these discrepancies by listening for statements that express these discrepancies, reflecting these statements back to the patient, and encouraging him or her to elaborate on these statements. Third, the clinician avoids argumentation whenever possible, because this approach typically reduces the likelihood that patients will engage in behavior change. More specifically, if a clinician argues for a specific change, this often elicits an argument from the patient against the recommended change, particularly if the patient is not yet ready to make such a change. Fourth, a clinician working within a motivational interviewing framework rolls with resistance, meaning that he or she switches strategies as needed to avoid argumentation. This tactic might involve taking a different approach to interacting with the patient, such as reframing or restating something the patient has said to convey an understanding of the patient's perspective. Such an approach helps to ensure that the clinician and the patient remain on the same "side" of the discussion, rather than creating opposition between the clinician and patient. Finally, the clinician attempts to support self-efficacy, or the patient's belief in his or her ability to do a specific task or behavior. This support can be accomplished by making statements and asking questions that increase the patient's feelings of hope and optimism that it is possible to make the desired change.

The motivational interviewing approach assumes that people differ with respect to the degree to which they are ready to engage in adaptive behavioral changes and is consistent with a previously developed model of stages of behavioral change [34]. This model purports that when people change from maladaptive to adaptive behaviors, they move through a series of stages, each accompanied by specific challenges that must be overcome before moving onto the next stage. These stages include precontemplation, contemplation, preparation, action, maintenance, and possibly relapse. During the precontemplation stage, an individual is not considering making any behavioral change and is often resistant to change when suggested by others. The contemplation stage involves recognizing a problem or a need to change, actively thinking about making a change, and weighing the pros and cons of changing behavior. The preparation stage involves making a commitment to change and taking the initial steps toward behavior change. After making this commitment, the individual enters the action stage. During this stage, the individual engages in specific behaviors that are consistent with the desired change. An individual in the maintenance stage works on continuing with any changes made during the action stage. If an individual is not able to sustain these changes over time, he or she enters the relapse stage and can re-enter the stages of change at any point.

Given that a particular patient may be in any of one these stages of change when presenting for treatment, assessing his or her readiness to change in relation to a specific behavior or problem is integral to the success of motivational strategies. Indeed, a primary goal of this approach is to "meet the patient where he or she is at" by matching an intervention to an individual's particular stage of change. For instance, it would not be helpful to develop a plan for behavioral change with a patient who is in the precontemplation stage; doing so would likely generate resistance on the part of the patient and undermine the clinician's goals of assisting the patient in making desired changes. Instead, clinicians can target their interventions to address the specific challenges inherent in a particular stage of change to maximize the likelihood that the patient will progress to the next stage.

The timing of motivational interventions is important for facilitating behavior change. Consequently, the clinician's goals will differ depending on a patient's stage of change [29,33]. For a patient in the precontemplation stage, the clinician attempts to raise doubt by increasing the patient's awareness of the risks and problems associated with current behaviors. During the contemplation stage, the clinician seeks to "tip the balance" by eliciting statements from the patient about the reasons to change and the costs associated with not changing, as well as strengthening the patient's sense of self-efficacy that change is possible. Clinician goals during the preparation stage include assisting the patient in determining the most appropriate course of action to bring about the desired behavioral changes. During the action stage, the clinician helps the patient make steps toward change, whereas clinician goals for the maintenance stage include reviewing progress and helping to renew motivation and commitment to change as needed. If a patient relapses into prior maladaptive behaviors, the clinician reviews with the patient the process of contemplation, preparation, and action to determine how to address obstacles that might have led to relapse. The clinician also helps the patient from becoming overly discouraged in response to relapse by indicating that making behavioral changes often requires multiple attempts.

Motivational interviewing was initially developed to address problems related to addiction and substance use [32]. Because these intervention strategies focus on enhancing motivation to change behaviors and not on a specific type of problem or disorder (eg, substance use), they also have been used to address an array of physical and mental health problems that involve behavioral components. A recent meta-analysis of controlled trials of motivational interviewing and adaptations of this treatment indicates that this approach has shown a significant effect for problems involving alcohol use, drug use, exercise, diet, and several physiologic indicators (ie, total blood cholesterol, systolic blood pressure) [35,36]. A unique strength of motivational interviewing interventions is that they can be effective even when they are brief. Meta-analytic findings indicate that motivational interviewing interventions as brief as 15 to 20 minutes can have a significant effect on patient outcomes [36]. Additionally, psychologists and physicians have obtained effects using motivational interviewing strategies in the majority of controlled trials conducted by these professionals [36], suggesting that these interventions may have wide-ranging applications within the health care field.

To date, only one published study has examined the efficacy of a motivational interviewing approach for addressing chronic pain problems [37]. In that study, 78 persons with chronic pain were randomly assigned to a two-session intervention or control condition. The intervention condition consisted of one assessment session and one feedback session that were both conducted using a motivational interviewing approach. These sessions focused on readiness to engage in self-management strategies for pain and sought to increase the participant's motivation to engage in these strategies. In contrast, the first session of the control condition consisted of a "treatment as usual" pain assessment, and the second session involved feedback about this assessment. At the end of the second session in both conditions, participants were offered the opportunity to participate in a series of pain management workshops that focused on a variety of pain self-management topics (ie, exercise, activity pacing, relaxation, cognitive strategies, and medication use). The results indicated that participants in the motivational interviewing condition were significantly more likely to attend the pain management workshops than were participants in the control condition (74% versus 41%). Moreover, participation in the pain management workshops was unrelated to any of the other pretreatment factors assessed (eg, a variety of demographic, medical, and psychologic variables), suggesting that the motivational interviewing intervention was a primary factor that influenced subsequent participation in the pain management program. The results of this study provide preliminary and promising support that motivational interviewing may be useful in increasing the likelihood that persons with chronic pain will engage in pain management treatment.

Motivational interviewing strategies are particularly appropriate when the patient needs to engage in a specific behavior to improve (eg, start and maintain a regular exercise program, manage his or her diet to lose weight, take a specific medication regimen as prescribed), yet the patient may be ambivalent about that behavior. Determining whether this applies to any one of the patient cases described in the introductory article requires, first, a specific treatment plan and, second, some indication that the patient is less than enthusiastic about following through with this plan. Of the four cases described, the patient with fibromyalgia (Case 3) is most likely to meet these criteria. Current standards of fibromyalgia treatment include participation in a regular exercise program, yet many patients with fibromyalgia find that exercise can result in significant discomfort, at least in the short term.

Because making behavioral changes is an important component of pain rehabilitation, a motivational interviewing approach is a natural complement to the interventions used to address chronic pain problems. Rehabilitation professionals can use several simple motivational strategies in their work with patients to address pain problems. One can begin a dialog with patients about their readiness to change a particular behavior related to chronic pain (eg, participating in an exercise program) by asking patients to rate how important it is to them to work toward a specific pain management goal, and how confident they are that they will be able to succeed in making a change if they chose to do so (ratings are made on a scale of 0 to 10). Clinicians can then ask patients to discuss why they are at a particular point along each continuum and not at a lower level, as well as what would need to happen in order for them to perceive the goal as being more important or to feel more confident about their ability to make a change [38]. In doing so, patients will naturally discuss: (1) the reasons they might have for engaging in the new adaptive response, (2) the reasons why they believe engaging in that response is possible for them, and (3) a tentative plan for making an important behavioral change. This straightforward method for eliciting "change talk" leads to increased motivation and opportunities for adaptive behavior change [33].

Another strategy for enhancing patient motivation involves offering patients a number of options for ways to address a particular problem. Offering patients choices when discussing behavioral changes can empower them and provide them with a greater sense of control, enhancing their commitment to change. This approach also avoids the common scenario of the clinician suggesting a specific course of action and eliciting resistance in a patient who is not ready to make a particular change. Additionally, clinicians should avoid lecturing, arguing, or engaging in power struggles with patients about pain-related issues whenever possible, because each of these behaviors are likely to reduce patient motivation to change. If the clinician realizes that he or she is engaging in any of these behaviors, he or she should switch gears and engage in empathic listening and reflecting to convey an understanding of the patient's experience and to strengthen rapport with the patient. Listening is a cornerstone of the motivational approach and can provide the clinician with useful information about whether patients are ready to change, what they value, and why they might want to change. All of this information can be used to bolster patient readiness to change and their motivation to make and maintain pain-related behavioral changes. More detailed descriptions of specific motivational interventions that can be used during different stages of change have been outlined by Miller and Rollnick [33] and further elaborated by Jensen [29] with respect to addressing chronic pain problems specifically.

Summary

As a biopsychosocial understanding of chronic pain has become more sophisticated during recent decades, a variety of psychologically based treatment approaches have been developed and empirically validated for helping people better manage their pain. These approaches to pain management have much to offer persons with chronic pain in terms of enhancing quality of life and pain-related coping, as well as reducing disability and pain-related interference with functioning. Although some treatments, like hypnotic analgesia, may require referral to a specialized provider, several of the principles of other psychologically based treatment approaches for pain management (eg, operant behavioral therapy, cognitive-behavioral therapy, motivational interviewing) can easily be integrated into work with persons with pain in a rehabilitation setting. Rehabilitation providers who are interested in incorporating these treatment strategies into their clinical work who do not have prior exposure to these approaches are encouraged to review the suggested references and to seek out related training opportunities.

References

[1] Novy DM, Nelson DV, Francis DJ, et al. Perspectives of chronic pain: an evaluative comparison of restrictive and comprehensive models. Psychol Bull 1995;118(2):238–47.
[2] Loeser JD. What is chronic pain? Theor Med 1991;12:213–25.
[3] Turk DC, Monarch ES. Biopsychosocial perspective on chronic pain. In: Turk DC, Gatchel RJ, editors. Psychological approaches to pain management: a practitioner's handbook. 2nd edition. New York: Guilford Press; 2002. p. 3–29.
[4] Turk DC, Gatchel RJ, editors. Psychological approaches to pain management: a practitioner's handbook. 2nd edition. New York: Guilford Press; 2002.
[5] Morley S, Eccleston C, Williams A. Systematic review and meta-analysis of randomized controlled trials of cognitive behaviour therapy and behaviour therapy for chronic pain in adults, excluding headache. Pain 1999;80(1–2):1–13.
[6] Loeser JD. Multidisciplinary pain programs. In: Loeser JD, Butler SH, Chapman CR, et al, editors. Bonica's management of pain. 3rd edition. Philadelphia: Lippincott, Williams, & Wilkins; 2001. p. 255–64.
[7] Fordyce WE. Behavioral methods for chronic pain and illness. St.Louis: Mosby Year Book; 1976.
[8] Fordyce WE, Fowler RS Jr, Lehmann JF, et al. Some implications of learning in problems of chronic pain. J Chronic Dis 1968;21(3):179–90.
[9] Novy D. Psychological approaches for managing chronic pain. J Psychopath Behav Assess 2004;26(4):279–88.
[10] Sanders SH. Operant conditioning with chronic pain: back to basics. In: Turk DC, Gatchel RJ, editors. Psychological approaches to pain management: a practitioner's handbook. 2nd edition. New York: Guilford Press; 2002. p. 128–37.
[11] Roelofs J, Boissevain MD, Peters ML, et al. Psychological treatments for chronic low back pain: past, present and beyond. Pain Rev 2002;9:29–40.
[12] Jensen MP, Turner JA, Romano JM, et al. Coping with chronic pain: a critical review of the literature. Pain 1991;47(3):249–83.
[13] Jensen MP, Romano JM, Turner JA, et al. Patient beliefs predict patient functioning: further support for a cognitive-behavioural model of chronic pain. Pain 1999;81(1–2):95–104.
[14] Moseley GL. Evidence for a direct relationship between cognitive and physical change during an education intervention in people with chronic low back pain. Eur J Pain 2004;8(1): 39–45.
[15] Thorn BE. Cognitive therapy for chronic pain. New York: Guilford Press; 2004.
[16] Winterowd C, Beck AT, Gruener D. Cognitive therapy with chronic pain patients. New York: Springer Publishing; 2003.
[17] Turk DC. A cognitive-behavioral perspective on treatment of chronic pain patients. In: Turk DC, Gatchel RJ, editors. Psychological approaches to pain management: a practitioner's handbook. 2nd edition. New York: Guilford Press; 2002. p. 138–58.
[18] DeGood DE, Tait RC. Assessment of pain beliefs and pain coping. In: Turk DC, Melzack RD, editors. Handbook of pain assessment. 2nd edition. New York: Guilford Press; 2001. p. 320–45.
[19] Rainville P, Duncan GH, Price DD, et al. Pain affect encoded in human anterior cingulate but not somatosensory cortex. Science 1997;277(5328):968–71.

[20] Hofbauer RK, Rainville P, Duncan GH, et al. Cortical representation of the sensory dimension of pain. J Neurophysiol 2001;86(1):402–11.
[21] Lang EV, Benotsch EG, Fick LJ, et al. Adjunctive non-pharmacological analgesia for invasive medical procedures: a randomised trial. Lancet 2000;355(9214):1486–90.
[22] Barber J. Hypnosis and suggestion in the treatment of pain: a clinical guide. New York: WW Norton & Company; 1996.
[23] Barber J. Rapid induction analgesia: a clinical report. Am J Clin Hypn 1977;19(3):138–45.
[24] Barber J. Hypnotic analgesia: mechanisms of action and clinical applications. In: Price DD, Bushnell MC, editors. Progress in pain research and management, vol. 29. Seattle (WA): IASP Press; 2004. p. 269–300.
[25] Patterson DR, Jensen MP. Hypnosis and clinical pain. Psychol Bull 2003;129(4):495–521.
[26] Jensen MP, Hanley MA, Engel JM, et al. Hypnotic analgesia for chronic pain in persons with disabilities: a case series. Int J Clin Exp Hypn 2005;53(2):198–228.
[27] Turk DC. Customizing treatment for chronic pain patients: who, what, and why. Clin J Pain 1990;6(4):255–70.
[28] Turk DC, Rudy TE. Neglected topics in the treatment of chronic pain patients: relapse, noncompliance, and adherence enhancement. Pain 1991;44:5–28.
[29] Jensen MP. Enhancing motivation to change in pain treatment. In: Turk DC, Gatchel RJ, editors. Psychological approaches to pain management: a practitioner's handbook. 2nd edition. New York: Guilford Press; 2002. p. 71–93.
[30] Jensen MP, Nielson WR, Kerns RD. Toward the development of a motivational model of pain self-management. J Pain 2003;4(9):477–92.
[31] Kerns RD, Bayer LA, Findley JC. Motivation and adherence in the management of chronic pain. In: Block AR, Kremer EF, Fernandez E, editors. Handbook of pain syndromes: biopsychosocial perspectives. Mahwah (NJ): Lawrence Erlbaum; 1999. p. 99–121.
[32] Miller WR, Rollnick S. Motivational interviewing: preparing people to change addictive behavior. New York: Guilford Press; 1991.
[33] Miller WR, Rollnick S. Motivational interviewing: preparing people for change. 2nd edition. New York: Guilford Press; 2002.
[34] DiClemente CC, Prochaska JO. Self-change and therapy change of smoking behavior: a comparison of processes of change in cessation and maintenance. Addict Behav 1982; 7(2):133–42.
[35] Burke BL, Arkowitz H, Menchola M. The efficacy of motivational interviewing: a meta-analysis of controlled clinical trials. J Consult Clin Psychol 2003;71(5):843–61.
[36] Rubak S, Sandbaek A, Lauritzen T, et al. Motivational interviewing: a systematic review and meta-analysis. Br J Gen Pract 2005;55(513):305–12.
[37] Habib S, Morrissey S, Helmes E. Preparing for pain management: a pilot study to enhance engagement. J Pain 2005;6(1):48–54.
[38] Rollnick S. Readiness, importance, and confidence: critical conditions of change in treatment. In: Miller WR, Heather N, editors. Treating addictive behaviors. 2nd edition. New York: Plenum Press; 1998. p. 49–60.

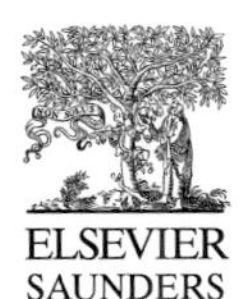
ELSEVIER
SAUNDERS

Phys Med Rehabil Clin N Am
17 (2006) 435–450

PHYSICAL MEDICINE
AND REHABILITATION
CLINICS OF
NORTH AMERICA

Multidisciplinary and Interdisciplinary Management of Chronic Pain

Steven Stanos, DO[a,b,*], Timothy T. Houle, PhD[c]

[a]*Department of Physical Medicine and Rehabilitation, Northwestern University, Feinberg Medical School, Ward Building, 3-130, 303 E. Chicago Avenue, Chicago, IL 60611, USA*

[b]*Chronic Pain Care Center, Rehabilitation Institute of Chicago, 1030 N. Clark, Suite 320-D, Chicago, IL 60610, USA*

[c]*Department of Anesthesiology, Wake Forest University School of Medicine, Wake Forest University Health Sciences, Medical Center Boulevard, Winston-Salem, NC 27157, USA*

The cost of chronic pain and related impairment and disability ranges from $70 to $120 billion dollars annually. Population studies have found that persistent pain conditions are common, and that the probability of resolution after 1 year is approximately 50%, with a strong relationship between persistence of pain and the presence of a psychologic disorder [1]. A recent study found psychosocial variables to predict strongly long-term and short-term disability, health care visits in patients with low back pain, provocative diskography, and physical examination findings [2]. These data emphasize the need for consideration of a broad group of factors in treating pain.

In Case 4 in the introductory article to this issue, which particularly underscores the importance of such a broad approach, the injured worker who sustained an L1 compression fracture has no objective evidence of a "pain generator" despite ongoing subjective reports of pain and presumed affective distress and loss of quality of life. A comprehensive assessment should help to identify more appropriately causes of ongoing pain and pain-related disability. Specifically, some helpful inquiries could explore broader domains such as the patient's own cognitions, maladaptive thoughts, and expectations regarding his pain condition.

The current International Association for the Study of Pain (IASP) defines pain as "an unpleasant sensory and emotional experience associated with actual or potential tissue damage, or described in terms of such damage" [3].

* Corresponding author. Chronic Pain Care Center, Rehabilitation Institute of Chicago, 1030 N. Clark, Suite 320-D, Chicago, IL 60610.

E-mail address: sstanos@ric.org (S. Stanos).

1047-9651/06/$ - see front matter
doi:10.1016/j.pmr.2005.12.004

When compared with acute pain, chronic pain serves little to no protective homeostatic mechanism. This lack of utility underscores the importance of understanding the complex aspects of chronic pain. Often, maladaptive responses and cognitions develop in response to persistent pain, and these responses fall under the influence of factors not subsumed in the traditional biomedical model. A multidisciplinary approach seems prudent in effectively assessing and treating pain and restoring physical and psychosocial functioning after "acute" or unimodal treatments have failed.

This article focuses on understanding the complexities of the chronic pain patient, with particular emphasis on the conceptual factors related to the physical, psychologic, and social changes that may perpetuate chronic pain and disability, and the outcomes and issues related to multidisciplinary and interdisciplinary treatment programs. Effective assessment and treatment of chronic pain conditions and related suffering necessitates a thorough appreciation for this subjective multidimensional phenomenon.

Multidisciplinary treatment and the biopsychosocial model

Formal investigation into the variety of influences on pain probably began during World War II, when Beecher observed that injured soldiers removed from a fierce battle requested significantly less morphine as compared to those patients later seen in civilian practice with similar degrees of injuries. In 1959 Beecher published a landmark work describing how the contextual nature of pain or other influences could affect how pain is perceived [4]. This idea was greatly advanced with the 1965 publication of Melzack and Walls' Gate Control Theory of pain [5]. The theory championed a convergent view of pain processing, highlighting the dorsal horn as no longer a passive conduit of pain processing but a "gating" mechanism acting as an active transmission system that could inhibit or facilitate pain transmission on the basis of the pattern of afferent impulses reaching it and descending impulses from supraspinal centers. Since that time, empirical evidence has been steadily accruing illustrating what Beecher understood in 1946, that is, the perception of pain is influenced by many factors, biology being only one.

Traditional biomedical models purport that pain, like other biologically mediated phenomena, is directly related to the biology of the organism. In the case of pain, the medical model would predict that the greater the injury or nociceptive input, the greater the pain intensity experienced by the organism. Although this assumption is intuitively valid and anecdotally supported, empirical support is often limited. Knowledge of the extent or degree of sustained injury or physiologic insult remains a poor predictor of reported chronic pain. Over the past 40 years, a broader biopsychosocial model that accounts for a host of influences has been used to better account for the experience of pain [6,7].

The biopsychosocial model can be summarized as considering the bidirectional relationships among biologic (physiologic), psychologic (behavioral), and social (environmental) factors in the explanation of disease and illness [8]. This multifactorial model attempts to bridge the centuries-old gap between the mind and body, yet goes further to emphasize the importance of societal influences. The model necessitates the consideration of factors beyond the existing physiologic pathology in the study and treatment of illness.

The evolution of the biopsychosocial model has been profound. In the years since its formal inception, it has been widely used in the treatment of many disorders, including cardiovascular diseases, cancer, gastrointestinal disorders, and infectious diseases, among many others [8,9]. Use of the biopsychosocial model has advanced our understanding of the etiologies and course of many diseases, emphasizing that physiologic pathology accounts for only a portion of the relevant factors in illness.

In particular, the treatment of chronic pain has been revolutionized with application of the biopsychosocial model. Two decades of research have largely supported the utility of this approach in treating chronic pain and have led to the creation of multidisciplinary and interdisciplinary pain treatment centers on which this article is focused [10–15].

Treatment models for chronic pain: multidisciplinary versus interdisciplinary

Multidisciplinary and interdisciplinary treatment models are part of a continuum of medical care ranging from unimodal patient care to completely integrative care. These models include in order of increasing comprehensiveness and philosophical complexities: parallel, collaborative, coordinated, multidisciplinary, interdisciplinary, and integrative approaches [16]. For example, in an emergency room setting, parallel practice may be used with acute cardiac chest pain management whereby several physicians and ancillary staff provide care independently. Often, in the early management of work-related injuries, collaborative and coordinated models may include practitioners acting independently and sharing patient records, with facilitation by a case manager.

The terms *multidisciplinary* and *interdisciplinary*, although sometimes used interchangeably, represent two distinct models along a continuum of more collaborative approaches. Although the interdisciplinary approach is an extension of a more general multidisciplinary approach, both models use the biopsychosocial model to address the multifactorial causes of suffering. The next section describes the similarities and differences between the two.

Multidisciplinary pain treatment

Multidisciplinary treatment often involves one or two specialists (ie, a surgeon, pain interventionalist, and nurse) directing the services of a number of team members, often having independent goals. The concept of multidisciplinary management traces its development to the experiences of physicians working with persistent pain states following World War II. Anesthesiologist Dr. John Bonica and neurosurgeon Dr. Benjamin Crue both recognized that patients with persistent and complex pain conditions responded more ideally to a comprehensive biopsychosocial assessment and treatment delivered by several different medical specialists and health care providers. Nevertheless, a distinction can be made between the philosophies of these two revolutionary physicians.

Bonica has been described as a "peripheralist" in that he viewed chronic pain as a manifestation of peripheral input. As might be expected, this peripheral focus led to the creation of treatments primarily focused on disrupting peripheral input via surgical interventions and nerve blocks as well as incorporating behavioral treatments. In contrast, Crue has been described as a "centralist," because he emphasized the brain as the central player in pain modulation. This approach led to the creation of treatments primarily focused on psychotherapeutic approaches and unconscious emotions related to chronic pain and suffering. Both physicians were credited with the organization of pain treatment programs in the 1960s [17].

The growth of multidisciplinary pain treatment has been substantial, leading to the need for development of standards and accreditation processes. A committee on standards for pain treatment facilities was established by the American Pain Society in the early 1980s, and a process was subsequently developed to accredit multidisciplinary pain centers (MPCs) by the Commission on Accreditation of Rehabilitation Facilities (CARF). Non-CARF accredited programs also exist. Furthermore, the IASP has delineated four levels of pain programs [18]: MPCs, multidisciplinary pain clinics, pain clinics, and modality-oriented clinics. Multidisciplinary pain clinics and centers include similar clinical approaches; however, the MPCs are usually associated with major health science institutions with an additional focus on pain-related research and outcomes.

Interdisciplinary pain treatment

Incorporation of the cognitive and behavioral approaches adapted in the 1970s and 1980s led to the development of interdisciplinary models under the more general "multidisciplinary" umbrella. Interdisciplinary pain programs provide outcome-focused, coordinated, goal-oriented interdisciplinary services. The interdisciplinary model has been used effectively in several other specialties and conditions, including palliative care, anticoagulation, diabetes, and asthma management. An interdisciplinary team model is characterized by team members working together for a common goal, making collective therapeutic decisions, and having face-to-face meetings and patient team conferences to facilitate communication and consultation. Interdisciplinary teams may be led by a physician, psychologist, or nurse and include comprehensive assessment (including physical medicine, pain psychology, and vocational rehabilitation), goal setting, and treatment, usually provided in one facility. These programs have also been referred to as biopsychosocial functional restoration type programs. Work hardening/functional restoration programs are often modeled on this approach. Formal programs vary in intensities but include 3- to 8-week, 4- to 8-hours per day programs, with tailored group and individual therapies usually provided in an outpatient setting.

Multidisciplinary assessment and the chronic pain patient

Chronic pain patients are typically subject to failed interventions and therapies. As a result, the patient is frequently demoralized and turns from an active participant in their care to a more passive individual, often with great affective distress. This reaction only serves to perpetuate subjective disability and learned helplessness. If we are to treat these individuals successfully, knowledge of the issues that shape their presentation is essential. Not surprisingly, multidisciplinary treatment requires multidisciplinary assessment of potential treatment targets. The following sections describe a group of domains that should be considered in treatment planning.

The physiatric assessment

The physiatrist may serve as the team leader, assessing patients at the initial evaluation focusing on a comprehensive musculoskeletal examination including assessing compensatory postural and muscular imbalances that may help perpetuate ongoing pain and dysfunction. The physiatrist, in conjunction with the evaluating pain psychologist and vocational counselor, must also assess and document observed pain behavior and the level of affective distress, motivation, and readiness and expectancies for treatment, and discuss issues related to return to work and previous levels of functioning.

In many cases, disability behaviors are thought to be perpetuated by financial, vocational, and psychologic rewards related to not working or "being sick." This concept of "secondary gain" may be erroneously equated with malingering. In fact, it is more appropriate to relate secondary gain to more complex psychosocial issues (Box 1) [19]. The works of Gatchel, Fishbain, and Kwan have described these important related and evolving concepts of "secondary gain and loss" and "tertiary gain and loss" (Box 2) [19]. In this regard, "losses" or "gains" associated with illness and disability may affect the patient and the patient's family or work colleagues [19–22]. Examples of secondary losses are as follows [20]:

Economic loss
Loss of social relationships at work and support network
Loss of community approval
Social stigma of being disabled

Box 1. Common secondary gains

Internal

Gratification of pre-existing unresolved dependency strivings or affiliation needs
Gratification of pre-existing unresolved revengeful strivings
Attempt to elicit care giving, sympathy, and concern from family or friends
Obtain one's entitlement for years of struggling
Ability to withdraw from unpleasant/unsatisfactory life roles and responsibilities
Adoption of "sick role"
Obtaining drugs

External

Obtain financial awards associated with disability
Protection from legal obligations
Job manipulation
Vocational retraining and skill upgrade

Negative sanctions from family
Guilt over disability
Loss of recreational activities
Loss of respect from family and friends

The physiatrist must develop trust and rapport with the patient to understand barriers to recovery (ie, contentious relationships involving the family, employer, case manager, and the legal system) that may potentially lead to delay of clinical improvement and case resolution.

Although analgesic medication management is usually the initial primary focus of acute pain pharmacotherapy, a more rational polypharmacy approach is employed in an MPC model to treat more effectively the multidimensional effects of chronic pain. This approach helps to simplify and coordinate the use of a number of medications with numerous mechanisms targeted at achieving analgesia, improved mood, and restorative sleep. Medication assessment and management should also include screening for aberrant use and possible titration of opioids and other dependency producing medications when appropriate.

Psychologic assessment and psychosocial influences

The patient's affective state should be assessed thoroughly. Emotional state has been shown to be related to pain sensitivity. Specifically, anxiety

Box 2. Examples of common tertiary gains and losses

Tertiary gains

Family member caretaker
- Gratification of altruistic needs
- Means of making ill person develop dependency on caretaker
- Gain sympathy from social network over the ill family member
- Financial gain

Professional caretaker (ie, physician, nurse, case manager)
- Gratification of altruistic needs
- Admiration and respect from patients or their support groups
- Financial rewards associated with increased client pool

Tertiary losses

- Family member caregiver
  - Increased responsibilities
  - Emotional effect of experiencing suffering of a loved one
  - Financial hardship
- Professional caregiver
  - Being viewed by one's colleagues or others as dishonorable or contributing to patients disability

has been shown to increase the amount of pain experienced [23–25]. Unpleasant affective states have been found to decrease pain thresholds, whereas positive affect may increase pain thresholds [26]. Depression has been found to be highly prevalent in chronic pain patients, and it has been demonstrated that the presence of depression leads to increased disability from pain [27]. The question of whether depression is a cause or effect of chronic pain disability has been widely researched [28].

Similarly, general anxiety has been shown to affect disability from pain [29], but pain-related anxiety or fear is more predictive of disability [30]. The perceived stress level has also been shown to impact the chronic pain outcome adversely, perhaps more in fibromyalgia than other pain disorders [31]. It is important to assess other mood states such as anger and hostility, because they have been found to have a role in pain outcome, perhaps playing a substantial role in chronic low back pain [32]. The emotional state is related not only to pain sensitivity but also to perceived disability from pain.

Psychologic influences have a role in the perception of pain and in the adjustment to pain. In 1968 and 1988, Fordyce made an important distinction between pain and suffering [33,34]. His groundbreaking works have attempted to explain why certain individuals are affected more by pain and are more disabled by it. Using a behavioral framework, he described how "pain behaviors," which are indicative of suffering, could be placed under stimulus control. This concept is akin to the notion that certain pain behaviors (ie, grimacing, limping, calling in sick) can actually be rewarded or punished, increasing or decreasing their use. While evaluating a patient, careful observation of their overt pain behaviors can lead to clues as to the type of reinforcement that they are receiving in regards to their pain. The reduction of pain behaviors is often a major treatment goal, and it is essential to gather information about a patient's repertoire of responses to pain.

The patient's healthy responses to pain should also be evaluated. Many factors have been demonstrated to alleviate suffering and can be used to help patients improve their functioning. Research has shown that the use of active coping styles such as relaxation [35], problem solving [36], and guided imagery [37] predicts lower pain intensity ratings, reduces disability from pain, and improves the overall level of functioning. The daily use of coping strategies, or coping efficacy, has been shown to affect daily pain intensity or adjustment to pain [38–43]. Daily activity level has been examined as a potential factor in daily pain and mood [44]. Positive and negative mood has been shown to covary with adjustment to chronic pain [38,45]. Perceived social support has been shown to buffer the daily effects of pain on mood [45]. Less disability from pain has been found in patients who use such strategies, and the ability to function has been shown to increase with the adoption of these strategies [46].

Cognitive aspects of pain coping should also be evaluated. Pain catastrophizing is characterized as the overestimation of negative consequences of pain and the underestimation of one's ability to cope [47]. Individuals who use catastrophic cognitions report greater pain intensity and poorer adjustment to chronic pain. A relationship between pain beliefs, such as controllability and predictability of pain, and an individual's adjustment to chronic pain has also been empirically demonstrated. The concepts of perceived control and self-efficacy reflect the belief that pain can be controlled and that one actually has the ability to do so. Both of these beliefs have been shown to be predictive of a better adjustment to chronic pain and have been identified as salient targets for cognitive-behavioral interventions [36]. Recently, the concept of acceptance of pain, characterized as shifting focus from cure focused to coping focused, has been shown to predict greater adjustment to pain and less disability from it [48].

Multidisciplinary and interdisciplinary team components

Treatment teams may include a physiatrist, a physical or occupational therapist, a pain psychologist, a relaxation (biofeedback) therapist, vocational and therapeutic recreational therapists, social workers, and nurses. Therapists work "interdependently," sharing common treatment philosophies and goals fostered by ongoing communication between disciplines, leading to more effective monitoring of program progress and adjustment of patient goals. An interdisciplinary model helps facilitate a clear, concise, and consistent therapeutic message that focuses on patients' assuming a more active role in self-management, flare-up management, and exercise progression. A list of common treatment goals is presented in Box 3.

Let us consider the injured worker in Case 4 (lumbar vertebral fracture) who complains of ongoing thoracolumbar pain despite multiple interventional procedures and a number of "failed" physical therapy sessions. He is adamant that any thoracolumbar movement causes "too much pain" and is reluctant to participate in physical therapy. Ongoing relative guarding of normal spinal motion and a heightened fear of movement contribute to compensatory musculoskeletal impairments, subjective pain, and additional myofascial dysfunction. Progress in any additional active physical or occupational treatment may be limited by ongoing catastrophic thinking and increased fear avoidance related to normal spinal motion. An interdisciplinary physical therapy focus could incorporate more whole body techniques (ie, aquatic and creative movement therapies) focusing on improving upper limb and hip girdle range of motion, in turn, leading to a gradual decrease in pain-related fear and improvement in thoracolumbar motion.

Incorporating relaxation techniques (ie, deep breathing, progressive muscle relaxation) with therapeutic stretching could help the patient progress in the exercise program and improve activity tolerance. Biofeedback is a treatment that has been shown to be effective in the management of pain [49]. It helps patients become more aware of their physiologic responses to pain or other stressors. Originally thought to reduce physiologic arousal, biofeedback may primarily serve to enhance a patient's sense of self-efficacy or perceived ability to manage pain effectively. At the conclusion of formal treatment, patients should be independent, with self-management

Box 3. Team concepts of multidisciplinary and interdisciplinary treatment

Goals of treatment
Decrease pain intensity
Increase physical activity
Decrease reliance on pain medication
Improve psychosocial functioning
Return to work and previous leisure pursuits/interests
Reduce use of health care services

Commonalities of treatment
Reconceptualize patient's pain
Foster optimism and combat demoralization
Active patient participation and responsibility
Specific training in specific skills
Encourage feelings of success, self-control, and self-efficacy

techniques including a daily home exercise and aerobic program, relaxation techniques, and pacing.

Outcomes of multidisciplinary and interdisciplinary treatment

Two systematic reviews have examined the efficacy of multidisciplinary treatment programs. Flor and coworkers [13] reviewed controlled and non-controlled studies and concluded that MPCs were effective, although the methodologic quality of many of the studies was lacking. In comparison with no treatment or unimodal care, treated patients were functioning better than 75% of controls and had significant improvements regarding function, pain intensity, pain behaviors, and medical use. Cutler and coworkers [50] combined MPC treatment with other nonsurgical approaches for low back pain and concluded that MPCs were effective at returning patients to work.

A recent review of ten randomized controlled studies examined the efficacy of MPC treatment for low back pain [14]. Programs fell into two broad categories: (1) daily intensive (more than 100 hours) and (2) once- or twice-weekly programs (less than 30 hours of treatment). There was strong evidence that intensive MPCs with functional restoration improved function and decreased pain when compared with inpatient or outpatient nonmultidisciplinary treatment, yet contradictory evidence was found regarding vocational outcomes. Insurance providers have shown some reluctance to cover the cost of multidisciplinary and cognitive-behaviorally based pain treatment programs owing to apparent "lack of evidence"; however, randomized controlled trials examining cognitive-behavioral treatments have repeatedly demonstrated efficacy for chronic pain [51–53].

Return to work

Studies have suggested that patients receiving workers' compensation generally engage in more pain behavior, report higher levels of pain, and experience more pain-elated disability than do patients who do not receive compensation for their pain [54]. Psychologic variables are strong predictors of success in treatment for all pain populations but perhaps especially so for patients receiving workers' compensation [55]. Elevated hysteria and depression scores predicted greater improvements at discharge. Return to work rates for treated patients may fluctuate, and rates vary widely in primarily work hardening–based and more extensive cognitive-behaviorally based MPCs between 31% and 81% [56–59].

Although several systematic reviews and meta-analyses have demonstrated that MPCs improve psychosocial function, decrease pain, and return patients to work [58–61], other studies have suggested conflicting results with longer term outcomes. In general, follow-up studies on return to work are limited to less than 1 year posttreatment. Robinson and coworkers conducted a telephone survey evaluating clinical and disability status 3.0 and 4.6 years after patients underwent multidisciplinary treatment versus evaluation only. With a response rate of 50%, the analyses showed no difference in disability status, pain intensity, or functional and work status. It was proposed that the discrepancy in outcomes as compared with other positive ones in MPC treatment might have been due to the retrospective methodology, loss of subjects to follow-up, publication bias, and the use of workers' compensation claimants rather than other chronic pain cohorts. Also, patients were referred on average at 3 years of pain onset, highlighting the importance of early intervention based on recovery curves suggesting that aggressive intervention should be considered no later than 3 to 6 months [62,63]. Unfortunately, some workers' compensation patients with recalcitrant pain are referred for MPC treatment only as a last resort. In many instances, injured workers are referred to document disability and to obtain case closure or be deemed at maximum medical improvement, contributing negatively to outcomes research.

Cost-effectiveness

Studies have suggested that treatment in MPCs may produce billions of dollars in savings as related to health care expenditures and indemnity costs [10]. A recent study of the 3-year outcome of MPC treatment demonstrated cost-effectiveness for improving health and increasing return to work in a female blue-collar and service workers cohort [64]. Skouen and coworkers [65] examined the relative cost-effectiveness of treating work-related chronic low back pain with an average of 3 months' sick leave. The study compared a "light" multidisciplinary program intervention (physical therapy, psychologic treatment, and educational programming), an "extensive" multidisciplinary treatment program (4 week, 6-hours per day treatment with cognitive-behavioral treatment, education, exercise, and occupational therapy), and control management or "usual care" (medical treatment by a general practitioner). Men, not women, with low back pain returned to work more often in the light program when compared with patients in the treatment as usual group. Interestingly, a marked increase in return to work was noted in men in the light treatment group around 10 to 11 months. This increase may be related to the fact that in the country where the study was performed (Norway), work-related disability benefits are reduced by 40% after 12 months on sick leave. Women did not benefit from either type of program. It was proposed that women, when compared with men, had lower relative incomes, less education, and occupations more often associated with higher levels of musculoskeletal problems (ie, nursing assistants and cleaners), which may have adversely impacted the motivation for return to work. At-risk patient groups may more readily respond to multidisciplinary programs that emphasize treating illness behavior, psychosocial stressors, and individual job factors [65].

A randomized controlled study of patients with musculoskeletal pain on sick leave (at least 8 months) categorized patients into three groups based on the prognosis for return to work (good, medium, and poor) based on screening of psychologic, motivational, and physical findings. Patients were randomized to three treatment programs based on levels of intensity (ordinary treatment, light multidisciplinary, and extensive multidisciplinary). Patients in the good prognosis group did equally well in all three programs. The patients with a medium prognosis benefited equally from the two MPCs. The patients with a poor prognosis returned to work to a lesser extent than did patients with a good prognosis independent of treatment. The poor prognosis group receiving extensive MPC treatment returned to work at a higher rate than did poor prognosis patients receiving ordinary treatment. The poor prognosis subgroup was characterized by patients with psychosocial problems and more generalized muscular versus localized pain complaints. In general, the screening assessment (good, medium, poor prognosis) was able to predict the correct level of treatment. A cost-benefit analysis demonstrated that an appropriate combination of screening and assignment of treatment based on prognosis screening results was economically beneficial [66].

Efforts by insurers to "carve out" certain treatment components as a cost-savings measure may compromise overall outcomes. Robbins and coworkers [67] examined 1-year outcomes of interdisciplinary treatment. "Carve outs" did not receive physical therapy as part of the interdisciplinary program and exhibited significantly worse functioning and vocational status. Dropouts were twice as likely to be taking opioid medications and less likely to be taking antidepressants, underscoring additional inadequate treatment of comorbid depression, a condition associated with a significant percentage of chronic pain suffers [67].

Future directions: examining process

Recently, in an attempt to better understand the process behind the well-documented treatment gains, studies have been conducted examining the "active ingredients" of treatment. These studies have identified cognitive changes, in particular changes in pretreatment versus posttreatment levels of catastrophizing, as crucial predictors of outcome [68,69]. Other studies have identified changes in pain-related fear as predictors of outcome [70]. Work is now beginning at the authors' center to examine the effects of secondary gain (ie, workers' compensation status) on treatment gains. These designs have begun to suggest the importance of processes associated with successful treatment of chronic pain; however, at the time of this writing, even quantifying changes in these variables accounts for only a portion of the total variance observed in treatment gains. Clearly, there is more occurring in treatment than is currently understood.

Future research will examine more of the treatment process to better elucidate the necessary elements of treatment from the nonspecific elements. For instance, can the number of treatment modalities be reduced and achieve the same beneficial outcomes? Growing evidence suggests that certain groups of patients may benefit from multidisciplinary treatment more than others do. Patients involved in the workers' compensation system or in third-party litigation have been shown to have reduced benefit from treatment [63]. Many questions remain.

Formal multidisciplinary and interdisciplinary treatment is part of one end of the continuum of comprehensive pain management. Only a small number of patients may have access to formal treatment programs close to home. Physiatrists may still manage patients with a similar biopsychosocial model. Communication and collaboration between participating team members (ie, physical and occupational therapists, pain psychologists, social workers, nurse educators, and physicians) may include different offices at different sites. Understanding ongoing psychosocial, familial, and vocational issues while developing an open rapport and mutual respect among the patient, physician, and case manager will lead to improved outcomes, decreased pain and suffering, and an improved quality of life.

References

[1] Gureje O, Simon GE, Von Korff M. A cross-national study of the course of persistent pain in primary care. Pain 2001;92(1–2):195–200.

[2] Caragee EJ, Alamin TF, Miller JL, et al. Discographic MRI and psychosocial determinants of low back pain disability and remission: a prospective study in subjects with benign persistent back pain. Spine J 2005;5:24–35.

[3] Mersky H, Bogduk N. Classification of chronic pain. IASP Task Force on Taxonomy. 2nd edition. Seattle (WA): IASP Press; 1994. p. 209–14.

[4] Beecher H. Measurement of subjective responses. New York: Oxford University Press; 1959.

[5] Melzack R, Wall PD. Pain mechanisms: a new theory. Science 1965;50:971–9.

[6] Engel GL. The need for a new medical model: a challenge for biomedicine. Science 1977;196: 129–36.

[7] Gatchel RJ, Turk DC. Psychological approaches to pain management: a practitioner's handbook. New York: Guilford Press; 1996.

[8] Camic P, Knight SJ. Clinical handbook of health psychology. Seattle (WA): Hogrefe & Huber; 1988.

[9] Belar CD, Deardorff WW. Clinical health psychology in medical settings: a practitioner's guidebook. Washington (DC): American Psychological Association; 1995.

[10] Turk DC, Okifuji A. Psychological factors in chronic pain: evolution and revolution. J Consult Clin Psychol 2002;70(3):678–90.

[11] Nielson WR, Weir R. Biopsychosocial approaches to the treatment of chronic pain. Clin J Pain 2001;17(4 Suppl):S114–27.

[12] Jensen MP, Turner JA, Romano J. Correlates of improvement in multidisciplinary treatment of chronic pain. J Consult Clin Psychol 1994;62(1):172–9.

[13] Flor H, Fydrich T, Turk DC. Efficacy of multidisciplinary pain treatment centers: a meta-analytic review. Pain 1992;49:221–30.

[14] Guzman J, Esmail R, Karjalaninen K. Multidisciplinary rehabilitation for chronic low back pain: systematic review. BMJ 2001;322:1511–6.

[15] Turk DC, Flor H. Chronic pain: a biobehavioral perspective. In: Gatchel RJ, Turk DC, editors. Psychosocial factors in pain: critical perspectives. New York: Guilford Press; 1999.
[16] Boon H, Verhoef M, O'Hara D, et al. From parallel practice to integrative health care: a conceptual framework. BMC Health Serv Res 2004;4(1):15.
[17] Past President's perspective: an interview with Benjamin Crue, MD. American Pain Society Bulletin 2005;(Winter):3.
[18] Loeser JD. Desirable characteristics for pain treatment facilities. In: Bond MR, Charlton JE, Woolf CJ, editors. Pain research and clinical management, vol. 4. Amsterdam: Elsevier; 1991. p. 411–5.
[19] Dersh J, Polatin PB, Leeman G, et al. The management of secondary gain and loss in medicolegal settings: strengths and weaknesses. J Occup Rehab 2004;14(4):267–79.
[20] Fishbain D. Secondary gain concept: definition problems and its abuse in medical practice. Am Pain Soc J 1994;3(4):263–4.
[21] Gatchel RJ. Psychosocial factors that can influence the self-assessment of function. J Occup Rehab 2004;14:197–206.
[22] Kwan O, Ferrari R, Friel J. Tertiary gain and disability syndromes. Med Hypotheses 2001; 57(4):459–64.
[23] Sternbach RA. Pain: a psychophysiological analysis. New York: Academic Press; 1968.
[24] Graffenried B, Adler R, Abt K, et al. The influence of anxiety and pain sensitivity on experimental pain in man. Pain 1978;4:253–63.
[25] Glynn CJ, Lloyd JW, Folkhard S. The effects of reported arousal, anxiety, aggression, and depression on the diurnal variation of reported intractable pain. Pain 1981;S74:74–89.
[26] Meagher MW, Arnau RC, Rhudy JL. Pain and emotion: effects of affective picture modulation. Psychosom Med 2001;63(1):79–90.
[27] Banks S, Kerns RD. Explaining high rates of depression in chronic pain: a diathesis-stress framework. Psychol Bull 1996;119(1):95–110.
[28] Kuch K. Psychological factors and the development of chronic pain. Clin J Pain 2001;17(4): S33–8.
[29] McCracken LM, Gross RT, Aikens J, et al. The assessment of anxiety and fear in persons with chronic pain: a comparison of instruments. Behav Res Ther 1996;34(11–12):927–33.
[30] McCracken LM, Faber SD, Janeck AS. Pain-related anxiety predicts non-specific physical complaints in persons with chronic pain. Behav Res Ther 1998;36(6):621–30.
[31] Davis MC, Zautra AJ, Reich JW. Vulnerability to stress among women in chronic pain from fibromyalgia and osteoarthritis. Ann Behav Med 2001;23(3):215–26.
[32] Burns JW. Anger management style and hostility: predicting symptom-specific physiological reactivity among chronic low back pain patients. J Behav Med 1997;20(6):505–22.
[33] Fordyce WE, Fowler RS, DeLateur B. An application of behavior modification technique to a problem of chronic pain. Behav Res Ther 1968;6:105–7.
[34] Fordyce WE. Pain and suffering: a reappraisal. Am Psychol 1988;43(4):276–83.
[35] Carlson H. Efficacy of abbreviated progressive muscle relaxation training: a quantitative review of behavioral medicine research. J Consult Clin Psychol 1993;61:1059–67.
[36] Lorig KR, Sobel DS, Ritter PL, et al. Effect of a self-management program on patients with chronic disease. Eff Clin Pract 2001;4(6):256–62.
[37] Hadhazy VA, Ezzo J, Creamer P, et al. Mind-body therapies for the treatment of fibromyalgia: a systematic review. J Rheumatol 2000;27(12):2911–8.
[38] Keefe FJ, Affleck GA, Lefebvre JC, et al. Pain coping strategies and coping efficacy in rheumatoid arthritis: a daily process analysis. Pain 1997;69:35–42.
[39] Jensen M, Turner J, Romano J, et al. Coping with chronic pain: a critical review of the literature. Pain 1991;47:249–83.
[40] Affleck G, Tennen H, Urrows S, et al. Neuroticism and the pain-mood relation in rheumatoid arthritis: insights from a prospective daily study. J Consult Clin Psychol 1992;60:119–26.
[41] Affleck G, Urrows S, Tennen H, et al. Daily coping with pain from rheumatoid arthritis: patterns and correlates. Pain 1992;51:221–9.

[42] Affleck G, Tennen H, Keefe FJ, et al. Everyday life with osteoarthritis or rheumatoid arthritis: independent effects of disease and gender on daily pain, mood, and coping. Pain 1999;83:601–9.
[43] Keefe FJ, Salley AN, Lefebvre JC. Coping with pain: conceptual concerns and future directions. Pain 1992;51:131–4.
[44] Vendrig AA, Lousberg R. Within-person relationships among pain intensity, mood and physical activity in chronic pain: a naturalistic approach. Pain 1997;73:71–6.
[45] Feldman SI, Schaffer-Neitz R, Downey G. Pain, negative mood, and perceived support in chronic pain patients: a daily diary study of people with Reflex Sympathetic Dystrophy Syndrome. J Consult Clin Psychol 1999;67(5):776–85.
[46] Kroenke K, Swindle R. Cognitive-behavioral therapy for somatization and symptom syndromes: a critical review of controlled clinical trials. Psychother Psychosom 2000;69(4):205–15.
[47] Severeijns R, Vlaeyen JW, Van den Hout MA, et al. Pain catastrophizing predicts pain intensity, disability, and psychological distress independent of the level of physical impairment. Clin J Pain 2001;17(2):165–72.
[48] McCracken LM. Learning to live with the pain: acceptance of pain predicts adjustment in persons with chronic pain. Pain 1998;74(1):21–7.
[49] Astin JA. Mind-body therapies for the management of pain. Clin J Pain 2004;20(1):27–32.
[50] Cutler RB, Fishbain DA, Rosomoff HL, et al. Does nonsurgical pain center treatment of chronic pain return patients to work? A review and meta-analysis of the literature. Spine 1994;19:643–52.
[51] McCracken LM, Turk D. Behavioral and cognitive-behavioral treatment for chronic pain: outcome, predictors of outcome, and treatment process. Spine 2002;27(22):2564–73.
[52] Morley S, Eccleston C, Williams A. Systematic review and meta-analysis of randomized trials of cognitive behavior therapy and behavior therapy for chronic pain in adults, excluding headache. Pain 1999;80:1–13.
[53] Van Tulder MW, Ostelo R, Vlaeyen JW, et al. Behavioral treatment for chronic low back pain: a systematic review within the framework of the Cochrane Back Review Group. Spine 2001;26(3):270–81.
[54] Kleinke CL, Spanger AS. Predicting treatment outcome of chronic back pain patients in a multidisciplinary pain clinic: methodological issues and treatment implications. Pain 1988;33:41–8.
[55] Krause N, Dasinger L, Deegan L, et al. Psychosocial job factors and return-to-work after compensated low back injury: a disability phase-specific analysis. Am J Ind Med 2001;40:374–92.
[56] Richardson IH, Richardson PH, Williams AC, et al. The effects of a cognitive-behavioral pain management programme on the quality of work and employment status of severely impaired chronic pain patients. Disabil Rehabil 1994;16(1):26–34.
[57] Norrefalk JR, Svensson O, Ekholm J, et al. Can the back-to-work rate of patients with long-term non-malignant pain be predicted? Int J Rehabil Res 2005;28(1):9–16.
[58] Lanes TC, Gauron EF, Spratt KF, et al. Long-term follow-up of patients with chronic back pain treated in a multidisciplinary rehabilitation program. Spine 1995;20(7):801–6.
[59] Gatchel RJ, Mayer TG, Hazard RG, et al. Functional restoration: pitfalls in evaluating efficacy. Spine 1992;17(8):988–95.
[60] Hazard RG, Fenwick JW, Kalisch SM, et al. Functional restoration with behavioral support: a one-year prospective study of patients with chronic low-back pain. Spine 1989;14(2):157–61.
[61] Jensen IB, Bodin L. Multimodal cognitive-behavioural treatment for workers with chronic spinal pain: a matched cohort study with an 18-month follow-up. Pain 1998;76(1–2):35–44.
[62] Cheadle A, Franklin G, Wolfhagen C, et al. Factors influencing the duration of work-related disability: a population-based study of Washington State workers' compensation. Am J Public Health 1994;84(2):190–6.

[63] Robinson JP, Fulton-Kehoe D, Franklin GM, et al. Multidisciplinary pain center outcomes in Washington State Workers' Compensation. J Occup Environ Med 2004;46(5):473–8.
[64] Jensen IB, Bergstrom G, Ljungquist T, et al. A 3-year follow-up of a multidisciplinary rehabilitation programme for back and neck pain. Pain 2005;115(3):273–83.
[65] Skouen JS, Grasdal AL, Haldorsen EM, et al. Relative cost-effectiveness of extensive and light multidisciplinary treatment programs versus treatment as usual for patients with chronic low back pain on long-term sick leave. Spine 2002;9:901–10.
[66] Haldorsen EM, Gradsal AL, Skouen JS, et al. Is there a right treatment for a particular patient group? Comparison of ordinary treatment, light multidisciplinary treatment, and extensive multidisciplinary treatment for long-term sick listed employees with musculoskeletal pain. Pain 2002;95:49–63.
[67] Robins H, Gatchel RJ, Noe C, et al. A prospective one-year outcome study of interdisciplinary chronic pain management: compromising its efficacy by managed care policies. Anesth Analg 2003;97:156–62.
[68] Burns JW, Glenn B, Bruehl S, et al. Cognitive factors influence outcome following multidisciplinary chronic pain treatment: a replication and extension of a cross-lagged panel analysis. Behav Res Ther 2003;41:1163–82.
[69] Burns JW, Kubilus A, Bruehl S, et al. Do changes in cognitive factors influence outcome following multidisciplinary treatment for chronic pain? A cross-lagged panel analysis. J Consult Clin Psychol 2003;71:81–91.
[70] Vlaeyen JW, de Jong J, Geilen M, et al. Graded exposure in vivo in the treatment of pain-related fear: a replicated single-case experimental design in four patients with chronic low back pain. Behav Res Ther 2001;39(2):151–66.

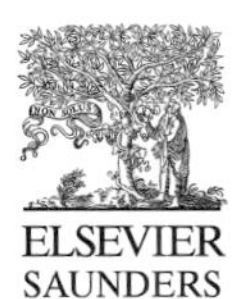
ELSEVIER
SAUNDERS

Phys Med Rehabil Clin N Am
17 (2006) 451–472

PHYSICAL MEDICINE
AND REHABILITATION
CLINICS OF
NORTH AMERICA

Complementary Medicine in Chronic Pain Treatment

Charles A. Simpson, DC

Complementary Healthcare Plans, Inc., 6600 SW 105th Avenue, Suite 115, Beaverton, OR 97008, USA

Identifying and defining alternative approaches to health and healing have been problematic for decades. The emergence of organized medicine in the last century, by exclusion, defined a large number of existing healing disciplines. Fifty years ago Brian Inglis [1] developed a model of *Fringe Medicine* that, in part, consigned nonstandard approaches to healing to the periphery of science and the health care system. Eisenberg's [2] seminal study in 1993 looked at "un-orthodox" medicine in exclusionary terms: what it is not taught in medical schools, not available in hospitals, and not generally considered "real" medicine.

Both of these perspectives fail to provide meaningful distinctions. Neither bears up to careful scrutiny of the current state of complementary and alternative medicine (CAM). As research on the use of CAM accumulates, it is apparent that the volume of health care delivered outside of the orthodox mainstream equals that of conventional care provided in physician offices—hardly an image of a peripheral factor in the overall picture of health care. The popularity of complementary medicine with the public has not gone unnoticed by conventional medicine (CM) institutions either. Health insurance plans and hospitals have integrated, to some extent, nontraditional health care providers and therapies largely for market-driven reasons. Complementary medicine topics are being integrated into medical school curricula.

More recently, the emergence of complementary medicine on the national research scene through the National Institutes of Health National Center for Complementary and Alternative Medicine (NCCAM) promises to develop the academic and intellectual infrastructure that can explore evidence that demonstrates the utility of complementary therapies. There are currently more than 1200 randomized, controlled trials (RCTs) and 150 Cochrane Collaboration reviews of alternative therapies. As noted several

E-mail address: Csimpson@chpplans.us

1047-9651/06/$ - see front matter
doi:10.1016/j.pmr.2005.11.006

years ago in a *New England Journal of Medicine* editorial [3], in the future, medicine will be divided into those approaches to health and healing that are backed by scientific evidence and those that are not. A recent Institute of Medicine report on complementary medicine emphasizes, "The committee recommends that the same principles and standards of evidence of treatment effectiveness apply to all treatments, whether currently labeled as conventional medicine or CAM" [4]. This evidence-based perspective will erode the barriers between health care that is provided in the tradition of western scientific medicine and healing disciplines that, in some instances, predate modern medicine by 3,000 years.

Yet there clearly are differences between health care available in physician offices, clinics, and hospitals and that provided by CAM practitioners. Three features of CAM distinguish it from conventional medicine. CAM therapies are individualized to each patient. CAM almost universally incorporates a philosophy of health that emphasizes and leverages an innate capacity for healing in every individual. And finally, CAM tends to acknowledge the existence of properties of living systems that are resistant to understanding by contemporary reductionistic scientific methods of inquiry.

These distinguishing features present significant challenges to research and assembling meaningful evidence. They also create opportunities to develop more effective, efficient, and humanizing care for a very difficult population of patients—those with chronic pain. A recent observation by Cicerone [5] on evidence-based practice and the limits of rational rehabilitation points out that "...we need to acknowledge the subjective meanings of illness and disability to the patients we serve. Any efforts to build our practice based on the best available systematic evidence are unlikely to succeed unless we include patients' values and beliefs and incorporate this perspective into our rehabilitation research. This aspect of evidence-based rehabilitation raises important questions about our fundamental roles and how we will choose to practice and define our field in the future."

Individualized treatment is a hallmark of most CAM therapies. For example, an acupuncture practitioner may evaluate two patients, both with the same conventional medicine diagnosis, but develop two radically different treatment plans based on the Oriental medicine examination findings and assessment. This approach seems to work well for patients. Studies of patients who obtain care from CAM practitioners reveal high levels of satisfaction with the practitioners and the outcome of the therapies. CAM providers spend time with their patients and they are successful in explaining to patients the nature of their health problems. Treatment planning tends to be a collaboration between therapist and patient. Interventions are developed that are consistent with each patient's needs and preferences.

Philosophy of care is not something that most conventional medicine practitioners ponder extensively. However, philosophical discourse underlies many CAM therapies. Chiropractic for example contains an extensive literature that can only be described as "philosophy." Beginning with the founder, D.D. Palmer, chiropractic thinkers have historically focused on not so much the rational scientific underpinnings of this healing art, but on the art itself. "Innate intelligence" is posited by Palmer and his successors as a fundamental life force; when fully expressed without interference, the ultimate expression of health occurs, naturally and without need of intrusion from outside agents. In this chiropractic philosophic world view, the aim of the chiropractor is to locate and correct interferences with this natural expression of the life force. Identified as "chi" in Oriental medicine, "prana" in yoga, "doshas" in Aruvedic medicine, "vix medica naturae" in naturopathic medicine, each discipline has elaborated some measure of a conceptual life force that guides and propels healing and health.

CM with its intellectual traditions anchored in western scientific thought is understandably skeptical of notions of innate intelligence, chi, or other conceptualization of a putative life force. Finding no testable hypotheses to investigate a possible life force, conventional medicine has largely dismissed such philosophical musing. Oschman [6] provides a comprehensive review of this seeming "impenetrable intellectual barrier" between CAM and CM world views.

There is considerable diversity in CAM practices;deciding which discipline to include under the rubric "CAM" and which to exclude can be problematic. Eisenberg [2] for example limited his survey inquiries to 16 "commonly used interventions" but included "relaxation therapy…lifestyle diets, spiritual or religious healing by others." Eisenberg does note a categoric difference however between CAM therapies that are delivered by a "professional," such as massage, and those that are largely self-administered without the involvement of a provider, such as lifestyle diets and intercessory prayer. NCCAM has categorized CAM in five "domains": alternative medical systems, mind-body interventions, biologically based treatments, manipulative and body-based methods, and energy therapies [7].

For this discussion, CAM therapies are limited to those commonly accessible in the community to chronic pain patients and, for the most part, administered under the guidance of licensed health care professionals. Although this approach may exclude some valuable and frequently used therapies, it does encompass CAM therapies that are in regular use by chronic pain patients, are at least somewhat institutionalized, have been used or referred to by CM providers and are capable of being integrated clinically and administratively into conventional medical care of chronic pain.

CAM therapies are categorized further by their intellectual and philosophic nature as being either essentially biologically based or energy based. Biologically based therapies are explained and practiced fundamentally in ways that are familiar to practitioners trained in the conventional medical model of western scientific inquiry. Clinical conditions are mostly described in terms of disturbed anatomy and physiology. Treatment interventions are categorized by their physiologic effects. Outcomes are measured in objective terms. These disciplines, such as chiropractic and natural medicine, often view themselves as being within the context of orthodox scientific thought. Many of these therapies have been rigorously scrutinized through the lens of western medical scientific investigation. The disciplines themselves are developing intellectual, administrative, and physical infrastructure to conduct research.

In contrast, energy-based therapies are most often founded on putative notions of natural systems of "invisible energetic relations and connections that govern living form and function" [6]. Although some of these energy-based therapies have undergone scientific inquiry, most notably acupuncture, the fundamental world view of energy-based healers has not been altered to conform to the understandings offered by rational reductionistic methods. For example, science has attempted to understand the physiologic basis of acupuncture. However few acupuncture practitioners endorse or, more importantly, practice within this intellectual context, preferring instead to explain what they do in the language of Oriental medicine, such as the flow of chi.

Why consider complementary and alternative medicine therapies in physical medicine practice?

CM physicians, especially in the challenging field of pain medicine, might want to better understand CAM therapies. Their patients are probably already using at least one CAM therapy concurrently with CM treatments. Potential complications arise with the combination of CAM and CM therapies. And perhaps most significantly, CAM therapies can improve the quality of care for chronic pain patients.

More than 60 million Americans suffer from chronic pain; about 40% of them fail to achieve adequate relief [8]. Surveys of CAM users note a high prevalence of chronic conditions, including chronic pain. Observers of the CAM scene note that "consumers will continue to use CAM, particularly in chronic conditions, in which patients struggle to find any treatment that may cure their condition or improve their quality of life" [9].

Most CAM interventions are "low-tech high-touch." They are often perceived as inherently safe and natural by patients and practitioners. However there is a growing body of evidence that illuminates adverse reactions to commonly used CAM therapies either by themselves or when combined with conventional medicine. Drug-herb interactions for example present potential challenges to patient safety and compromises of therapeutic intent. Eisenberg [2] noted that patients use CAM and CM concurrently for the same condition upward of 83% of the time. What is potentially more troublesome is that CAM users failed to disclose CAM use to CM physicians, Subsequent investigation indicates that this failure to disclose has not improved over time [10]. Better understanding by both CM and CAM practitioners of risks can modify the potential for adverse outcomes.

Avoiding adverse CM-CAM interactions can obviously improve patient care. Inquiring about CAM use, especially from an objective and evidence-based perspective, can enhance patient communication. The cultural competency of nonjudgmental acknowledgment of CAM use, particularly when reinforced by objective evidence of safety and effectiveness, can reinforce a productive therapeutic relationship between patient and physician. It is well recognized that effective physician-patient communication is a critical element predicting better patient satisfaction and compliance [11]. Moreover, as reliable evidence of CAM effectiveness emerges, CM physicians may be in a position to integrate evidence-based CAM approaches in an active manner rather than passively accepting what chronic pain patients may already be attempting to integrate on their own.

Evidence-based complementary and alternative medicine therapies

Assessing the evidence about CAM therapies for chronic pain is problematic from a number of perspectives. CAM therapies are often inherently resistant to analysis by commonly used clinical research methods. For example, in the hierarchy of evidence, the RCT is considered to be the gold standard. Yet many argue that this methodology, while well suited to the study of drugs, may not be the best research design to study complex, individualized treatments routinely offered by CAM practitioners [12,13]. For instance, trials of manipulative therapy have been plagued by the difficulty in developing a "sham" manipulation and concurrently controlling for the "nonspecific" effects of the hands-on practitioner-patient interaction with the sham treatment.

Evidence about any treatment for chronic pain is further confounded by the complex nature of the condition itself. Patient selection is often a significant challenge to study validity. Lumping a wide variety of patients with low back pain, for example, into a conceptually uniform study group ignores the wide variety of conditions that may fall into this population. It is no wonder that such trials frequently come up with equivocal results for almost any intervention whether conventional or complementary and fail to reveal significant differences in effectiveness between treatments. The challenges of applying evidence of this nature to the practical realities of treating patients have been increasingly recognized [14]. Fortunately, the research community, particularly in the CAM fields, is actively developing research strategies that are more appropriate both for the individualized nature of CAM interventions and the complex, multifactorial nature of chronic conditions such as chronic pain.

Finally, publication and indexing biases are obstacles to assembling reliable evidence about CAM therapies [15]. As in CM, studies with positive results are more likely to be submitted for publication. Many studies of CAM are in foreign language journals, thus limiting their exposure to English-speaking audiences. A more subtle bias also is observed in CM-published research on CAM. As one CAM researcher put it, "A negative study of acupuncture concludes that 'acupuncture doesn't work.' The analogue would be a negative drug trial that concluded 'medicine does not work'" (R. Hammarschlag, personal communication, June 2005).

Complementary and alternative medicine therapies

Biophysiologic therapies

These therapies are based mainly on concepts of biology and physiology commonly accepted in conventional biomedicine. These therapies rely on clinical theories, therapeutic approaches, and rationales that are couched in terms consistent with current scientific understanding of biology and physiology familiar to conventional medicine.

Manipulation

Manipulation is the most widely used CAM therapy . It is widely practiced by a variety of specialties including doctors of chiropractic (DC), osteopathic physicians (DO), medical physicians, physical therapists and some lay practitioners. It is estimated that DCs deliver over 90% of all manipulative therapy [16]. Chiropractic training in manipulative techniques is arguably the most extensive among manipulation practitioners.

Manipulation is thought to improve pain by locating and treating disturbed joint and muscle function described as dysfunction, subluxation, fixation, and other terminology that may vary by discipline, training, and technique. Of the CAM therapies, manipulation has been studied the most extensively. NCCAM has identified 537 clinical trials of manipulative and other bodywork therapies such as massage. While the results are often and predictably ambivalent, there is clear evidence that manipulation is superior to sham treatment and equivalent to other conservative interventions for acute spinal pain problems [17]. More recent investigations show long-term benefit for neck pain [18], headaches [19], and chronic mechanical spine pain [20].

Natural medicine therapies

A number of CAM practices use nutritional supplements and herbs (known collectively as nutraceuticals) in the treatment of chronic pain. While these natural medicine approaches are most commonly identified with doctors of naturopathic medicine (ND), herbs and supplements are frequently used by acupuncture/Oriental medicine and chiropractic providers as well.

Natural medicine can be used directly as analgesics (eg, white willow bark), antispasmodics (eg, valerian, passiflora), and tissue regeneraltion (eg, Boswellia, Zingiber curcuma). Nutritional and herbs interventions are most commonly applied to modify perceived underlying physiologic disturbances such as fibromyalgia, depression, osteoarthritis, and rheumatoid arthritis. Of commonly used nutritional approaches, glucosamine and chondroitin sulfate have been most extensively studied. Glucosamine has been shown to slow cartilage deterioration and relieve pain in knee osteoarthritis.

Many nutraceutical interventions are thought to modify disturbed metabolism, which underlies chronic pain conditions such as fibromyalgia. Although much nutraceutical information on the internet is proprietary and commercial, there are a number of evidence-based sources of information.

Body awareness therapy

A number of approaches to chronic pain treatment involve the idea of improved postural coordination by using conscious processes to alter automatic postural coordination and ongoing muscular activity. These body awareness therapies may be practiced by physical and occupational therapists, massage therapists as well as nonlicensed body-work professionals. Two common therapies are described, Alexander technique and Feldenkrais.

Alexander Technique is described as "…a method that works to change (movement) habits in our everyday activities. It is a simple and practical method for improving ease and freedom of movement, balance, support and coordination. The technique teaches the use of the appropriate amount of effort for a particular activity, giving you more energy for all your activities. It is not a series of treatments or exercises, but rather a reeducation of the mind and body" [21].

A systematic review of Alexander Technique revealed few high quality RCTs but noted promising results with Parkinson's and back pain [22].

Feldenkrais is said to improve function by "expanding the self-image through movement sequences that bring attention to the parts of the self that are out of awareness and uninvolved in functional actions. Better function is evoked by establishing an improved dynamic relationship between the individual, gravity, and society" [23]. Jain and colleagues [24] provide a recent review of the method, its use, and the relevant research and research gaps concerning these body awareness therapies.

Therapeutic massage

Massage therapy encompasses more than 150 named body work systems and perhaps thousands of variations and individual techniques. Therapeutic, clinical, or medical massage is engaged to treat specific clinical conditions. The physiologic effects of massage are well documented, including muscular relaxation, improved blood and lymph circulation, and neurohormonal-immunologic effects. There are more than 20 clinical trials of massage for pain. Physical Medicine & Rehabilitation Clinics of North America reviewed therapeutic massage in 1999 [25]. A more recent Cochrane review of massage for low back pain concluded, "Massage might be beneficial for patients with subacute and chronic non-specific low-back pain, especially when combined with exercises and education" [26].

Breath pattern retraining

In 1975, Lum [27] introduced the concept of disordered breathing patterns as the underlying cause of "a collection of bizarre and unrelated symptoms" including cardiovascular, neurologic, respiratory, gastro-intestinal, musculoskeletal, psychologic, other syndromes. More recently, Chaitow [28] has emphasized disturbed breathing patterns as the cause of chronic pain. Proposed mechanisms are summarized as "respiratory alkalosis, leading to reduced oxygenation of tissues (including the brain), smooth muscle constriction, heightened pain perception, speeding up of spinal reflexes, increased excitability of the corticospinal system, hyperirritability of motor and sensory axons, changes in serum calcium and magnesium levels, and encouragement of myofascial trigger points." Breath pattern retraining therapists note that the respiratory mechanism is the only physiologic function that is under both autonomic and voluntary control.

A recent RCT [29] revealed equivalent improvement from 12 sessions of breath therapy on visual analogue pain scale (VAS), Roland Scale and short form-36 (SF-36) when compared with high-quality, extended physical therapy. Breath therapy was found to be safe.

Prolotherapy

The use of proliferation therapy (prolotherapy) has waxed and waned for nearly a century. Often provided by CM practitioners, prolotherapy is also frequently in the therapeutic armamentarium of naturopathic physicians. After an injury, failure of adequate tendon or ligament healing is thought to result in instability, connective tissue insufficiency, or lack of tensile strength. Normal use of these compromised structures causes pain. Prolotherapy consists of injections of an array of substances intended to trigger growth factors in local connective tissue and restart the repair sequence that results in more normal and functional tissue.

A recent critical review of prolotherapy retrieved over 30 studies of prolotherapy for spinal pain. These reflected wide variation in treatment protocols and concluded that "clinical studies published to date indicate that it may be effective at reducing spinal pain" [30]. A Cochrane review concluded that, "If used alone, prolotherapy injections do not have a role in the treatment of chronic low-back pain. When combined with other treatments, they may give prolonged partial relief of pain and disability" [31].

Trigger point manipulation

Travell and Simons [32] offered an early treatise on myofascial trigger points (TrP) which were defined originally as "a hyperirritable spot in skeletal muscle that is associated with a hypersensitive palpable nodule in a taut band. The spot is tender when pressed and can give rise to characteristic referred pain, motor dysfunction, and autonomic phenomena."

The understanding of the causet of trigger points has evolved. Current thinking has been summarized as "TrPs are evoked by the abnormal depolarization of motor end plates... presynaptic, synaptic, and postsynaptic mechanisms of abnormal depolarization (ie, excessive release of acetycholine [ACh], defects of acetylcholinesterase, and upregulation of nicotinic ACh-receptor activity, respectively)" [33].

No objective diagnostic tests for trigger points are available. Trigger points are diagnosed by manual palpation to identify a tender nodule, often at characteristic locations in muscle that produce characteristic radiating pain when stimulated. Despite this "low-tech" diagnostic method, TrP detection has good test-retest reliability [34]. Various approaches to treating trigger points have been elaborated including manual compression, "spray and stretch," injection, dry needling and modalities (ultrasound, electric stimulation, low level laser). Trigger point treatment is often rendered by certain CM physical medicine practitioners, but most frequently by chiropractors, acupuncturists, massage practitioners, and other CAM providers.

Energy-based therapies

Energy medicine is a domain in CAM that deals with energy fields of two types: veritable, which can be measured, and putative, which have yet to be measured.

The veritable energies include mechanical vibrations (such as sound) and electromagnetic forces, including visible light, magnetism, monochromatic radiation (such as laser beams), and rays from other parts of the electromagnetic spectrum. These veritable energy-based therapies involve the use of specific, measurable wavelengths and frequencies to treat patients.

In contrast, putative energy fields are based on the concept that human beings are infused with a subtle form of energy. This vital energy or life force is known under different names in different cultures and traditions, such as qi in traditional Chinese medicine (TCM), ki in the Japanese Kampo system, doshas in Ayurvedic medicine, and elsewhere as prana, etheric energy, fohat, orgone, odic force, mana, and homeopathic resonance. Vital energy is believed to flow throughout the material human body, but it has not been unequivocally measured by means of conventional instrumentation. Nonetheless, therapists claim that they can work with this subtle energy, see it with their own eyes, and otherwise sense its presence and quality and then use it to effect changes in another's physical body to influence health.

Veritable energy therapies

Magnetic therapy

Magnetic therapy has a long and controversial history in medicine. It has recently regained popularity in the marketplace. Application is by way of electromagnetic coils, in connection with acupuncture treatment and by way of static magnets. Magnetic therapy is typically applied to the skin overlying the affected area. The popular press indicates the use of magnets for treating a wide variety of chronic pain problems such as migraine, osteoarthritis, and injury to muscles, ligaments, and tendons. Contraindications are few but do include pregnancy, pediatrics, and implantable electronic devices.

Contemporary clinical trials of magnet therapy have produced conflicting results. A study of carpal tunnel syndrome in 2002 found no statistically significant difference between magnets and placebo. But the investigators did note, "Although this study did not show magnets to be more effective than the placebo, the reduction in pain with this simple intervention was remarkable" [35]. In a double-blind, placebo-controlled trial, static magnets produced statistically significant ($P < .05$) short-term pain relief in osteoarthritis of the knee [36]. Systematic reviews of magnet therapy are scarce, and evidence-based medicine reviews are lacking.

Microcurrent stimulation

Microcurrent has been used in CM for the treatment of nonunion fracture and delayed healing. The exact mechanism of action is unknown but may involve intracellular regulation of calcium. Microcurrent has found application in the treatment of soft tissue disorders as well.

McMakin has published three studies of this modality, which is termed frequency-specific microcurrent, in chronic pain patients. The studies are case series reports involving head, neck and face pain [37], chronic low back pain [38], and fibromyalgia associated with cervical spine trauma [39]. In the most recent study, McMakin and colleagues [39] began to explore the mechanisms of frequency-specific microcurrent. Their subjects revealed reductions in inflammatory cytokines, increase in β endorphins as well as subjective reports of pain relief in fibromyalgia.

Low-level laser therapy

Low-level laser therapy is a form of phototherapy that involves the application of low-power laser light to areas of the body to stimulate healing. It is also known as cold laser, soft laser, or low-intensity laser. It is hypothesized that photons are absorbed in the mitochondria. The light energy is converted to chemical energy within the cell that affects the permeability of the cell membrane, which in turn produces various physiologic effects. These physiologic changes affect a variety of cell types including macrophages, fibroblasts, endothelial cells, and mast cells.

Low-level laser therapy is widely used in physical therapy, chiropractic, and other physical medicine practice. Although reportedly safe, the modality is relatively new and is still controversial with respect to its effectiveness. A MedLine search retrieves over 500 citations. A recent systematic review of the literature of low-level laser therapy for acute and chronic neck pain concluded "Significant positive effects were reported in four of five trials" [40].Cochrane reviews of low-level laser therapy used in osteoarthritis and rheumatoid arthritis revealed, "Conflicting evidence of benefit...for the treatment of osteoarthritis" [41]. Low-level laser therapy for rheumatoid arthritis is somewhat more positive in that the therapy "provides short-term pain relief for patients with rheumatoid arthritis" [42]. Significantly, both reviews noted positive therapeutic results and called for more high-quality research on low-level laser therapy.

Putative energy therapies

Acupuncture and oriental medicine

Among the "putative energy" therapies, none have received the notice and scrutiny of acupuncture. The practice of oriental medicine itself includes a range of systems, interventions, schools of thought, and techniques. TCM, one such system, is widely taught and practiced in the United States. TCM encompasses herbs, massage, qigong, and acupuncture.

In the TCM view, the body is a delicate balance of two opposing and inseparable forces: yin and yang. Yin represents the cold, slow, or passive principle, whereas yang represents the hot, excited, or active principle. Among the major assumptions in TCM are that health is achieved by maintaining the body in a "balanced state" and that disease is due to an internal imbalance of yin and yang. This imbalance leads to blockage in the flow of qi (or vital energy) and of blood along pathways known as meridians. TCM practitioners typically use herbs, acupuncture, and massage to help unblock qi and blood in patients in an attempt to bring the body back into harmony and wellness [43]. These therapies are intended to balance the flow of qi and not to produce a specific physiologic effect.

Although not synonymous with TCM, needle acupuncture has received the most attention in the research and clinical communities. It is the most commonly performed Oriental medicine treatment in the United States. Acupuncture describes a family of procedures involving stimulation of anatomic locations on the skin by a variety of techniques. A number of approaches to diagnosis and treatment in American acupuncture incorporate medical traditions from China, Japan, Korea, and other countries. The most studied mechanism of stimulation of acupuncture points uses penetration of the skin by thin, solid, metallic needles, which are manipulated manually or by electrical stimulation [44]. The body of research literature on acupuncture is robust. A search on PubMed for "acupuncture" returned more than 9000 citations. Limiting the search terms to "acupuncture and chronic pain" returned 500 articles. The Cochrane Collaboration lists 123 reviews for "acupuncture" and 18 evidence-based medicine reviews specifically for "acupuncture and chronic pain." A comprehensive review of this literature base is well beyond the scope of this article, but there is conclusive evidence of the effectiveness and safety of this therapy.

It is clear that acupuncture is widely used by chronic pain patients. A telephone survey reported by Breivik and colleagues [45] found that 13% of chronic pain patients in Europe use acupuncture. Research methodology challenges in the investigation of acupuncture stubbornly persist. Meta-analyses frequently conclude that although acupuncture can be shown to be effective for pain relief, the therapy itself has not been shown to be superior to other therapies [46].

Craniosacral therapy

Craniosacral therapy developed from the work of an American osteopath, Dr. William Sutherland in the early 1900s. It is founded on the notion of the primary respiratory mechanism that involves intrinsic motions of the cranial bones, the dura, and the flow of cerebrospinal fluid. Rhythmic motions are said to be measurable with instruments, but in clinical practice, it is by palpation that a craniosacral therapy practitioner identifies disturbed cranial rhythms and applies corrective gentle manipulations. Restricted motion of the cranial bones at the sutures is thought to impede CSF flow and lead to disordered function and disease.

Craniosacral therapy is known in the osteopathic profession preferentially as cranial osteopathy. The chiropractic profession has a technique that encompasses much of craniosacral therapy, and others as well, known as sacro-occipital technique (SOT). CST is also practiced by a variety of other hands-on practitioners including physical and massage therapists, dentists, and lay practitioners.

Craniosacral therapy is included under the "putative" energy category in that the motions of the primary respiratory mechanism have not been irrefutably demonstrated. Skeptics and critics inside [47] and outside [48] of the osteopathic medicine profession have challenged the existence of these subtle rhythms. Reliability studies of the manual diagnosis of disturbed cranial rhythms have been disappointing [49]. The Cochrane Collaboration contains no evidence-based medicine reviews of craniosacral therapy. A systematic review of this approach "found insufficient evidence to support craniosacral therapy" [50].

Homeopathy

Homeopathy is a system of diagnosis and treatment founded by Samuel C. Hahnemann in Germany in the late eighteenth century. Homeopathy is currently practiced widely in Europe and Great Britain and by many practitioner types in the United States including MD, DO, DC, NDm and lay providers. Clinical evaluations include detailed history interviews that lead to individualized treatment regimens, depending on a host of physical, emotional, and psychologic factors. The therapies include the use of homeopathic remedies, which are derived from plant, mineral, and other extracts that have been serially diluted, often to the point where, statistically at least, no physical molecules of the original substance remain.

This fact of course challenges fundamentally the notions of science and the physical universe that underlie conventional medicine. Most CM practitioners simply cannot accept the idea that a substance that has nothing physically "there" can have any real effect beyond that attributable to placebo. Nonetheless, a number of studies in reliable scientific journals report the apparent effectiveness of the medicine.

There is an extensive literature on homeopathy. A MedLine search, 1996–2005 for "homeopathy" returned over 1300 citations. Many of these are foreign language publications. A strictly nonscientific sampling of these abstracts indicates that pain and chronic pain conditions have not typically been studied. A search of the British journal *Homeopathy* for "pain" retrieved only 14 abstracts. As with natural medicine approaches to pain treatment, a homeopathic practitioner is more likely to be evaluating and treating underlying causes of pain rather than treating pain itself.

Ayurvedic medicine

"Ayurveda, which literally means "the science of life," is a natural healing system developed in India. Ayurvedic texts claim that the sages who developed India's original systems of meditation and yoga developed the foundations of this medical system. It is a comprehensive system of medicine that places equal emphasis on the body, mind, and spirit, and strives to restore the innate harmony of the individual. Some of the primary Ayurvedic treatments include diet, exercise, meditation, herbs, massage, exposure to sunlight, and controlled breathing. In India, Ayurvedic treatments have been developed for various diseases (eg, diabetes, cardiovascular conditions, and neurologic disorders). However, a survey of the Indian medical literature indicates that the quality of the published clinical trials generally falls short of contemporary methodologic standards with regard to criteria for randomization, sample size, and adequate controls" [51].

"In the prebiblical Ayurvedic origins, every creation inclusive of a human being is a model of the universe. In this model, the basic matter and the dynamic forces (Dosha) of the nature determine health and disease, and the medicinal value of any substance (plant and mineral). The Ayurvedic practices (chiefly that of diet, life style, and the Panchkarama) aim to maintain the Dosha equilibrium. Despite a holistic approach aimed to cure disease, therapy is customized to the individual's constitution (Prakruti). Numerous

Ayurvedic medicines (plant derived in particular) have been tested for their biological (especially immunomodulation) and clinical potential using modern ethnovalidation, and thereby setting an interface with modern medicine" [52].

A MedLine search for "Ayurvedic medicine" retuned 66 results. A systematic review of ayurvedic medicine for treatment of rheumatoid arthritis (RA) concluded that, "There is a paucity of RCTs [randomized clinicial trials] of Ayurvedic medicines for RA. The existing RCTs fail to show convincingly that such treatments are effective therapeutic options for RA" [53]. However, as with other many CAM therapies, especially the energy-based modalities, the issues raised by double-blind methodologies and placebo effects have not been thoroughly accounted for. The "spiritual strength" of the Ayurvedic healer and the utility of the placebo effect are both acknowledged and considered significant in many non-western healing traditions [54].

Touch therapies

Touch is a fundamental human sense. The skin is arguably the largest sensory organ of the body. The power of human touch has been recognized throughout the history of medicine. Therapeutic Touch (TT) and its derivatives are energy-based therapies that have become common in some hospitals and other clinical settings:

> Therapeutic Touch is a contemporary healing modality drawn from ancient practices and developed by Dora Kunz and Dolores Krieger. The practice is based on the assumptions that human beings are complex fields of energy, and that the ability to enhance healing in another is a natural potential.
>
> TT is used to balance and promote the flow of human energy. It is taught in colleges around the world and has a substantial base of formal and clinical research. This research has shown that TT is useful in reducing pain, improving wound healing, aiding relaxation, and easing the dying process. It can be learned by anyone with a sincere interest and motivation toward helping others [55].

A Medline search for "therapeutic touch and pain" returned three citations. A Cochrane Review of TT for acute wound healing found insufficient evidence that TT enhances wound healing [56]. However, a pilot trial of TT in a cognitive behavioral therapy program found chronic pain patients who received TT in addition to relaxation and cognitive behavioral therapy fared better in terms of enhanced self-efficacy and unitary power, as well as having lower attrition rates than patients who only received relaxation training and cognitive behavioral therapy.

A study [57] at the University of Wisconsin-Eau Claire studied another touch therapy (Tellington Touch) in patients about to undergo venipuncture. The intervention is described as "gentle physical touch and consisting of four components: a mental attitude of openness, use of the hands and fingers, breath awareness, and moderate finger/hand pressure." Analysis of qualitative descriptions by patients and the phlebotomist-nurse demonstrated that this massage-like, caring touch promoted relaxation and produced a helpful distraction in patients about to undergo a potentially painful procedure. While further study is warranted, the implications for physicians and others who have hands-on contact with patients of any sort, and chronic pain patients in particular, seem obvious. The development of these skills may be of significant benefit to patients.

Reiki and energy healing therapies

Reiki (pronounced RAY-kee) is Japanese for a universal life energy. It is derived from rei, meaning "free passage" or "transcendental spirit" and ki, meaning "vital life force energy" or "universal life energy." Reiki is based on the belief that when spiritual energy is channeled through a Reiki practitioner, the patient's spirit is healed, which in turn heals the physical body [58,59]. Reiki practice usually involves no direct physical ontact between practitioner and recipient. By the practitioner holding the hands over the patient's body, the recipient is said to draw energy from the universal life force through the practitioner.

In the late 1800s, Dr. Mikao Usui developed modern reiki from ancient Asian healing traditions said to be thousands of years old. Introduced to the West in the 1970s, reiki has become a popular CAM therapy in the United States. Reiki and other energy healing (EH) therapies have also attracted the attention of conventional medicine practitioners and researchers [60]. A recent review noted, "The National Institutes of Health is funding numerous EH studies that are examining its effects on a variety of conditions, including temporomandibular joint disorders, wrist fractures, cardiovascular health, cancer, wound healing, neonatal stress, pain, fibromyalgia, and AIDS. Several well-designed studies to date show significant outcomes for such conditions as wound healing and advanced AIDS, and positive results for pain and anxiety, among others. It is also suggested that EH may have positive effects on various orthopaedic conditions, including fracture healing, arthritis, and muscle and connective tissue. Because negative outcomes risk is at or near zero throughout the literature, EH is a candidate for use on many medical conditions" [61].

Reiki is practiced by a variety of licensed health care practitioners including CM and CAM physicians, allied health care providers (RN, PT, OTR), psychotherapists, massage practitioners, as well as nonlicensed reiki "masters." Although reiki and other EH therapies are not without their critics [62], these high-touch, low-tech interventions are being adopted by hospitals, clinics, and physician offices as useful adjuncts to patient care [63,64]. Higher patient satisfaction, improved clinical outcomes, and lower costs are ascribed to implementing reiki and other EH therapies.

Summary

Far from being on the fringes of modern health care, many CAM therapies have been in regular and frequent use by many chronic pain patients. Increasingly these unconventional therapies are subjected to the same rigorous investigation that is expected of all contemporary evidence-based medical practices. Arguably, many CAM therapies hold up very well to this scrutiny and certainly as well as many commonly prescribed conventional medical therapies.

The fact that they are in common use by chronic pain patients suggests the need to better understand them. The emerging evidence that they are safe, clinically effective, and cost-effective when appropriately rendered further recommends them. That CAM therapies explicitly incorporate the power of awareness and intentions in the human interaction of the healing encounter may well be the key in achieving a more individualized, sensitive, and humanized approach to the treatment of a most difficult and challenging patient population—those with chronic pain.

Addendum: case histories

Because of the diversity of CAM procedures and CAM practitioners, it is not feasible to describe how CAM practitioners in general might evaluate the representative patients described elsewhere in this issue. Instead, the vignettes for these patients were presented to four different practitioners of CAM. Their responses are given below.

Case presentation #1: Peter R. Martin, LAc, Portland, OR

The assessment of the case sounds appropriate from a western medicine perspective. An acupuncture and Oriental medicine evaluation would further inquire as to the history and current symptoms incorporating the "10 questions" common to most acupuncture evaluations. These are similar to a system review in conventional medicine with inquiry about gastro-intestinal, genitourinary (GU), and other systemic issues, sensitivities to heat and cold, sleep patterns, diet, and exercise. In addition, the usual tongue and pulse diagnosis would add to the findings to develop the syndrome differentiation. The syndrome in this case would likely be a stagnation of blood and chi due to trauma. Pain is also a presumed stagnation of blood, chi, or both.

Acupuncture treatment would be directed to moving blood and chi in affected channels. Needle techniques along affected channels in the affected areas and at points distal to the affected areas are intended to activate the flow throughout the entire channel. In this case, scalp acupuncture would be an attractive option due to the head injury and intracranial vascular damage. Areas of the brain map to specific sites on the scalp that would be ripe for stimulation.

A typical acupuncture treatment plan would start with three treatments per week. The duration expected would vary depending on the stage of recovery. The case scenario does not specify the length of time since the injury. Scalp acupuncture works best in stroke cases for example within 6 months of the event. Were this case still fairly fresh, some positive result would be evident in a matter of weeks. More chronic, longstanding cases would warrant treatment plans ranging over a period of months.

Case presentation #2: Carolyn McMakin, DC, Vancouver, WA

Additional workup should include a detailed sensory examination along with a complete medication and nutraceutical history. Repeat sensory evaluation should be conducted at the beginning and end of each treatment session to document patient progress at each session and over the course of treatment.

Treatment protocols specific for diabetic neuropathy use an alternating DC current generator at frequencies thought to address acute and chronic inflammation and fibrosis of the nerves and blood vessels common in diabetic neuropathy. Current levels vary from 100 to 200 mAs. Each treatment session lasts 40 to 60 minutes and is concluded with 15 minutes of positive polarized DC current thought to reduce inflammation in the nerves and improve secretion of nerve trophic factors.

Typical treatment plans involve three to six sessions over a 1- to 4-week interval, depending on the severity and chronicity of the peripheral neuropathy. Nutritional supplementation known to improve neural function should be considered including essential fatty acids-EPA/DHA, phosphatidyl, serine, vitamin B-6, B-12 and folate. If this post-MI patient is on statins, discontinuation should be considered to ameliorate their known deleterious effect on neural function. In their place, 200 to 1000 mg of Co-Q 10 should be considered. Statins might be reintroduced at the successful conclusion of treatment as long as improved neural function is maintained.

This treatment generally produces notable improvement in sensation after each session. At the conclusion of the treatment plan, improvement lasts from 1 to 2 weeks and reapplication of treatment every 1 to 2 weeks is necessary to maintain normal sensation.

Case presentation #3: Marian Fish, DC, Portland, OR

This case is the classic picture of post-traumatic fibromyalgia syndrome (FMS). This occurs in upward of one in five trauma patients. Risk factors for developing post-traumatic fibromyalgia include a family history of rheumatic disease and a personal history of chronic fatigue or frequent muscle aches and soreness. Inquiry about difficulty sleeping, pain while "holding positions" as in shopping, food preparation, sitting behind a desk, sewing, driving long distances, or other sedentary activities both serve to confirm the diagnosis but also may identify markers for functional improvement over a course of treatment.

Additional physical evaluation would usually include motion palpation to identify spinal or peripheral joint hypermobility as this frequently attends fibromyalgia. Skin rolling techniques will isolate skin and subcutaneous tissues that feel adherent to the underlying fascia.

Treatment would involve a combination of physical modalities, dietary modification, nutritional supplementation, and exercise. Physical therapy modalities such as electrical muscle stimulation are useful to facilitate muscular relaxation that in turn helps increase circulation to bring more oxygen and nutrients to the tissues. FMS patients have poor circulation and thus poor oxygenation to their tissues. Myofascial release is directed to tender areas identified with skin rolling.

FMS patients often have food sensitivities, which may be associated with a lack of digestive enzymes. Without adequate enzymes, food cannot be digested and used to make all the myriad hormones, buffering compounds, enzymes, and so forth, that the liver makes for normal metabolism. Delivery of nutrients to the muscle cells is a key factor, and relaxing the vasculature so the nutrients can be delivered is also axiomatic. Magnesium malate is given to relax the muscles and blood vessels. It improves sleep quality immensely in most people who are sleep deficient. This simple regimen appears to help most of these patients.

If the patient is not improved, free form amino acids are added as an alternative to or in addition to digestive enzymes to bolster digestion and subsequent biochemical events. Also stimulants, soda drinks, and refined sugar should be removed from the diet. Carbonated drinks especially create too much phosphorus, which can interfere with ATP activity. Most FMS patients are fatigued. Many patients improve when the soda drinks are eliminated. They also improve when common food intolerances such as dairy products and wheat are eliminated.

The patient needs to do 30 minutes or more of aerobic exercise daily, and do upper body strengthening with weights, preferably circuit weight training.

All but the truly recalcitrant will improve markedly or experience a complete remission.

Case presentation #4: Kevin Wilson, ND, Hillsboro, OR

Given the history of a fall from a height and with the presence of an L1 compression fracture, evaluation of ligamentous instability is appropriate. Static and motion palpation are the best tools to identify segmental hypermobility. Stress radiographs also could detect excessive vertebral motion, although stress radiography does not reliably identify instability.

Diagnostic injections at the thoracolumbar junction did not identify a pain generator. This may mean that levels above, below, or lateral to the fracture site may prove to be the source of pain. Similarly, ligamentous instability may well be not at the site of the fracture but at adjacent levels. The prolotherapy injections are diagnostic in that relief indicates both proper localization and tissue diagnosis.

This patient is a good candidate for prolotherapy or mesotherapy. A common prolotherapy protocol involves a cocktail of 12.5% solution glucose, 1% procaine, 10% glucosamine sulfate. These substances are safe and well tolerated by most patients. More aggressive combinations are also used including combinations of glucose, glycerin, and phenol. Mesotherapy involves shallow (2- and 4-mm) intradermal injections of therapeutic agents (eg, NSAIDs, salmon calcitonin) that migrate into underlying synovium, producing the therapeutic effect.

A typical treatment plan for prolotherapy to a weight-bearing area, such as the thoracolumbar junction, is injection at 2- to 4-week intervals for a total of four to10 injections. A typical trial of four injections will demonstrate the effectiveness of the therapy. One or two injections after the patient is completely asymptomatic seem to enhance effectiveness and promote long-term pain relief.

References

[1] Inglis B. Fringe Medicine. London: Faber and Faber; 1964.

[2] Eisenberg D. Unconventional medicine in the United States—prevalence, cost, and patterns of use. N Engl J Med 1993;328:426–525.

[3] Angell M, Kassirer JP. Alternative medicine–the risks of untested and unregulated remedies. N Engl J Med 1998;339:839–41.

[4] Committee on the Use of Complementary and Alternative Medicine by the American Public Board on Health Promotion and Disease Prevention. Institute of Medicine of the National Academies. Complementary and alternative medicine in the United States. Washington, DC: The National Academies Press; 2005.

[5] Cicerone KD. Evidence-based practice and the limits of rational rehabilitation. Arch Phys Med Rehabil 2005;86:1073–4.

[6] Oschman J. Energy medicine in therapeutics and human performance. Edinburgh: Butterworth-Heinman; 2003.

[7] National Center for Complementary and Alternative Medicine. What is complementary and alternative medicine? NCCAM Publication No. D156. Available at: http://nccam.nih.gov. Accessed February 8, 2006.

[8] Whitten CE, Evans CM, Cristobal K. Pain management doesn't have to be a pain: working and communicating effectively with patients who have chronic pain. Permanente J 2005;5(2): 41–8.

[9] Lundgren J, Ugalde V. The demographics and economics of complementary alternative medicine. Phys Med Rehabil Clin N Am 2004;15(4):955–61.

[10] Studdert D, Eisenberg D, Miller F, et al. Trends in alternative medicine use in the United States. 1990–1997: results of a follow-up national survey. JAMA 1998;280:1569–75.

[11] Hirsh AT, Atchison J, Berger J, et al. Patient satisfaction with treatment for chronic pain: predictors and relationship to compliance. Clin J Pain 2005;21(4):302–10.

[12] Paterson C, Dieppe P. Characteristic and incidental (placebo) effects in complex interventions such as acupuncture. BMJ 2005;330:1202–5.

[13] Sullivan MD. Placebo controls and epistemic control in orthodox medicine. J Med Philos 1993;18(2):213–31.

[14] Cicerone K. Evidence-based practice and the limits of rational rehabilitation. Arch Phys Med Rehabil 2005;86(6):1073–4.
[15] Shekell P, Morton S, Suttorp M, et al. Challenges in systematic reviews of complementary and alternative medicine topics. Ann Int Med 2005;142:1042–7.
[16] Shekelle PG, Adams AH, Chassin MR, et al. Spinal manipulation for low back pain. Ann Intern Med 1992;117:590–8.
[17] Assendelft W, Morton S, Yu E, et al. Spinal manipulative therapy for low back pain: A meta-analysis of effectiveness relative to other therapies. Ann Intern Med 2003;138:871–81.
[18] Bronfort G. The effectiveness of cervical adjustment for acute and chronic neck pain: excerpts from a systematic review and best evidence synthesis. J Am Chiro 2003;40(7):42.
[19] McCrory D, Penzein D, Hasselblad V, et al. Evidence report: Behavioral and physical treatments for tension-type headache. Durham (NC): Duke University Evidence-based Practice Center; 2001.
[20] Muller R, Giles LGF. Long-term follow-up of a randomized clinical trial assessing the efficacy of medication, acupuncture, and spinal manipulation for chronic mechanical spinal pain syndromes. J Manip Phys Ther 2005;29(1):3–11.
[21] Rickover R, Rickover A. What is Alexander technique? Available at: http://www.alexandertechnique.com/at.htm. Accessed February 8, 2006.
[22] Erntst E, Canter PH. The Alexander technique: a systematic review of controlled clinical trials. Forsch Komplementarmed Klass Naturheilkd 2003;10(6):325–9.
[23] Feldenkrais Educational Foundation of North America. Standards of practice. Available at: http://www.feldenkrais.com/method/standards/index.html#what. Accessed February 8, 2006.
[24] Jain S, Janssen K, DeCelle S. Alexander technique and Feldenkrais method: a critical overview [review]. Phys Med Rehabil Clin N Am 2004;15(4):811–25.
[25] Braverman DL, Schulman RA. Massage techniques in rehabilitation medicine. Phys Med Rehabil Clin N Am 1999;10(3):631–49, ix.
[26] Furlan AD, Brosseau L, Imamura M, et al. Massage for low-back pain. The Cochrane Database of Systematic Reviews 2006;1. Available at: http://www.cochrane.org/reviews/en/ab001929.html. Accessed February 8, 2006.
[27] Lum LC. Hyperventilation: the tip of the iceberg. J Psychosomatic Res 1975;19:375–83.
[28] Chaitow L. Breathing pattern disorders, motor control and low back pain. J Osteo Med 2004;7(1):34–41.
[29] Mehling WE, Hamel K, Acree M, et al. Randomized, controlled trial of breath therapy for patients with chronic low back pain. Altern Ther Health Med J 2005;11(4):44–52.
[30] Dagenais S, Haldeman S, Wooley JR. Intraligamentous injection of sclerosing solutions (prolotherapy) for spinal pain: a critical review of the literature. Spine J 2005;5(3):310–28.
[31] Yelland MJ, Del Mar C, Pirozzo S, et al. Prolotherapy injections for chronic low-back pain. The Cochrane Database of Systematic Reviews 2006;1. Available at: http://www.cochrane.org/reviews/en/ab004059.html. Accessed February 8, 2006.
[32] Travell JG, Simons DG. Myofascial pain and dysfunction: the trigger point manual: the upper extremities, vol. 1. Baltimore, MD: Williams & Wilkins; 1983.
[33] McPartland J. Travell trigger points–molecular and osteopathic perspectives. J Am Osteopath Assoc 2004;104(6):244–9.
[34] Al-Shenqiti AM, Oldham JA. Test-retest reliability of myofascial trigger point detection in patients with rotator cuff tendonitis. Clin Rehabil 2005;19(5):482–7.
[35] Carter R, Hall T, Aspy CB, Mold J. The effectiveness of magnet therapy for treatment of wrist pain attributed to carpal tunnel syndrome. Fam Pract 2002;51(1):38–40.
[36] Wolsko PM, et al. Double-blind placebo-controlled trial of static magnets for the treatment of osteoarthritis of the knee: results of a pilot study. Altern Ther Health Med J 2004;10(2):36–43.
[37] McMakin C. Microcurrent treatment of myofascial pain in the head, neck and face. Top Clin Chiro 1998;5(1):29–35.

[38] McMakin C. Microcurrent therapy: a novel treatment for chronic low back myofascial pain. J Bodywork Movement Ther 2004;8:143–53.
[39] McMakin C, Gregeory W, Phillips T. Cytokine changes with microcurrent treatment of fibromyalgia associated with cervical trauma. Journal of Bodywork and Movement Therapies 2005;9:169–76.
[40] Chow RT, Barnsley L. Systematic review of the literature of low-level laser therapy (LLLT) in the management of neck pain. Lasers Surg Med 2005;37(1):46–52.
[41] Brosseau L, Gam A, Harman K, et al. Low level laser therapy (Classes I, II and III) for treating osteoarthritis. The Cochrane Database of Systematic Reviews 2006;1. Available at: http://www.cochrane.org/reviews/en/ab002026.html. Accessed February 8, 2006.
[42] Brosseau L, Robinson V, Wells G, et al. Low level laser therapy (Classes I, II and III) for treating rheumatoid arthritis. The Cochrane Database of Systematic Reviews 2006;1. Available at: http://www.cochrane.org/reviews/en/ab002049.html. Accessed February 8, 2006.
[43] National Center for Complementary and Alternative Medicine. Acupuncture. NCCAM Publication No. D003. Available at: http://nccam.nih.gov/health/backgrounds/wholemed.htm#tcm. Accessed February 8, 2006.
[44] Acupuncture. NIH consensus statement online. 1997;15(5):1–34.
[45] Breivik H, Collett B, Ventafridda V, et al. Survey of chronic pain in Europe: prevalence, impact on daily life, and treatment. Eur J Pain 2005, in press.
[46] Manheimer E, White A, Berman B, et al. Meta-analysis: acupuncture for low back pain. Ann Intern Med 2005;142(8):651–63.
[47] Bledsoe BE, Licciardone JC. The elephant in the room: does OMT have proved benefit? J Am Osteopath Assoc 2004;104:405–6.
[48] Barrett S. Craniosacral therapy. Available at: http://www.quackwatch.org/01QuackeryRelatedTopics/cranial.html. Accessed February 8, 2006.
[49] Moran RW, Gibbons P. Intraexaminer and interexaminer reliability for palpation of the cranial rhythmic impulse at the head and sacrum. J Manipulative Physiol Ther 2001;24:183–90.
[50] Green C, Martin CW, Bassett K, Kazajian H. A systematic review of craniosacral therapy: biological plausibility, assessment reliability and clinical effectiveness. Comp Ther Med 1999;7(4):199–270.
[51] National Center for Complementary and Alternative Medicine. Whole medical systems: An overview. CCAM Publication No. D236. Available at: http://nccam.nih.gov/health/backgrounds/wholemed.htm#am. Accessed February 8, 2006.
[52] Chopra A, Doiphole VV. Ayurvedic medicine. Core concept, therapeutic principles, and current relevance. Med Clin N Am 2002;86(1):75–89, vii.
[53] Park J, Ernst E. Ayurvedic medicine for rheumatoid arthritis: a systematic review. Semin Arthr Rheumatism 2005;34(5):705–13.
[54] Jonas WB, Levin JS. Essentials of complementary and alternative medicine. Baltimore: Lippincott, Williams and Wilkins; 1999. p. 210.
[55] Pumpkin Hollow Foundation. Therapeutic touch defined. Available at: http://therapeutictouch.org/whatistt.html. Accessed February 8, 2006.
[56] O'Mathuna DP, Ashford RL. Therapeutic touch for healing acute wounds. Cochrane Database Systematic Rev 2003;4:CD002766.
[57] Wendler M. Effects of Tellington Touch in healthy adults awaiting venipuncture. Research in Nursing and Health 2003;26:40–52.
[58] National Center for Complementary and Alternative Medicine. What is complementary and alternative medicine? Available at: http://nccam.nih.gov/health/whatiscam/index.htm#d11. Accessed February 8, 2006.
[59] International Cyber Business Services, Inc. What is reiki? Available at: http://www.holistic-online.com/reiki/hol_reikiintroduction.htm. Accessed February 8, 2006.
[60] Chu DA. Tai chi, qi gong and reiki. Phys Med Rehabil Clin N Am 2004;15(4):773–81, vi.

[61] Dinucci EM. Energy healing: a complementary treatment for orthopaedic and other conditions. Orthop Nurs 2005;24(4):259–69.
[62] Jarvis W. Reiki. Available at: http://www.ncahf.org/articles/o-r/reiki.html. Accessed February 8, 2006.
[63] Sawyer J. The first Reiki practitioner in our OR. AORN Journal. March 1998.
[64] Rand W. Reiki in hospitals. Available at: http://www.reiki.org/reikinews/reiki_in-hospitals.htm. Accessed February 8, 2006.

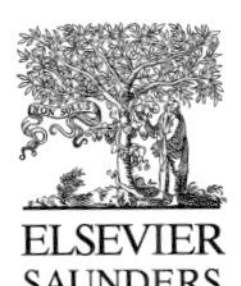

ELSEVIER
SAUNDERS

Phys Med Rehabil Clin N Am
17 (2006) 473–490

PHYSICAL MEDICINE
AND REHABILITATION
CLINICS OF
NORTH AMERICA

Traumatic Brain Injury and Pain

Kristen Brewer Sherman, PhD,
Myron Goldberg, PhD*, Kathleen R. Bell, MD

Department of Rehabilitation Medicine, University of Washington School of Medicine, 1959 NE Pacific Street, Box 356490, Seattle, WA 98195-6490, USA

This article considers the evaluation and treatment of chronic pain conditions in patients with traumatic brain injury (TBI). The emergence of significant pain problems in cases of TBI is quite common [1–3]. This high co-occurrence rate stems in large part from the nature of accident-related events and forces (eg, causing multi-trauma) as well as changes in brain functioning that affect sensory and motoric functioning and, perhaps, perception of pain stimuli. While affecting the emergence and course of pain, these trauma-related biologic factors are often not sufficient to account for the persistence of pain into chronic states in all cases. Often psychologic (eg, cognitive, emotional) and social factors also need to be considered to understand the persistence of pain complaints, prompting the need for use of a biopsychosocial approach in the evaluation and treatment of chronic pain conditions in patients with TBI.

Although widely cited in the literature as a distinct factor affecting management and outcome [4], the co-existence of TBI and pain has not actually received much well-controlled, systematic study in terms of its epidemiology, course, evaluation, treatment, or effects on functional outcome. However, what is well known in the clinical setting is that the co-occurrence of pain and TBI offers unique conceptual, diagnostic, and treatment challenges for the practitioner. This article focuses on chronic pain in patients with TBI, with the following aims: (1) to provide an overview of the extent and nature of the co-morbid problem; (2) to highlight the clinical challenges that are unique; and (3) to discuss specific evaluation and treatment approaches for two of the more frequent pain conditions in patients with TBI, namely headache and pain arising from spasticity.

Supported in part by the National Institute of Disability and Rehabilitation Research, U.S. Department of Education (grant no. H133A020508).

* Corresponding author.

E-mail address: goldbm@u.washington.edu (M. Goldberg).

doi:10.1016/j.pmr.2005.11.007 ***pmr.theclinics.com***

Background

Several pain conditions are common among patients with TBI, including headache and neuropathic pain, as well as pain arising from such conditions as spasticity, heterotopic ossification, deep venous thrombosis, genitourinary and gastrointestinal disorders, and orthopedic trauma (ie, fractures and other musculoskeletal injuries) [5]. Despite their common appearance in clinical practice, these chronic pain conditions in patients with TBI have received little attention in the literature from an epidemiologic standpoint. Moreover, the few studies that are present in the literature have largely had a narrow focus (ie, examined only one or a small number of pain conditions) and differed in methodologic approaches, such as sample selection. Therefore, our knowledge about frequency, nature, and course of the co-morbid problem remains rather limited, given the nature of the literature to date.

Research-based estimates of the overall prevalence of chronic pain and TBI are quite high, though variable. In a recent prospective study of patients who had been hospitalized on an acute rehabilitation unit for TBI, Hoffman and colleagues [3] found that at 1-year post injury 72.6% of individuals complained of pain of some form, with 47.2% reporting mild pain and 25.4% reporting moderate to severe pain. Being female, having a lower functional status, and being depressed were associated with increased pain severity. Lahz and Bryant [1] found that slightly over half of a sample of consecutive patients referred to an outpatient brain injury clinic reported a chronic pain problem, with similar pain report rates obtained for those with mild TBIs (58%) and those with moderate to severe TBIs (52%). Other studies have found similarly high pain report rates but a negative relationship between injury severity and pain report frequency. For example, in a retrospective chart review involving patients seen in an outpatient brain injury clinic, Uomoto and Esselman [6] reported that 95% of patients with mild TBI and only 22% of patients with moderate to severe TBI identified some form of pain problem. A similar negative relationship between injury severity and pain report frequency occurred in a study by Beetar and colleagues [2], which involved a TBI outpatient sample referred for a neuropsychologic examination. This study is also noteworthy in that a comparison in pain report rates was made between their TBI sample and a sample of outpatients with non-TBI, neurologic disorders (eg, stroke, brain tumor). Notably, patients with TBI were 2 1/2 times more likely than their non-TBI, neurologic counterparts to report some form of pain.

Prevalence rates by pain type (eg, musculoskeletal, neuropathic) in patients with TBI have simply not yet been well established in the literature. A few studies have looked at pain location. Perhaps as might be expected, the head is the most common location of pain and is consistently found to be a more frequent site among mild TBI cases [7], with half to three quarters of most samples reporting significant headache, as compared with about a third of those with moderate to severe TBI [1,6,8]. Notably, different types or locations of pain often co-occur in the same patient, especially among those with less severe brain injury. For example, Uomoto and Esselman [6] found that 60% of their sample with mild TBI reported more than one pain location.

As noted previously, mild TBI groups, in general, have been found to report pain, especially headache, more frequently than those with more severe injuries. This negative relationship between TBI severity and pain may, at first glance, seem counterintuitive. One hypothesis to explain this apparent paradox is that patients with the most severe TBIs are often treated with paralytic agents and bed rest, allowing for healing of cervical injuries, whereas those with milder injuries continue to use potentially damaged muscles and ligaments in their necks, interfering with healing [9,10]. However, providers may be less aware of pain among those more severely injured because there are other more pressing concerns that require attention, and those with more severe injuries may have more difficulty communicating their pain.

Little is known about the course of pain in TBI populations, as there are few studies that have looked systematically at trends. One exception is a study by Olver and colleagues [11], which found an increase in reported pain problems from 2 to 5 years post-injury. Clinically, the course varies widely, with many patients improving, but with others having very chronic, at times debilitating, pain problems. As noted previously, in cases where little improvement in or worsening of the pain condition occurs over time, it is especially important to take a biopsychosocial approach to evaluation and treatment of mechanisms or factors that might be involved in the maintenance of the pain condition.

In summary, studies to date, although containing potential methodologic limitations (eg, subject selection), provide a consistent picture of a rather high co-occurrence rate of TBI and chronic pain. Additionally, findings from a few studies suggest that the prevalence rate for pain may be significantly higher for TBI than other neurologic brain disorders and, in those patients with TBI, is negatively related to brain injury severity. Clearly, however, additional well-designed, epidemiologic-based studies are needed, as our information regarding the actual prevalence as well as course of pain in persons with TBI is incomplete.

Evaluation and treatment strategies

Challenges

The co-occurrence of TBI and chronic pain presents a number of conceptual, diagnostic, and treatment challenges that need to be considered and managed by the rehabilitation clinician. Conceptually, the challenge for the clinician in treating a patient with TBI and pain is best described by the following question: "Does the pain condition complicate the TBI condition or does the TBI condition complicate the pain condition?" This "background-foreground" discrimination task is made more complex for the clinician by the likelihood that the effects of cognitive and behavioral impairment and pain on a patient's functional status vary over time. This dynamic situation requires a readiness on the part of clinicians to recalibrate their view of causal factors as well as the focus of treatment at any given time. Moreover, and as with many co-morbid conditions, TBI and pain do not simply act as independent factors, but often function in an interactive manner that results in increases in symptom intensity associated with each condition and, in turn, level of disability. How the clinician works through this conceptual challenge posed by the co-occurrence of TBI and pain is not a mere intellectual exercise, as the perception can influence impressions and treatment decision-making over the course of care.

The diagnostic challenges can, to some degree, be broken down by TBI severity. For patients with moderate to severe TBI, even determining whether a significant pain problem is present may be the primary challenge. Often verbal communication ability is severely compromised in these patients, an impairment that prevents or significantly degrades the primary means on which clinicians typically rely to identify the presence of pain. In such situations, the presence of pain must then be inferred by less reliable methods (eg, observations of nonverbal behaviors which may be indicative of pain, such as agitation). Even when communication ability is well preserved, the types and extent of cognitive functioning impairment experienced by patients with moderate to severe TBI can affect the reliability and validity of clinicians' efforts to identify the presence of pain. For example, in cases in which severe executive dysfunction is present, patients are at risk to "over-focus" or perseverate on salient stimuli, like pain, leading to the possibility of intensifying their experience of pain. Memory disturbance in patients with moderate to severe TBI is another cognitive deficit that, in many cases, can prevent conveyance of accurate information on such parameters as frequency, pattern, and activities that increase pain [4], which assist the clinician in determining the type of treatment approach to be followed as well as when to initiate, change, or terminate treatment.

Dealing effectively with these diagnostic challenges is essential in caring for patients with moderate to severe TBI, as pain that is inadequately managed has the potential to compromise recovery, by interfering with a patient's ability to participate and benefit from other rehabilitation treatments as well as negatively impact their emotional status. Additionally, poorly managed pain can act as an internal antecedent stimulus (or trigger) for difficult-to-manage behavioral problems, like restlessness and agitation, for which patients with moderate to severe TBI are already at risk. Clinically, our experience tells us that adequate evaluation of pain in cases of moderate to severe TBI depends on a combination of patient supplied information and external sources of information. In terms of the patient, the clinician needs to often and keenly take notice of nonverbal expressions of pain, like grimacing, agitation, or guarding. In some cases, patients who are not able to verbally communicate effectively about pain may be able to use a simple visual analog scale, with anchors including facial expression. External sources of information can prove to be invaluable and include caregivers and rehabilitation staff who are typically able to spend more time with the patients. In particular, these external sources can often provide useful information about the temporal relationships between certain activities and pain indicators. In the end, in moderate to severe TBI cases in which there is a reasonable question about the presence of pain, it is likely best to assume its presence, given what we know about prevalence rates.

The diagnostic challenge in cases of mild TBI and pain is somewhat different. In this instance, the common dilemma facing the clinician is determining the factors contributing to the cognitive, emotional, and behavioral changes that follow the injury. Pain, by itself, has been shown to have the capacity to significantly interfere with neuropsychologic functioning in people without any known brain injury in several studies [12–14], with attention and speed of mental processing being perhaps the two most vulnerable cognitive abilities affected [12]. Disentangling the relative contribution of pain and TBI on cognitive functioning can be an arduous task, regardless of brain injury severity, but one accentuated particularly in mild TBI cases. However, the impressions that the clinician reaches regarding etiology can have an enormous impact on treatment decisions as well as education of patients regarding factors impacting their functional status and sense of well being.

The treatment challenge is multifold. As highlighted by Ivanhoe and Hartman [5], a guiding principle in traumatic brain injury rehabilitation should be the promotion of cognitive recovery. With this principle in mind, one challenge for the clinician is selecting treatments that strike the optimal balance between reducing pain and preserving or enhancing cognitive functioning. This balancing act is particularly relevant when pharmacologic management of pain is part of the equation, as many medications, especially in the opioid and antidepressant classes, can have deleterious cognitive side effects [15]. Patients with TBI are conceivably even more vulnerable than other patients to the cognitive side effects of certain analgesic medications, although this has not been systematically studied. Because of this, the use of nonsedating analgesics (eg, acetaminophen, nonsteroidal anti-inflammatory drugs, and transdermal lidocaine patches) should be a first line in treating pain in patients with TBI.

Another treatment challenge is that cognitive functioning impairments are likely to affect adherence to treatment recommendations (eg, home exercise program, medications) and safety precautions. Memory difficulty and executive dysfunction (eg, difficulties with initiation or behavioral impulsiveness) are the most notable types of cognitive problems that could affect adherence. In such cases, the clinician needs to determine early in the course of treatment the extent to which the patient can be responsible for his/her care and, in turn, whether supervision is needed. In a related matter, patients with moderate to severe cognitive problems may not be able to reliably request pain medications in a timely manner, before pain becomes overly intense and disabling. It is often advantageous (for the patient and caregiver alike) to use a scheduled, rather than as-needed, dosing of pain medication. Aside from their potential impact on pharmacologic interventions, cognitive difficulties also have the potential to interfere with the effectiveness of nonpharmacologic pain management approaches, including physical therapy and psychotherapy. Compensatory methods (eg, mediset, detailed written instructions for patients and caregivers) for these difficulties need to be incorporated on a routine to basis increase the chances of therapeutic success.

Lastly, behavioral and emotional factors common to TBI and pain can complicate treatment decisions and outcome. Psychopathology, especially mood disorder, occurs frequently in patients with chronic pain disorders [16] and those with traumatic brain injury [17]. In particular, mood disturbance and anxiety problems have been shown to affect patients' experience of pain and interfere with the quality and consistency of cognitive functioning [18–20]. By the same token, pain and effects of TBI can impact emotional functioning, creating a feedback loop that has the potential to lead to further disability. Therefore, treatment decision-making in many cases will depend on thorough consideration not only of pain and TBI-related factors but also of emotional functioning.

Clearly, comorbid pain and TBI offer a number of challenges to the rehabilitation clinician. Next, the article focuses on more specific issues and recommendations for evaluation and treatment. Based on what is seen clinically, the focus is particularly on pain related to spasticity and headache.

Pain and severe traumatic brain injury: spasticity

As noted earlier, pain can originate from a number of sources in patients with severe TBI. However, spasticity and related conditions occur commonly in this population and result in diagnostic and management dilemmas that may be different from other populations with spasticity. Spasticity in patients with severe TBI tends to be associated with both rigidity and dystonic-type posturing. The spastic rigidity noted with decerebrate and decorticate posturing can result in the rapid progression of joint contracture, particularly in young males. The co-occurrence of spasticity and rapidly developing contracture can result in painful positioning and resistance to joint stretching.

Early evaluation and management of spasticity and contracture in this group is complicated by the frequent inability of the patient to cooperate fully with a comprehensive musculoskeletal examination and the presence of musculoskeletal co-morbidities such as occult fractures, peripheral nerve injuries, and heterotopic ossification. The presence of pain in these patients and the contribution of pain to increasingly severe levels of spasticity are often overlooked in the context of severe TBI [21]. As noted earlier, the patient with severe TBI is often unable to communicate effectively, so the clinician must use observational means to diagnose pain in this context. Although the presence of muscle spasms can be painful in the absence of other conditions, spasticity leads to the formation of joint contracture, tendonitis, skin breakdown, and postural abnormalities, contributing further to the likely presence of pain. Painful or noxious stimuli can further aggravate muscle spasm, thereby contributing to the persistence of musculoskeletal pain.

Evaluation

The evaluation for spasticity and other painful musculoskeletal conditions may have to be completed in several sessions because of the patient's limited ability to cooperate and to minimize discomfort. It may be useful to premedicate with analgesics or to use heating pads or warmed blankets to relax the limbs before the examination. In extreme cases of spasticity, conscious sedation or even general anesthesia may be needed to fully examine a spastic, contracted limb. Distinguishing elevated degrees of spasticity from joint contracture may also be simplified through the use of anesthetic peripheral nerve injections, temporarily reducing spastic muscle tone. A physical examination for spasticity should always be performed in the resting/supine position and in the weight-bearing position (sitting or standing) as the intensity of spasticity may change markedly in different positions.

Typically, plain radiographs of limbs with significant spasticity and joint contractures are necessary to rule out occult fractures and heterotopic ossification. Bone scans may also be helpful both to stage heterotopic ossification, if present, and to perform a general survey of the skeleton.

Treatment: the stepped approach to the treatment of spasticity

The mere presence of spasticity or elevated muscle tone in a limb is not reason enough to initiate treatment. In some cases, spasticity can perform a useful function (eg, maintaining muscle bulk, assisting the patient in standing). However, if spasticity and the associated motor disorders of rigidity and dystonia cause pain, limit mobility, or interfere with caregiving, treatment should be undertaken.

In general, the treatment for spasticity is approached in a stepped or graduated manner (Fig. 1). Simpler or less invasive methods should be tried first in most situations. Management techniques with greater potential risk or expense would be used if less complex or invasive methods are not sufficient to relieve discomfort or optimize function. However, it is often necessary to combine methods to achieve the desired outcomes. For instance, in

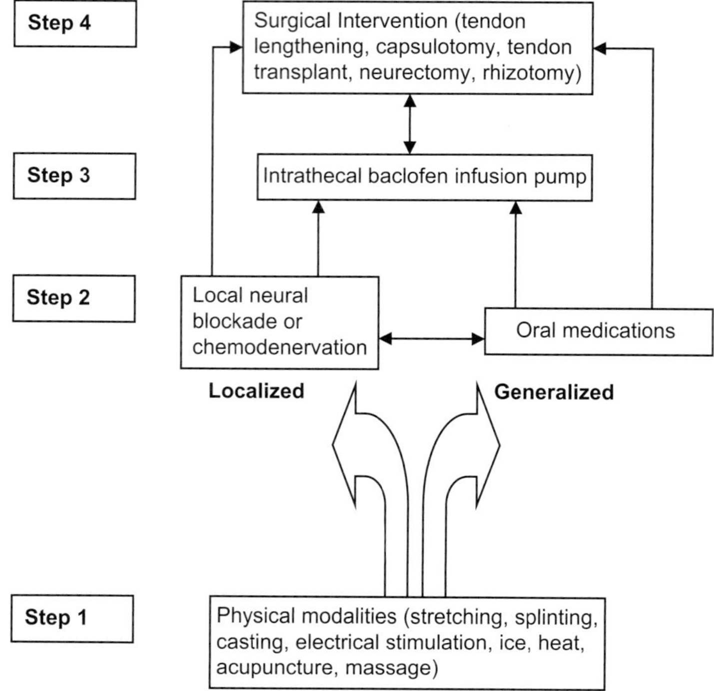

Fig. 1. The stepped approach to the management of spasticity.

a patient with spastic tetraplegia, splints, local neural blockade, and oral medications may be used simultaneously. In all instances, the goal is to optimize function and comfort without compromising cognitive function.

Physical approaches are the first techniques indicated in the treatment of spasticity. These might include removing or treating noxious or painful stimuli, daily splinting to maintain functional joint position, and regular stretching of involved muscles. Ice application to an affected muscle can be used before therapy to decrease muscle reactivity to stretch [22,23]. Casting a joint is a very effective means of controlling tone and stretching affected joints but requires skill to prevent skin breakdown [24–26]. Alternative physical treatments to control pain and spasticity may be explored. Massage is quite useful for pain relief and temporary muscle relaxation and can be used on a regular basis for those with adequate funding but there is little if any literature detailing its effect on spasticity [23]. Acupuncture has not been studied specifically for this purpose. There is evidence that acupuncture is helpful in the short-term treatment of some chronic painful musculoskeletal conditions [27,28].

If spasticity is more generalized, as in tetraplegia, or these physical maneuvers are insufficient to control spasticity, then other methods are used including oral medication, chemodenervation, implantation of intrathecal pumps for the administration of low-dose baclofen, or orthopedic surgery to reduce contracture [21,29].

In treating musculoskeletal pain and spasticity in patients with TBI, pharmacologic intervention should address both problems and can be used on a short-term basis to, for example, facilitate physical interventions or on a long-term basis in combination with other treatments (Box 1). Adequate treatment of pain before physical therapy sessions involving painful muscle stretching or the use of uncomfortable splints can decrease agitation and improve cooperation. Analgesics such as acetaminophen and nonsteroidal anti-inflammatory drugs have no effect on cognition and are quite effective for low to mid-levels of musculoskeletal pain. Narcotics, of course, can be sedating and should be used sparingly but are indicated for temporary or acute use for higher levels of pain. All spasticity-specific medications have some sedating effects, limiting their usefulness in people with significant cognitive impairment. Dantrolene sodium probably has the least effect on cognition, acting primarily on the muscle membrane, rather than on the central nervous system, and is probably the first-line drug to be considered in persons with TBI [21].

For more localized problems, the use of chemodenervation techniques can greatly contribute to management of pain and spasticity. Both neurolytic injections (phenol, alcohol) and botulinum toxin injections can be used, depending on the circumstance. For treatment early after TBI or for very localized problems, botulinum toxin is preferred because it has few potentially long-term effects [30]. Botulinum toxin is very expensive, has an upper limit for dosing to prevent systemic weakness, and must be repeated every 8 to 12 weeks. For people with more widespread, severe spasticity issues, neurolytic blocks can be very helpful in combination with botulinum

Box 1. Medications used to treat spasticity and pain

Nonspecific analgesics
Acetaminophen
Nonsteroidal anti-inflammatory drugs
Transdermal lidocaine
Narcotic analgesics[a]
Spasticity-specific medications
Dantrolene sodium
Baclofen
Tizanidine
Diazepam[a]

[a] Indicates choices with significant cognitive effects usually avoided in this population.

toxin injections in preserving functional limb positions. Although literature concerning the occurrence of adverse effects is sparse, the use of phenol blocks at nerves with minimal sensory distribution (eg, musculocutaneous, obturator, or even tibial) is unlikely to result in significant dysesthesia, and the amount of permanent axonal loss in a well-localized block is minimal [31–34]. Anesthetic peripheral nerve blocks can also be used as an adjunct to casting a limb to allow better positioning during the procedure.

Continuous intrathecal baclofen infusion via implanted pumps can also be very useful in controlling spasticity and pain and in improving function, particularly in those with more prominent lower limb spasticity. However, due to the expense, potential for adverse outcome, and the need for commitment to pump maintenance on the part of the patient and caregivers, this option is generally reserved for those in whom other treatment modalities have failed [35].

As noted earlier, spasticity and the loss of motor control can result in localized painful conditions such as subluxation, tendonitis, and capsulitis. There is limited evidence that intra-articular steroid injections for shoulder capsulitis and subacromial steroid injections for rotator cuff tendonitis have some benefit [36,37]. Electrical stimulation is another modality that has been used with success in shoulder pain associated with hemiplegia and spasticity [38–40]. Transdermal lidocaine preparations may be useful in providing local pain relief. Use of these techniques may allow decreased use of potentially sedating analgesic medications.

Education for nursing and therapy staff is essential in providing adequate pain relief for people with severe TBI and limited communication and cognitive abilities. Pain assessment in these individuals is essential as pain may compromise cognition (by impacting sleep or by increasing distraction) and motor recovery. When painful musculoskeletal conditions are noted, consideration should be given to scheduled analgesia before therapy sessions and comfort measures such as icing and heat packs should be used after stretching. Local blocks should be considered early, even during the intensive care stay, in patients with very severe spasticity to control pain and maintain good limb and joint positioning.

Pain and mild traumatic brain injury: headache

Pain is a salient feature for people with mild TBI and those with post-concussion syndrome, especially for those injuries associated with motor vehicle accidents. The most common persisting symptoms after such an injury are headache and neck pain [6,41]. These painful conditions may occur in combination with cognitive complaints such as reduced attention, memory impairment, and slowed processing speed, completing the picture of persistent post-concussion syndrome. It is often difficult to sort out which set of complaints came first. Painful conditions can result in sleep disturbance and depression, affecting cognitive efficiency while undiagnosed cognitive disorders give rise to depression and anxiety, which can enhance painful conditions.

Headache after TBI is poorly characterized. The International Headache Society describes the following types of post-traumatic headaches: (1) acute post-traumatic headache (moderate-severe or mild), (2) chronic post-traumatic headache (moderate-severe or mild), (3) acute headache attributed to whiplash, (4) chronic headache attributed to whiplash, (5) headache attributed to intracranial hematoma, (6) headache attributed to other head or neck trauma, and (7) post-craniotomy headache. These headaches, however, may have a variety of characteristics and may resemble migraines, cluster headaches, or tension-type headaches [42].

Although there are a variety of conditions that can result in headache after TBI (Box 2), migraine and tension-type headaches are the most frequent. Much of the literature on post-traumatic headache does not differentiate migraine-type headache. Trauma may trigger a first episode of migraine or may trigger more frequent or severe migraine in susceptible individuals [43,44]. Migraines can occur independently, or against a backdrop of chronic daily headache, and will have important implications for treatment. The lack of clarity in the description of headaches after TBI is reflected in studies that describe the epidemiology and natural history, diagnosis, and management. Often, this confusion results in inadequate diagnosis and a reliance on psychologic mechanisms as an explanation for headache after mild TBI. However, more recent publications are beginning to shed light on this complex subject and support a more nuanced examination of the patient with post-traumatic headache. For instance, a Swiss group closely analyzed the headache phenomenology in a group of 112 patients with chronic post-traumatic headache. In this group, 37% met the criteria for tension-type headache, 27% for migraine, and 18% for cervicogenic headache. Eighteen

Box 2. Types of headache encountered after traumatic brain injury

Tension-type
Migraine (common and other)
Basilar migraine headache
Cervicogenic (neuritic)
Dysautonomic
Intracranial and vascular
Increased intracranial pressure or hydrocephalus
Chronic subdural hematoma
Vascular injury (carotid or vertebrobasilar dissection, traumatic intracranial aneurysm)
Post-craniotomy infection

percent had headaches that overlapped classification [44]. Packard and Ham [45] note that the biochemical changes seen in mild TBI mirror in many ways the picture seen in migraine headaches: changes in extracellular K + and Na +, Ca + +, and Cl−, release of excitatory amino acids, altered levels of 5-HT, and changes in cerebral glucose use. This does not imply that psychologic factors do not play a part in chronic post-traumatic headache syndromes, particularly those cases in which severe functional impairment is seen in people in whom the mechanism of injury would seem to indicate a lesser degree of overall injury. Cultural mores, life stresses, litigation, and other factors undoubtedly contribute to the severity and chronicity of headache syndromes in a portion of the affected population [46].

Evaluation

In evaluating headache in the person with concussion or mild TBI, it is most often not necessary to obtain neuroimaging or laboratory studies although suspicion of cervicogenic or musculoskeletal origin would indicate a set of plain radiographs of the cervical spine. Signs and symptoms that might indicate such a need would be focal or progressive abnormal pathologic signs, altered consciousness, increasing severity, nausea or vomiting, or nighttime occurrence of headache. Headache history should include overall characterization (COLDER: Character, Onset, Location, Duration, Exacerbation, Relief), premorbid history, family history, frequency, and associated symptoms [47]. In addition, a history should examine factors that might contribute to the exacerbation of a headache syndrome such as insomnia, depression, and environmental triggers for headache (eg, caffeine consumption). Although most headaches occurring after mild TBI are primarily musculoskeletal or tension-type headaches, a number of other headache types may be observed (see Box 2). A thorough physical examination of the head, face, neck, and shoulder girdle area should be conducted including postural observations, auscultation of blood vessels, measurement of range of motion, palpation of the region, testing for reflexes, and cranial nerve examination.

Treatment

Treatment strategies for headache pain in mild TBI often must take into account multiple co-morbidities, including other types of pain, cognitive deficits, sleep disturbance, anxiety and mood disorders. Selecting treatments that can address multiple problems simultaneously is often possible. Treatment of headache pain can be frustrating to the patient and health care provider and initially requires frequent check-ins and documentation by the patient of treatment effectiveness. Clear instructions for the use of headache medications should be given to avoid the pitfall of overuse and rebound headaches from occurring. Basic headache "hygiene" measures should be taken: avoidance of caffeinated beverages or excess alcohol, daily exercise, consistent bedtime/awakening schedule, and avoiding possible dietary triggers. Examining the patient's expectations for treatment is helpful; headaches are extremely common in the general population and total freedom from headaches is rarely possible. Counseling patients can help them to have realistic expectations of treatment.

Although patients (and most physicians) typically expect headache treatment to be pharmacologic, addressing posture and muscle spasm even in migraine-type headaches can be helpful and is necessary for the successful treatment of tension-type and cervicogenic headaches. Teaching the patient self-management techniques (early intervention, adjunctive relaxation, and proper use of medications) is crucial to successful management of chronic headache syndromes.

Pharmacologic

Pharmacologic intervention should be selected after a headache type is identified. Treating early headaches aggressively may limit the chronicity and frequency of headache complaints. Over-the-counter medications (acetaminophen and nonsteroidal anti-inflammatories) can be used initially. Narcotic medications should be reserved for management of the acute, post-event pain and for severe, intermittent headaches. The concept of rebound headaches should be thoroughly discussed with the patient to avoid overuse of analgesic or migraine-abortive medications. Classes of medications for various headache types are listed in Box 3. For migraine-type headaches occurring less often than twice per week, abortive medications, such as the triptans, are indicated. These can be extremely effective in managing migraine headache but, since the various triptan medications have different biologic properties, more than one medication may need to be tried before success is obtained. For patients with more frequent migraine headaches, prophylactic medications are used, such as the tricyclic antidepressants or a variety of antiepileptic drugs. The topic of medical management of headache cannot be covered comprehensively in this articler; many excellent reviews of the topic can be found elsewhere [48–50].

Physical therapeutics

Physical interventions aimed at reducing muscle spasm and tightness can be beneficial even in patients with mixed headache pictures, although well-controlled trials are lacking [51]. Physical therapy (including range of motion, joint mobilization, muscle stretching, strengthening) appears to be effective for tension-type headaches; chiropractic manipulation may be somewhat less effective [52–54]. For migraine headache, physical therapy is most effective when combined with biofeedback, relaxation training, and exercise [52]. Physical therapy is most beneficial in all situations when

Box 3. Headache types and medication classes used in treatment

Musculoskeletal and cervicogenic headaches
Non-steroidal anti-inflammatory drugs (NSAIDs)
Analgesics
Tricyclic antidepressants

Migraine (abortive)
NSAIDs
Ergotamine/caffeine
Midrin
Fiorinal
Triptans
Dihydroergotamine
Steroids

Migraine (prophylactic)
Tricyclic antidepressants
Beta-blocking agents
Antiepileptic drugs (valproic acid, topiramate, gabapentin)
Calcium channel-blocking agents

mobilization or manipulation is combined with exercise, stretching, and training in good body mechanics [52]. Other physical modalities may include trigger point injections or dry needling. Injections with local anesthetics or steroids for headaches associated with occipital neuralgia may be beneficial [48]. There has been conflicting evidence to date regarding whether injection of botulinum toxin for headache is significantly better than placebo, at least for migraine headache [55]. However, in certain patients, botulinum toxin injections help to decrease the frequency of headaches.

Counseling and behavioral strategies

Psychologic methods for the treatment of chronic pain, including headache, are detailed elsewhere in this volume by Osborne et al and Stanos and Houle. This article focuses on how to adapt these treatments for the individual with TBI. In the acute phases of recovery from injury, pain treatment tends to focus on underlying physiologic causes. It is generally as pain becomes more chronic that psychologic or psychosocial treatment comes into play.

Interdisciplinary treatment or combination treatments (ie, medication plus cognitive-behavioral psychotherapy) tend to maximize functional outcomes [56]. Although many patients will welcome a referral to a psychologist or counselor, others may have misconceptions or biases, such as thinking such a referral means my physician believes "my pain is all in my head." It can greatly assist the therapeutic relationship and the likelihood that the patient will follow through on the referral if the referring practitioner provides information about how the psychologist might be able to assist in managing their pain problem, such as by learning strategies to improve their sleep and mood as well as skills to reduce stress and muscle tension.

Behavioral strategies are widely accepted as efficacious for tension-type and migraine headache in general [57] but are less studied specifically for post-traumatic headache. One notable exception is a recent study by Gurr and Coetzer [58], which reported encouraging results when adapting cognitive-behavioral treatment for post-traumatic headache.

It is usually beneficial to begin supportive counseling early after injury, preferably with a psychologist or other qualified professional well versed in treating both TBI and pain conditions. Pain can tax the most able person's coping skills. Cognitive difficulties render this an even greater challenge for the patient with a TBI. Applying effective pain coping skills relies substantially on efficient memory skills (eg, recall of newly learned coping strategies) and executive functions (eg, initiation of a coping strategy, shifting focus away from pain), two areas of cognitive functioning that are commonly affected by TBI. In addition, fatigue and sleep disturbance often persist after TBI, irrespective of pain, further diminishing one's ability to cope effectively. Therefore, in working with TBI patients, psychologists almost always need to adapt elements in their therapeutic approach to address diminished cognitive resources and intensified collateral symptoms, like fatigue and sleep disturbance, that affect the patient's pain experience.

Types of appropriate treatment depend on the individual and the particular symptom picture, but in general, psycho-educational, behavioral, and cognitive-behavioral approaches are recommended. Throughout treatment, but especially early on, it is helpful to provide information about the nature of the person's brain injury, the pain problem, and the biopsychosocial model, highlighting for patients and families the importance of addressing multiple areas to improve function. For example, many patients benefit from using sleep hygiene techniques at first to improve their sleep, but then may discover that improved sleep also helps pain, cognition, and mood. Increasing the patient's ability to cope with pain and factors that affect their pain experience should be another focus of treatment. It is here, especially, that the psychologist needs to recognize need for adapting his/her therapeutic approach with the patient. Such adaptations may include, for example, providing written summaries of sessions, including written homework, communicating recommendations to family members or caregivers, and asking other members of the treatment team to reinforce therapeutic messages. Each of these adaptations may improve the adherence and participation of the patients with cognitive impairments. Additionally, using cognitive rehabilitation techniques such as a memory book, either in conjunction with a speech therapist or as part of psychology sessions is often useful, if not essential in some cases. A memory book, for example, can be used to record dysfunctional thoughts as well as therapy homework. Lastly, repeated practice or rehearsal, beyond what is typical, is often required to promote accurate learning of a given coping strategy and facilitate subsequent recall of the strategy under demanding circumstances (eg, increases in stress or pain). Such practice is often done in a therapeutic session (eg, through 1:1 instruction and role playing) as well as through ample homework. Patients often do best with relatively strict coping routines, or scripts.

Group psychotherapy can add a useful element to the overall treatment program. Being part of a treatment group enables the patient to recognize that others are coping with similar problems and to shift some attention away from the self and ongoing symptoms. Often, patients can learn from each other, and at times, other patients may have more credibility than health care professionals. Likewise, it is often beneficial to invite family members to some sessions, both to inform the therapist of problems or successes occurring in the home or other environments and also to assist the patient in remembering and carrying out homework assignments. Providing families with information about pain and about brain injury can be very effective and can help family members change their own behaviors so that inadvertent reinforcement of pain-related behaviors is minimized or eliminated and, at the same time, promotion of improved function is maximized, explicitly and implicitly by what family members say and do.

References

[1] Lahz S, Bryant RA. Incidence of chronic pain following traumatic brain injury. Arch Phys Med Rehabil 1996;77(9):889–91.

[2] Beetar JT, Guilmette TJ, Sparadeo FR. Sleep and pain complaints in symptomatic traumatic brain injury and neurologic populations. Arch Phys Med Rehabil 1996;77(12):1298–302.

[3] Hoffman JM, Pagulayan KF, Zawaideh N, Bell KR. Pain after traumatic brain injury: predictors and correlates [poster presentation]. Chicago: American Congress of Rehabilitation Medicine; 2005.

[4] Whyte J, Hart T, Laborde A, Rosenthal M. Rehabilitation issues in traumatic brain injury. In: Delisa JA, editor. Physical medicine and rehabilitation: principles and practice. 4th edition. Philadelphia: Lippincott Williams & Wilkins; 2005. p. 1692–3.

[5] Ivanhoe CB, Hartman ET. Clinical caveats on medical assessment and treatment of pain after TBI. J Head Trauma Rehabil 2004;19(1):29–39.

[6] Uomoto JM, Esselman PC. Traumatic brain injury and chronic pain: differential types and rates by head injury severity. Arch Phys Med Rehabil 1993;74(1):61–4.

[7] Yamaguchi M. Incidence of headache and severity of head injury. Headache 1992;32(9): 427–31.

[8] Couch JR, Bearss C. Chronic daily headache in the posttrauma syndrome: relation to extent of head injury. Headache 2001;41(6):559–64.

[9] Zasler ND. Posttraumatic headache: caveats and controversies. J Head Trauma Rehabil 1999;14(1):1–8.

[10] Martelli MF, Zasler ND, Bender MC, Nicholson K. Psychological, neuropsychological, and medical considerations in assessment and management of pain. J Head Trauma Rehabil 2004;19(1):10–28.

[11] Olver JH, Ponsford JL, Curran CA. Outcome following traumatic brain injury: a comparison between 2 and 5 years after injury. Brain Inj 1996;10(11):841–8.
[12] Hart RP, Martelli MF, Zasler ND. Chronic pain and neuropsychological functioning. Neuropsychol Rev 2000;10(3):131–49.
[13] Dick B, Eccleston C, Crombez G. Attentional functioning in fibromyalgia, rheumatoid arthritis, and musculoskeletal pain patients. Arthritis Rheum 2002;47(6):639–44.
[14] Grigsby J, Rosenberg NL, Busenbark D. Chronic pain is associated with deficits in information processing. Percept Mot Skills 1995;81(2):403–10.
[15] Killen SA, Huntoon E. Drugs for pain management. Phys Med Rehabil Clin N Am 1997; 8(4):695–705.
[16] Ham LP, Andrasik F, Packard RC, Bundrick CM. Psychopathology in individuals with post-traumatic headaches and other pain types. Cephalalgia 1994;14(2):118–26 [discussion: 178].
[17] Koponen S, Taiminen T, Portin R, et al. Axis I and II psychiatric disorders after traumatic brain injury: a 30-year follow-up study. Am J Psychiatry 2002;159(8):1315–21.
[18] Ottowitz WE, Dougherty DD, Savage CR. The neural network basis for abnormalities of attention and executive function in major depressive disorder: implications for application of the medical disease model to psychiatric disorders. Harv Rev Psychiatry 2002;10(2):86–99.
[19] Rapoport MJ, McCullagh S, Shammi P, Feinstein A. Cognitive impairment associated with major depression following mild and moderate traumatic brain injury. J Neuropsychiatry Clin Neurosci 2005;17(1):61–5.
[20] Gallagher RM, Verma S. Managing pain and comorbid depression: A public health challenge. Semin Clin Neuropsychiatry 1999;4(3):203–20.
[21] Zafonte R, Elovic EP, Lombard L. Acute care management of post-tbi spasticity. J Head Trauma Rehabil 2004;19(2):89–100.
[22] Bell KR, Lehmann JF. Effect of cooling on h- and t-reflexes in normal subjects. Arch Phys Med Rehabil 1987;68(8):490–3.
[23] Gracies JM. Physical modalities other than stretch in spastic hypertonia. Phys Med Rehabil Clin N Am 2001;12(4):769–92 [vi.].
[24] Mortenson PA, Eng JJ. The use of casts in the management of joint mobility and hypertonia following brain injury in adults: a systematic review. Phys Ther 2003;83(7):648–58.
[25] Singer BJ, Singer KP, Allison GT. Evaluation of extensibility, passive torque and stretch reflex responses in triceps surae muscles following serial casting to correct spastic equinovarus deformity. Brain Inj 2003;17(4):309–24.
[26] Pohl M, Ruckriem S, Mehrholz J, et al. Effectiveness of serial casting in patients with severe cerebral spasticity: a comparison study. Arch Phys Med Rehabil 2002;83(6):784–90.
[27] Goddard G. Short term pain reduction with acupuncture treatment for chronic orofacial pain patients. Med Sci Monit 2005;11(2):CR71–4.
[28] Targino RA, Imamura M, Kaziyama HH, et al. Pain treatment with acupuncture for patients with fibromyalgia. Curr Pain Headache Rep 2002;6(5):379–83.
[29] Gormley ME Jr, O'Brien CF, Yablon SA. A clinical overview of treatment decisions in the management of spasticity. Muscle Nerve Suppl 1997;6:S14–20.
[30] Brashear A, Gordon MF, Elovic E, et al. Intramuscular injection of botulinum toxin for the treatment of wrist and finger spasticity after a stroke. N Engl J Med 2002;347(6):395–400.
[31] Bell KR. The use of neurolytic blocks for the management of spasticity. Phys Med Rehabil Clin N Am 1995;6(4):885–95.
[32] Bell KR, Williams F. Use of botulinum toxin type a and type b for spasticity in upper and lower limbs. Phys Med Rehabil Clin N Am 2003;14(4):821–35.
[33] Zafonte RD, Munin MC. Phenol and alcohol blocks for the treatment of spasticity. Phys Med Rehabil Clin N Am 2001;12(4):817–32 [vii.].
[34] Kirazli Y, On AY, Kismali B, Aksit R. Comparison of phenol block and botulinus toxin type a in the treatment of spastic foot after stroke: a randomized, double-blind trial. Am J Phys Med Rehabil 1998;77(6):510–5.

[35] Ivanhoe CB, Tilton AH, Francisco GE. Intrathecal baclofen therapy for spastic hypertonia. Phys Med Rehabil Clin N Am 2001;12(4):923–38 [viii–ix.].
[36] Alvarez CM, Litchfield R, Jackowski D, et al. A prospective, double-blind, randomized clinical trial comparing subacromial injection of betamethasone and xylocaine to xylocaine alone in chronic rotator cuff tendinosis. Am J Sports Med 2005;33(2):255–62.
[37] Carette S, Moffet H, Tardif J, et al. Intraarticular corticosteroids, supervised physiotherapy, or a combination of the two in the treatment of adhesive capsulitis of the shoulder: a placebo-controlled trial. Arthritis Rheum 2003;48(3):829–38.
[38] Price CI, Pandyan AD. Electrical stimulation for preventing and treating post-stroke shoulder pain. Cochrane Database Systematic Rev 2000;(4):CD001698.
[39] Turner-Stokes L, Jackson D. Shoulder pain after stroke: a review of the evidence base to inform the development of an integrated care pathway. Clin Rehabil 2002;16(3):276–98.
[40] Yu D. Shoulder pain in hemiplegia. Phys Medicine Rehabil Clin N Am 2004;15(3):683–97 [vi–vii].
[41] Kasch H, Stengaard-Pedersen K, Arendt-Nielsen L, Staehelin Jensen T. Headache, neck pain, and neck mobility after acute whiplash injury: a prospective study. Spine 2001; 26(11):1246–51.
[42] Headache Classification Subcommittee. The international classification of headache disorders. 2nd edition. Cephalalgia 2004;24(Suppl 1):9–160.
[43] Solomon S. John graham senior clinicians award lecture. Posttraumatic migraine. Headache 1998;38(10):772–8.
[44] Radanov BP, Di Stefano G, Augustiny KF. Symptomatic approach to posttraumatic headache and its possible implications for treatment. Eur Spine J 2001;10(5):403–7.
[45] Packard RC, Ham LP. Pathogenesis of posttraumatic headache and migraine: a common headache pathway? Headache 1997;37(3):142–52.
[46] Solomon S. Chronic post-traumatic neck and head pain. Headache 2005;45(1):53–67.
[47] Zafonte RD, Horn LJ. Clinical assessment of posttraumatic headaches. J Head Trauma Rehabil 1999;14(1):22–33.
[48] Bell KR, Kraus E, Zasler N. Medical management of post traumatic headache: pharmacological and physical treatment. J Head Trauma Rehabil 1999;14:34–8.
[49] Goadsby PJ. Headache (chronic tension-type). Clin Evidence 2003;10:1538–46.
[50] Oldman AD, Smith LA, McQuay HJ, Moore RA. Pharmacological treatments for acute migraine: quantitative systematic review. Pain 2002;97(3):247–57.
[51] Lenssinck ML, Damen L, Verhagen AP, et al. The effectiveness of physiotherapy and manipulation in patients with tension-type headache: a systematic review. Pain 2004;112(3): 381–8.
[52] Biondi D. Physical treatments for headache: a structured review. Headache 2005;45:738–48.
[53] Hammill JM, Cook TM, Rosecrance JC. Effectiveness of a physical therapy regimen in the treatment of tension-type headache. Headache 1996;36(3):149–53.
[54] Astin JA, Ernst E. The effectiveness of spinal manipulation for the treatment of headache disorders: a systematic review of randomized clinical trials. Cephalalgia 2002;22(8):617–23.
[55] Peloso P, Gross A, Haines T, et al. Medicinal and injection therapies for mechanical neck disorders. Cochrane Database Systematic Rev 2005;(2):CD000319.
[56] Martelli MF, Grayson RL, Zasler ND. Posttraumatic headache: Neuropsychological and psychological effects and treatment implications. J Head Trauma Rehabil 1999;14(1):49–69.
[57] Penzien DB, Rains JC, Lipchik GL, Creer TL. Behavioral interventions for tension-type headache: overview of current therapies and recommendation for a self-management model for chronic headache. Curr Pain Headache Rep 2004;8(6):489–99.
[58] Gurr B, Coetzer BR. The effectiveness of cognitive-behavioural therapy for post-traumatic headaches. Brain Inj 2005;19(7):481–91.

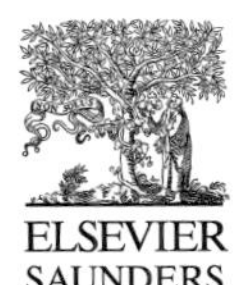
ELSEVIER
SAUNDERS

Phys Med Rehabil Clin N Am
17 (2006) 491–510

PHYSICAL MEDICINE
AND REHABILITATION
CLINICS OF
NORTH AMERICA

Treatment of Fibromyalgia, Myofascial Pain, and Related Disorders

Joanne Borg-Stein, MD

Rehabilitation Center, Spaulding Newton-Wellesley Rehabilitation Hospital, 65 Walnut Street, Wellesley, MA 02481, USA

A 35-year-old woman was rear ended in a motor vehicle accident 1 year ago. She initially complained of diffuse posterior neck pain but no discomfort in her shoulder girdle, midback, or low back, and no symptoms suggesting a cervical radiculopathy. A cervical MRI scan was negative for a disk herniation or compromise of neural elements. The patient was seen by an interventional pain physician who suspected a facet arthropathy; however, diagnostic medial branch blocks to anesthetize the C5-5 and C6-7 facet joints produced no pain relief, and the physician did not believe he had more to offer the patient. Since the time of the accident, the patient's pain has gradually spread such that it now involves essentially the entire spine. On examination, the patient appears to have trigger points involving the upper trapezius and levator scapulae muscles bilaterally. Also, she reports tenderness in 14 of the 18 sites designated by the American College of Rheumatology for the diagnosis of fibromyalgia.

Definition

Fibromyalgia syndrome (FMS) is a disorder defined as chronic widespread pain of at least 6 months' duration with widespread musculoskeletal aching accompanied by multiple widespread tender points. According to the 1990 American College of Rheumatology criteria, a patient must have pain in the axial skeleton, pain above and below the waist, and pain to palpation in at least 11 of 18 paired tender points throughout the body. The majority of patients (80%) are women [1].

Myofascial pain syndrome (MPS) is defined as pain that originates from myofascial trigger points (MTrPs) in skeletal muscle, either alone or in combination with other pain generators. MTrPs are discrete areas of focal

E-mail address: jborgstein@partners.org

doi:10.1016/j.pmr.2005.12.003 ***pmr.theclinics.com***

tenderness within a muscle that are characterized by hypersensitive palpable taut bands of muscle that are painful to palpation. Manual pressure over these points reproduces the patient's pain and refers pain in a characteristic pattern. Some clinicians prefer the term *regional soft tissue pain* as clinically useful, encompassing pain and localized tenderness not only in muscle but also in other contiguous soft tissues, such as ligaments and tendons [2].

Epidemiology

Fibromyalgia is present in 6 to 10 million Americans [3]. Chronic widespread musculoskeletal pain has been subjected to several epidemiologic studies during the last decade. According to these studies, 10% of the general population reports such complaints, clearly indicating chronic widespread musculoskeletal pain as a major health problem in the Western world. The prevalence of fibromyalgia is reported to be 3% to 5% with a significant female predominance [4]. Recent evidence suggests that fibromyalgia and related syndromes may share heritable pathophysiologic features. Serotonin and dopamine-related genes may have a role in the pathogenesis [5].

Myofascial pain has a high prevalence among individuals with regional pain complaints. The prevalence varies from 21% of patients seen in a general orthopedic clinic to 30% of general medical clinic patients with regional pain to as high as 85% to 90% of patients presenting to specialty pain management centers. Women and men are affected evenly [6–8].

Clinical presentation

The symptoms of fibromyalgia consist of musculoskeletal pain and stiffness in a widespread distribution, usually involving the neck, shoulder, and pelvic girdles as well as all of the extremities. Patients may present with pain predominantly in one or two regions (ie, the low back or neck are the most common areas), but direct questioning reveals pain in many other areas. Other common symptoms are general fatigue, poor sleep, and morning fatigue. Paresthesia is present in about one half of cases, usually in the extremities, and may mimic nerve root compression. Associated conditions such as migraine, irritable bowel syndrome, and restless legs syndrome are common [9].

The characteristic symptoms of myofascial pain may begin after a discrete trauma or injury or may be of insidious onset. Patients note localized or regional deep aching sensations, which can vary in intensity from mild to severe [10]. The MTrPs of each muscle have their own characteristic pain pattern; therefore, the distribution of pain can help identify which muscles may contain the responsible MTrP [11]. Frequently, associated autonomic dysfunction may occur, including abnormal sweating, lacrimation, dermal flushing, and vasomotor and temperature changes [12]. Cervical myofascial pain may be associated with neuro-otologic symptoms including imbalance, dizziness, and tinnitus [13]. Functional complaints include decreased work tolerance, impaired muscle coordination, stiff joints, fatigue, and weakness. Other associated neurologic symptoms include paresthesias, numbness, blurred vision, twitches, and trembling. Later stages can be compounded by sleep disturbance, mood changes, and stress [14–16].

Physical examination of the patient with fibromyalgia reveals pain to palpation over 11 of 18 characteristic tender points (Fig. 1). The pressure applied should just blanch the fingernail bed of the examining physician. Examination of the joints and nervous system is normal despite the symptom of a swollen feeling in the joints and numbness. Range of motion of the cervical and lumbar spines may be slightly restricted because of pain. Diffuse soft tissue tenderness on palpation of the cervical, thoracic, and lumbar spine areas (including ligaments and paraspinal muscles) may be present [17].

Physical examination of the patient with myofascial pain begins with a careful medical, neurologic, and musculoskeletal examination. Posture, biomechanics, and joint function should be analyzed to identify any underlying factors that may have contributed to the development of the local or regional pain. An active MTrP is usually associated with a painful restricted range of motion. The trigger point should be identified by gentle palpation across the direction of the muscle fibers. The examiner should appreciate a "ropelike" nodularity to the taut band of muscle. Palpation of this area is exquisitely painful and reproduces the patient's local and referred pain pattern [18].

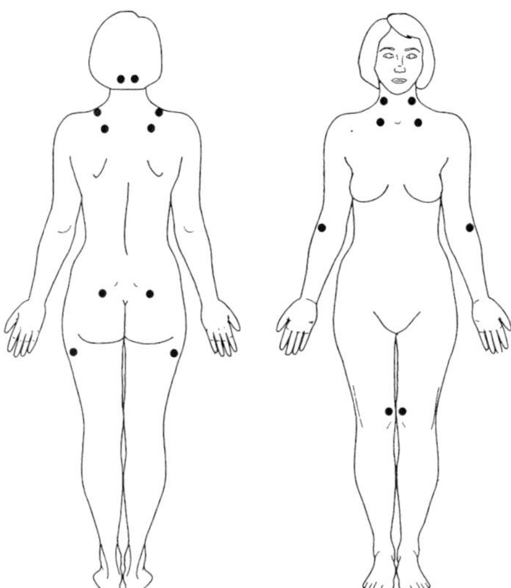

Fig. 1. 18 tender points of fibromyalgia. (*From* Freundlich B, Leventhal L. The fibromyalgia syndrome. In: Schumacher HR Jr, Klippel JH, Koopman WJ, editors. Primer on the rheumatic diseases. 10th edition. Atlanta: Arthritis Foundation; 1993. p. 247–9; with permission).

Laboratory tests

Routine laboratory tests such as a complete blood count, erythrocyte sedimentation rate, and chemistry profile are normal in FMS and MPS. Thyroid function tests are normal but may be helpful to exclude hypo- or hyperthyroidism in patients with muscle pain. Radiologic examinations (radiographs, CT scan, MRI) are normal; however, it is common to find coincidental osteoarthrosis or diskogenic changes. The treating clinician must determine the relevance of these findings to the patient based on the clinical scenario [19].

Well-controlled studies in patients with fibromyalgia and chronic muscle pain demonstrate normal muscle biopsy, electromyography, and nerve conduction studies [20]. Sleep electroencephalogram (EEG) studies may be requested to confirm a clinical suspicion of sleep disorders, such as periodic limb movement disorder, REM-behavior disorder, and sleep apnea. Alpha intrusion into stage 4 delta waves is seen in about 40% of patients, but these studies should be ordered only when there is clinical suspicion of the previously mentioned disorders [21].

Differential diagnosis

In clinical practice, there is often substantial overlap in the presentation of muscle pain disorders. The differences among myofascial pain, regional soft tissue pain, and widespread muscle pain are often indistinct. The differential diagnosis of muscle pain is broad. The following questions may be useful in distinguishing the contributions of different factors and may help the clinician develop an appropriate and specific treatment plan.

Is there regional myofascial pain, with trigger points present?

Is the myofascial pain the primary pain generator, or are there other co-existing or underlying structural diagnoses?

Is there a nutritional, metabolic, psychologic, visceral, or inflammatory disorder that may contribute to or cause the myofascial pain or regional muscle pain?

Is there widespread pain and other associated symptoms?

The differential diagnosis should include (but is not limited to) the following factors:

Joint disorders: zygoapophyseal joint disorder, osteoarthritis, loss of normal joint motion

Inflammatory disorders: polymyositis, polymyalgia rheumatica, rheumatoid arthritis

Neurologic disorders: radiculopathy, entrapment neuropathy, metabolic myopathy

Regional soft tissue disorders: bursitis, epicondylitis, tendonitis, cumulative trauma

Diskogenic disorders: degenerative disk disease, annular tears, protrusion, herniation
Visceral referred pain: gastrointestinal, cardiac, pulmonary, renal
Mechanical stresses: postural dysfunction, scoliosis, leg length discrepancy
Nutritional, metabolic, and endocrine conditions: deficiency in vitamins B_1, B_{12}, or folic acid; alcoholic and toxic myopathy; iron, calcium, magnesium deficiency; hypothyroidism
Psychologic disorders: depression, anxiety, disordered sleep
Infectious diseases: viral illness, chronic hepatitis, bacterial or viral myositis
Fibromyalgia or widespread chronic pain [2]

Pathophysiology of fibromyalgia and myofascial pain syndrome

Chronic muscle pain, regional myofascial pain, and fibromyalgia may be considered as a spectrum of clinical disorders. They share pathophysiologic mechanisms and often coexist in the same patient. The discussion herein is organized by neuroanatomic location; however, one should appreciate that these processes are interrelated and should be considered in an integrated fashion.

Motor end plate

An important finding in the pathophysiology of myofascial pain is a pathologic increase in the release of acetylcholine (Ach) by the nerve terminal of an abnormal motor end plate under resting conditions, an occurrence supported by electrodiagnostic evidence [22,23]. This abnormality is considered the primary dysfunction in the "integrated hypothesis" proposed by Simons and coworkers [11,18], which postulates a positive feedback loop (Fig. 2).

In support of the concept of the abnormal motor end plate, electrodiagnostic studies have demonstrated end plate noise (EPN) significantly more frequently in MTrPs than in the same end plate zone outside of the MTrP [23,24]. Because EPN is characteristic but not diagnostic of MTrPs, the significance of these findings remains disputed. An increase in EPN has been seen in

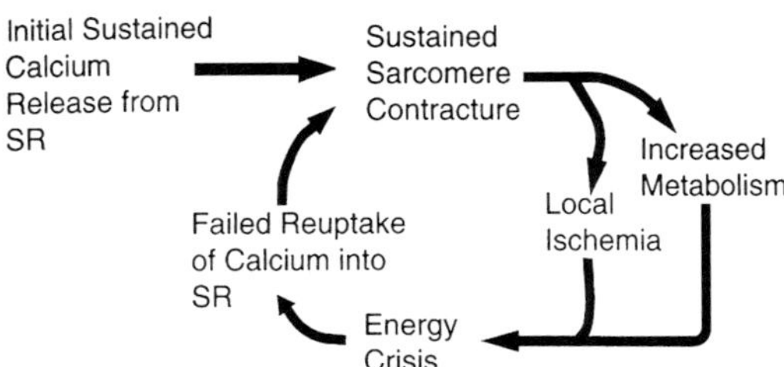

Fig. 2. "Integrated hypothesis," which postulates a positive feedback loop. (*From* Simons DG, Travell JG, Simons LS. Myofascial pain and dysfunction: the trigger point manual, Vol. 1. Upper half of body. 2nd edition. Baltimore: Williams & Wilkins; 1999, p. 71; with permission.)

response to many types of mechanical and chemical stimulation of the end plate structure and does not seem to be specific to myofascial pain [25,26].

Muscle fiber

It is hypothesized that increased Ach release could result in sustained depolarization of the postjunctional membrane of the muscle fiber and produce sustained sarcomere shortening and contracture. This maximally contracted sarcomere in the region of the motor end plate, referred to as a "contraction knot" by Simons [11], is diagrammed in Fig. 3. Compelling histologic support for this phenomenon is found in canine models of MTrPs. Longitudinal sections of dog trigger points demonstrate this sarcomere shortening, and cross-sections of dog and human MTrPs strongly suggest it as well [27,28].

One consequence of a chronically sustained sarcomere shortening may be greatly increased local energy consumption and reduction of local circulation, a combination that produces local ischemia and hypoxia. The unrelieved sustained tension of muscle fibers in the taut band produces an enthesopathy at the myotendinous junction that can be identified as an attachment MTrP. Muscle stretching techniques may be effective by equalizing sarcomere length throughout the affected muscle fibers and by breaking the feedback cycle.

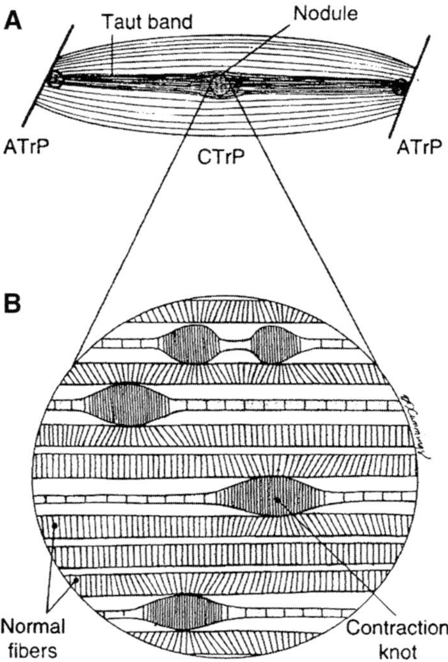

Fig. 3. Trigger point complex. (*From* Simons DG, Travell JG, Simons LS. Myofascial pain and dysfunction: the trigger point manual, Vol. 1. Upper half of body. 2nd edition. Baltimore: Williams & Wilkins; 1999, p. 70; with permission.)

The localized muscle ischemia stimulates the release of neurovasoreactive substances such as prostaglandins, bradykinin, capsaicin, serotonin, and histamine that sensitize afferent nerve fibers in muscle. These sensitized fibers may in turn account for local muscle tenderness [18]. The most recent research by Shah and coworkers [29] demonstrates increased concentrations of protons (H+), bradykinin, calcitonin gene-related peptide, substance P, tumor necrosis factor-alpha, interleukin-1 beta, serotonin, and norepinephrine in the biochemical milieu of human trapezius muscle in patients with neck pain and active MTrPs when compared with controls.

Central mechanisms: spinal and supraspinal

The referred pain resulting from trigger points arises from central convergence and facilitation. It is known from experimental data [18,30] that, under pathologic conditions, convergent connections from deep afferent nociceptors to dorsal horn neurons are facilitated and amplified in the spinal cord. Referral to adjacent myotomes occurs owing to spreading of central sensitization to adjacent spinal segments [31,32]. This pattern results in referred pain and expansion of the region of pain beyond the initial nociceptive region.

At the level of the central nervous system (CNS), spinal neuroplastic changes occur in the second order neuron pool of the dorsal horn owing to persistent pain. These changes produce a long lasting increase in the excitability of nociceptor pathways. Central sensitization results and is characterized by increased excitability of the neurons and expansion of the receptive pool of neurons. Neurotransmitters involved in the process of central sensitization include substance P, *N*-methyl-D-aspartate, glutamate, and nitric oxide [22]. In addition, there may be impairments in supraspinal inhibitory descending pain control pathways releasing inhibitory neurotransmitters such as gaba-aminobutyric acid, serotonin, and norepinephrine [33]. A recent study of cerebrospinal fluid levels of opioid peptides in fibromyalgia demonstrates that opioid dysfunction may contribute to pain [34].

In FMS, significant peripheral pathology is absent. Recent studies suggest central sensitization as the most important CNS aberration. Controlled studies have shown an increase in cerebrospinal fluid substance P (which mediates pain transmission) as well as a decrease in serum serotonin (which mediates pain inhibition) and CSF 5HIAA (a metabolite of serotonin). These findings may explain the amplified pain and decreased pain threshold in FMS [35,36]. Sleep abnormality has been objectively documented by EEG studies. Disturbed stage 4 sleep may explain the reported decrease in serum insulinlike growth factor-1 (which reflects the integrated secretion of growth hormone) [37,38].

FMS is not a psychiatric condition; however, a psychologic disturbance (anxiety, mental stress, depression) is present in 30% to 40% of patients (generally similar to rheumatoid arthritis). Psychologic factors seem to aggravate but not cause the pain. There is no correlation between psychologic status and other symptoms of FMS besides pain (eg, swollen feeling, paresthesia, number of tender points) [39].

Most recent fMRI studies of the brain demonstrate that fibromyalgia is characterized by cortical or subcortical augmentation of pain processing. These studies provide further evidence for a physiologic explanation for fibromyalgia pain [40,41].

Treatment of fibromyalgia and myofascial pain syndrome

The following discussion refers to management of muscle pain syndromes including FMS and MPS. Much of the research has been done on one or both of these overlapping populations of patients. When clinically relevant, techniques specific to MPS or FMS are noted.

Diagnosis and education

Make a firm diagnosis of FMS or MPS based on its characteristics; avoid unnecessary investigations.

Educate patients regarding FMS and MPS.

Reassure the patient the muscle pain does not cause tissue damage.

Demonstrate an attitude of understanding and empathy; this is crucial for success in management. Never imply that symptoms are "all psychologic."

Elucidate probable mechanisms of pain to the patient in simple language (neuroendocrine dysfunction equals a chemical imbalance). Explain low serotonin and how its deficiency causes pain. Significant psychologic factors, if present, should be explained as aggravating factors.

Recognize and address significant psychologic factors, such as depression, anxiety, mental stress (at home or work), and poor coping skills. A minority of patients will require referral to a psychiatrist for management of more severe psychiatric disease and psychopharmacologic consultation and management.

Inquire about all aggravating factors that vary from patient to patient and individualize management.

Help patients to have restful sleep.

Encourage cardiovascular fitness.

Provide physical therapy for management of regional musculoskeletal disorders.

Promote behavioral modification through education including cognitive behavioral concepts [9].

Pharmacologic management

Given the considerable clinical overlap among myofascial pain, fibromyalgia, regional soft tissue pain, and tension headache, agents beneficial in one syndrome may be useful in another. In the absence of controlled data specifically examining drug efficacy in each disorder, clinicians often generalize from these associated disorders.

Nonsteroidal anti-inflammatory drugs

Nonsteroidal anti-inflammatory drugs (NSAIDs) have minimal literature evaluating their use in chronic muscle pain. Several studies have found a small benefit of NSAIDs for management of pain in fibromyalgia if used in combination with alprazolam, amitriptyline, or cyclobenzaprine [42–44]. Interestingly, NSAIDs continue to be popular among patients, and in a recent study by Wolfe and coworkers [45], NSAIDs were considered more effective than acetaminophen for pain management by patients with fibromyalgia.

Tramadol

Tramadol is a combination of a weak opioid agonist and an inhibitor of the reuptake of serotonin and norepinephrine in the dorsal horn. There are no published controlled trials of tramadol for the treatment of myofascial pain; however, several studies support its efficacy in fibromyalgia, chronic low back pain, and osteoarthritis, all of which are commonly seen in association [46–50].

Antidepressants

Tricyclic antidepressants such as amitriptyline are effective for chronic tension-type headache, fibromyalgia, and intractable pain syndromes associated with muscle spasm [51–54]. Selective serotonin reuptake inhibitors (SSRIs) have not been specifically studied for myofascial pain, although efficacy has been documented in fibromyalgia for improving pain, sleep, and the global sense of well-being [51,55]. More recent studies support the use of dual reuptake inhibitors (serotonin and norepinephrine) for the treatment of fibromyalgia. Evidence supports the use of venlafaxine, milnacipran, and duloxetine [56–58].

Alpha-2 adrenergic agonists

The two major alpha-2 adrenergic agonists available for clinical use are clonidine and tizanidine. Tizanidine acts centrally at the level of the spinal cord to inhibit spinal polysynaptic pathways and to reduce the release of aspartate, glutamate, and substance P [59,60].

Anticonvulsants

To date, there is one controlled trial of pregabalin in the treatment of fibromyalgia that demonstrates reduction of pain, disturbed sleep, and fatigue when compared with a placebo [61]. One open label study of gabapentin in the treatment of chronic daily headache found possible efficacy [62].

Botulinum toxin

Botulinum toxin type A is emerging as a promising but expensive agent with efficacy in chronic MPS and chronic daily headache [63–65]. Cheshire and coworkers [66] performed a small randomized, double-blind, placebo-controlled trial of botulinum toxin type A and demonstrated a reduction of at least 30% in visual analogue pain scales, verbal pain descriptors, palpable muscle firmness, and pressure pain thresholds in the botulinum toxin group when compared with a placebo (saline) group. Fishman [67,68] has demonstrated improvement in patients with piriformis syndrome with injection of botulinum toxins (type A and type B). Porta [69] compared botulinum toxin A with steroid injection for the treatment of chronic myofascial pain and found greater improvement at 30 and 60 days posttreatment in the botulinum toxin treated group. By comparison, Wheeler and coworkers [70] were unable to demonstrate a statistically significant difference between botulinum toxin and placebo for the treatment of refractory unilateral cervicothoracic myofascial pain.

A peripheral and a central mechanism may explain the apparent efficacy of botulinum toxin in the treatment of chronic muscle pain. First, the blockade of Ach release at the neuromuscular junction reduces muscle hyperactivity, which, in turn, may decrease local ischemia. Second, if, as theorized, trigger points are sustained by excessive Ach release and sarcomere shortening, botulinum toxin may disrupt the abnormal neurophysiology of the trigger point. Evidence has also been found of retrograde uptake of botulinum toxin into the spinal cord and nucleus raphe, structures that modulate expression of neurotransmitters important in pain perception (eg, substance P, enkephalins) [71]. Additionally, botulinum toxin type A inhibits neurotransmitter release from primary sensory neurons in the rat formalin model. Through this mechanism, Botox inhibits peripheral sensitization in these models, which leads to an indirect reduction in central sensitization [72].

Nonpharmacologic treatment of muscle pain

Postural, mechanical, and ergonomic modifications

Although standard clinical practice and conventional wisdom includes efforts to correct postural and ergonomic abnormalities, there are limited direct data to support this approach in treating muscle pain. One study by Komiyama and coworkers [73] combined postural training and behavioral therapy in the treatment of myofascial oral pain and found that the subjects receiving the combination therapy were able to regain free unassisted mouth opening earlier than those treated with behavioral therapy alone; however, the differences in outcome were clinically minor.

The occupational medicine literature provides evidence that injuries are more common when workers are subjected to greater loads and have undesirable postures during their work [74]. Occupational muscle pain syndromes are theorized to occur as the result of repetitive microtrauma and myofascial shortening. Correction of awkward postures is a standard part of treatment of these disorders, although long-term efficacy studies are lacking [75].

Stress reduction

Stress reduction techniques, including cognitive-behavioral programs, meditation, progressive relaxation training, and biofeedback, are often incorporated into chronic pain rehabilitation programs. Studies specifically addressing the efficacy of these techniques for myofascial pain are few. Crockett and coworkers [76] compared a multifaceted relaxation program with physiotherapy with dental splinting and transcutaneous electric nerve stimulation (TENS) for management of chronic facial and masticatory myofascial pain. Equivalent results and good response were found among all treatment groups. Electromyographic biofeedback and meditation-based stress reduction programs are established as beneficial in fibromyalgia [77,78].

Acupuncture

A growing body of evidence supports the efficacy of acupuncture in myofascial pain and fibromyalgia. The limited amount of high-quality data suggest that real acupuncture is better than sham for relieving pain, improving global ratings, and reducing morning stiffness in fibromyalgia [79]. One exception to this is a recent randomized clinical trial of acupuncture compared with sham acupuncture in fibromyalgia that did not demonstrate any difference between the patients in the sham groups when compared with the treatment group [80]. The 1997 National Institutes of Health consensus statement on acupuncture [81] concluded that "acupuncture may be useful as an adjunct treatment or an acceptable alternative to be included in a comprehensive management program" in the treatment of fibromyalgia, myofascial pain, low back pain, osteoarthritis, and lateral epicondylitis. Birch and Jamison [82] found relevant acupuncture (over points relevant to myofascial neck pain) to be superior to NSAID treatment and irrelevant acupuncture (superficial needling not related to neck pain) in a group of 46 patients with chronic myofascial pain. Interestingly, a remarkably close correspondence has been described between acupuncture points and trigger points [83]. Questions that need to be answered in future randomized controlled trials include the true benefit of acupuncture in chronic muscle pain, the duration of benefit of acupuncture, the optimal acupuncture techniques, and the value of booster treatments for the treatment of muscle pain.

Massage, transcutaneous electrical nerve stimulation, and ultrasound

Studies suggesting the efficacy of massage as part of treatment for muscle pain are scant. In a study by Gam and coworkers [84], massage combined with stretching exercises was better than control treatment in reducing the number and intensity of MTrPs. There was only a mild reduction in neck and shoulder pain. Hernandez-Reif [85] found that massage therapy was effective in reducing pain, increasing serotonin and dopamine levels, and reducing symptoms associated with chronic low back pain; however, this study did not specify the etiology of the pain.

TENS treatment has shown mixed results in the treatment of myofascial pain. One single-blinded study [86] compared TENS with sham TENS in 10 patients for the treatment of myofascial pain and found no benefit for pain reduction; however, the study used subthreshold TENS parameters. By comparison, Graff-Radford and coworkers [87] compared four different TENS settings with a no-stimulation control in a double-blind study and found that high-frequency, high-intensity TENS reduced myofascial pain.

Ultrasound in combination with massage and exercise has been tested in a randomized controlled trial [84]. In that study, ultrasound, massage, and exercise had no additional benefit over sham ultrasound with massage and acupuncture for the treatment of MTrPs.

Exercise for fibromyalgia and myofascial pain

Exercise is one of the most important aspects of the rehabilitation and management of chronic muscle pain syndromes [88]. Reasons for this include optimization of flexibility, improvement of functional status, improvement of mood, self-efficacy, and reduction of pain.

Stretching exercises form the basis of treatment for myofascial pain. This treatment addresses the muscle tightness and shortening that are closely associated with pain in this disorder and permits gradual restoration of normal activity. Slow sustained stretch throughout the available range of motion is the most effective approach. Once muscle pain is decreased and range of motion restored, exercise to improve muscle strength and endurance should be instituted to maximize functional outcome. Aerobic exercise should also be included as part of an overall musculoskeletal and cardiovascular fitness program to prevent recurrence [89].

Patients should be encouraged to remain active but to perform daily activities in a gently lightly loaded manner. When a movement leads to pain, the patient should stop at that point and slowly and gently explore extending the movement just a little further to help release the muscle tightness. Clinical experience suggests that leaving a muscle in the shortened position aggravates MTrPs [2].

Trigger point injection for fibromyalgia and myofascial pain

In general, trigger points are the hallmark of MPS. Frequently, patients with generalized muscle pain, such as FMS, also have trigger points and painful shortened areas of muscle pain. These local areas may be treated with trigger point injections.

Stretching exercises are the mainstay of myofascial pain management, and injection therapy should be reserved to supplement or augment these exercises [89]. When MTrP injection is used as the primary therapy, patients are at risk for becoming dependent on this treatment for pain relief. Educating patients about the effectiveness of manual techniques and instruction in the specific techniques empowers patients to self-manage their symptoms. With increasing relief of pain and increasing function, resumption of normal activity helps to further inactivate MTrPs. Optimal results are obtained when injections are preceded and immediately followed by manual MTrP release techniques with patient training on how to perform a continuing home program [90].

When injection proves necessary for initiating therapy or dealing with a recalcitrant area of myofascial pain, a series of injections should be initiated, and the patient should be informed of the limited role of this treatment in the long-term management of myofascial pain. Often, three consecutive visits for injection are recommended in chronic myofascial pain, with reassessment after the third visit to evaluate the efficacy of the injections and to determine whether further injections are necessary.

MTrP injections may employ several medications, including no medication (dry needling), short- or long-acting anesthetics, steroids, and botulinum toxin. Injections may use several different techniques such as slow search [91], fast in–fast out, superficial dry needling, intramuscular stimulation, twitch-obtaining intramuscular stimulation, and needling and infiltration with preinjection blocks. Several theories exist regarding the mechanism of action of injections for myofascial pain.

Dry needling of the MTrP provides as much pain relief as injection lidocaine but causes more postinjection soreness [92]. The effectiveness of needling depends on the needle eliciting local twitch responses [92]. Presumably, the needle mechanically disrupts and terminates the dysfunctional activity of involved motor end plates, with or without injection. Longer-acting anesthetics are more myotoxic without a proven increase in MTrP pain relief. The effectiveness of injection of steroids in MTrPs is controversial and without a clear rationale, because little evidence exists to support an inflammatory pathophysiology for MTrPs. Injection of botulinum toxin is emerging as a good option for treatment of chronic muscle pain [93].

In a recent systematic review article on needling therapies for MTrPs, Cummings and White [94] concluded that, based on current medical evidence, the "nature of the injected substance makes no difference to the outcome and that wet needling is not therapeutically superior to dry needling." This treatment is clearly an area in which more research is needed.

Hong's fast in–fast out technique [92] elicits local twitch responses more quickly than other techniques and presumably reduces needle trauma to muscle fibers by the twitch movement. Baldry and coworkers [95] recommend superficial dry needling, which they speculate may inactivate MTrPs through stimulation of cutaneous A delta fibers. Chu [96], based on Gunn's work [97], has reported a technique in which neurogenically evoked muscle twitches relieve myofascial-type pain. The needling and infiltration technique described by Fischer and Imamura [98], who use a preinjection block, permits more thorough injection of the trigger point and taut band region with reportedly less patient discomfort.

All of these techniques rely on an accurate identification of MTrPs by means of palpation. There is no definitive evidence that one technique is superior to another in long-term outcome. Cummings and White [94] remark, "because no technique is better than any other, we recommend that the method safest and most comfortable for the patient should be used." Very slim acupuncture needles may have the advantage of minimizing tissue trauma, allowing the practitioner to needle four to six trigger points at one session.

Functional outcomes in chronic muscle pain

Outcome studies of myofascial pain and its treatment are few. In one study [99] of pain, disability, and psychologic functioning in chronic low back pain subgroups, patients with low back pain of myofascial origin demonstrated similar or slightly worse outcomes than those with disk herniation as measured by several standardized questionnaires on pain and disability. Patients with myofascial pain have less accurate beliefs regarding their pain symptoms, express more dissatisfaction with physician efforts to treat their pain, and report receiving a dearth of information from their physician [100]. A 1998 study by Heikkila and coworkers [101] investigated the outcome of a multidisciplinary rehabilitation program for patients with whiplash and myofascial pain. After the rehabilitation period, 49% of patients had improved their coping skills. This percentage rose to 63% after 2 years. In addition, 46% of patients had increased their life satisfaction. The myofascial pain group also decreased their sick-leave time [101].

In a national six-center longitudinal study, Wolfe and coworkers [102] determined the intermediate and long-term outcomes of fibromyalgia in patients seen in rheumatology centers that had a special interest in the syndrome. Although functional disability worsened slightly and health satisfaction improved slightly, measures of pain, global severity, fatigue, sleep disturbance, anxiety, depression, and health status were markedly abnormal at study initiation and were essentially unchanged over the study period.

Summary

Chronic muscle pain is a common clinical complaint among patients who seek care for musculoskeletal disorders. There is a spectrum of clinical presentation ranging from focal or regional complaints to widespread pain. Nevertheless, treatment paradigms overlap and are guided by the following major principles (as put forth by this author):

- Be a sympathetic provider.
- Make an accurate diagnosis of myofascial pain or fibromyalgia.
- Identify and treat any "peripheral pain generators" (eg, tendonitis, bursitis, radiculopathy), which decreases the peripheral nociceptive input to the CNS.

- Treat the CNS dysfunction with a balanced contemporary pharmacologic approach.
- Treat (or refer to another provider) the associated symptoms, such as disorders in sleep, mood, headache, and bowel, and fatigue.
- Engage all patients in a comprehensive exercise and functional rehabilitation program.
- Judicially offer injection techniques for local trigger points or other peripheral pain generators to reduce pain and facilitate rehabilitation.
- Educate all patients about the diagnosis and encourage self-management.
- Incorporate mind-body techniques for management of chronic pain.

Case management

In the case presented at the beginning of this article, the treating physician is presented with a patient who probably has the common combination of fibromyalgia and myofascial pain. Although there are many options for management, I might treat the patient as follows:

Begin with patient education about the diagnosis.

Use a CNS active agent at low doses in the evening around bedtime for aid with sleep and pain. For example, 10 mg of cyclobenzaprine or nortriptyline is a reasonable starting option.

Encourage an active aerobic exercise program.

Refer the patient to physical therapy for education in myofascial stretching techniques and a spine stabilization program.

On follow-up, if the nighttime medication is not adequate, consider the addition of a daytime antidepressant, such as the serotonin norepinephrine reuptake inhibitor venlafaxine (37.5 mg) or duloxetine (20 mg). Low doses are started initially with gradual upward titration based on clinical response.

On further follow-up, local trigger point injection might be used in the trapezius and levator scapulae if physical therapy and exercise do not diminish the local pain and dysfunction.

References

[1] Wolfe F, Smythe HA, Yunus MB, et al. The American College of Rheumatology 1990 criteria for classification of fibromyalgia: report of the Multicenter Criteria Committee. Arthritis Rheum 1990;33:160–72.

[2] Borg-Stein J, Simons DG. Myofascial pain. Arch Phys Med Rehabil 2002;83(Suppl 1): S40–7.

[3] Goldenberg DL. Office management of fibromyalgia. Rheum Dis Clin North Am 2002; 28(2):437–46.

[4] Gran JT. The epidemiology of chronic generalized musculoskeletal pain. Best Pract Res Clin Rheumatol 2003;17(4):547–61.

[5] Buskila D, Neumann L, Press J. Genetic factors in neuromuscular pain. CNS Spectr 2005; 10(4):281–4.
[6] Skootsky SA, Jaeger B, Oye RK. Prevalence of myofascial pain in general internal medicine practice. West J Med 1989;151:157–60.
[7] Gerwin RD. A study of 96 subjects examined both for fibromyalgia and myofascial pain. J Musculoskeletal Pain 1995;3(Suppl 1):121.
[8] Kaergaard A, Anderson JH. Musculoskeletal disorders of the neck and shoulders in female sewing machine operators: prevalence, incidence, and prognosis. Occup Environ Med 2000; 57:528–34.
[9] Borg-Stein J, Yunus M. Myofascial and soft tissue causes of low pain. In: Cole AJ, Herring SA, editors. The low back pain handbook. Philadelphia: Hanley & Belfus; 2003. p. 453–67.
[10] Fields HL. Pain. New York: McGraw-Hill; 1987. p. 210.
[11] Simons DG, Travell JG, Simons LS. Myofascial pain and dysfunction: the trigger point manual, Vol. 1. Upper half of body. 2nd edition. Baltimore: Williams & Wilkins; 1999.
[12] Fricton JR, Kroening R, Haley D, et al. Myofascial pain syndrome of the head and neck: a review of clinical characteristics of 164 patients. Oral Surg Oral Med Oral Path 1985;60: 615–23.
[13] Kraybak B, Borg-Stein J, Oas J, et al. Reduced dizziness and pain with treatment of cervical myofascial pain [abstract]. Arch Phys Med Rehabil 1996;77:939–40.
[14] Dohrenwend BP, Raphael KG, Marbach JJ, et al. Why is depression comorbid with chronic myofascial face pain? A family study test of alternative hypotheses. Pain 1999; 83:183–92.
[15] Gallagher RM, Verma S. Managing pain and comorbid depression: a public health challenge. Semin Clin Neuropsychiatry 1999;4:203–20.
[16] Schwartz RA, Greene CS, Laskin DM. Personality characteristics of patients with myofascial pain – dysfunction syndrome unresponsive to conventional therapy. J Dent Res 1979; 58:1435–9.
[17] Henriksson KG. Hypersensitivity in muscle pain syndromes. Curr Pain Headache Rep 2003;7(6):426–32.
[18] Mense S, Simons DG, Russell IJ. Muscle pain: understanding its nature, diagnosis, and treatment. Philadelphia: Lippincott, Williams & Wilkins; 2001.
[19] Yunus MB. Fibromyalgia and myofascial pain syndrome: clinical features, laboratory tests, diagnosis and pathophysiologic mechanisms. In: Rachlin ES, editor. Myofascial pain and fibromyalgia. St. Louis: Mosby; 1994. p. 3–29.
[20] Yunus MB, Kalyan-Raman UP, Masi AT, et al. Electron microscopic studies of muscle biopsy in primary fibromyalgia syndrome: a controlled and blinded study. J Rheumatol 1989;16:97–101.
[21] Yunus MB, Masi AT. Fibromyalgia, restless legs syndrome, periodic limb movement disorder and psychogenic pain. In: McCarty DJ Jr, Koopman WJ, editors. Arthritis and allied conditions: a textbook of rheumatology. Philadelphia: Lea & Febiger; 1992. p. 1383–405.
[22] Mense S. Pathophysiologic basis of muscle pain syndromes. Phys Med Rehabil Clin N Am 1997;8:179–96.
[23] Simons DG, Hong CZ, Simons LS. End plate potentials are common to midfiber myofascial trigger points. Am J Phys Med Rehabil 2002;81:212–22.
[24] Couppe C, Midttun A, Hilden J, et al. Spontaneous needle electromyographic activity in myofascial trigger points in the infraspinatus muscle: a blinded assessment. J Musculoskeletal Pain 2001;9:7–17.
[25] Liley AW. An investigation of spontaneous activity in the neuromuscular junction of the rat. J Physiol 1956;132:650–66.
[26] Heuser J, Miledi R. Effect of lanthanum ions on function and structure of frog neuromuscular junctions. Proc R Soc Lond Biol Sci 1971;179:247–60.

[27] Simons DG, Stolov WC. Microscopic features and transient contraction of palpable bands in canine muscle. Am J Phys Med 1976;55:65–88.

[28] Reitinger A, Radner H, et al. [Morphologic studies of trigger points.] Manuelle Med 1996; 34:256–62 [in German].

[29] Shah JP, Phillips TM, Danoff JV, et al. An in vivo microanalytical technique for measuring the local biochemical milieu of human skeletal muscle. J Appl Physiol 2005;99(5): 1977–84.

[30] Heheisel U, Mense S, Simons DG, et al. Appearance of new receptive fields in rat dorsal horn neurons following noxious stimulation of skeletal muscle: a model for referral of muscle pain? Neurosci Lett 1993;153:9–12.

[31] Vecchiet L, Vecchiet J, Giamberardino MA. Referred muscle pain: clinical and pathophysiologic aspects. Curr Rev Pain 1999;3:489–98.

[32] Bahr R, Blumberg H, Janig W. Do dichotomizing afferent fibers exist which supply visceral organs as well as somatic structures? A contribution to the problem of referred pain. Neurosci Lett 1981;24:25–8.

[33] Davidoff RA. Trigger points and myofascial pain: toward understanding how they affect headaches. Cephalalgia 1998;18:436–48.

[34] Baraniuk JN, Whalen G, Cunningham J, et al. Cerebrospinal fluid levels of opioid peptides in fibromyalgia and chronic low back pain. BMC Musculoskelet Disord 2004; 5(1):48.

[35] Russell IF, Littman B, Orr MD, et al. Elevated cerebrospinal fluid levels of substance P in patients with the fibromyalgia syndrome. Arthritis Rheum 1994;37:1593–601.

[36] Russell IF, Michalek JE, Vipraio GA, et al. Platelet 3H-imipramine uptake receptor density and serum serotonin levels in patients with fibromyalgia/fibrositis syndrome. J Rheumatol 1992;19:104–9.

[37] Moldofsy H, England R, Scarisbrick P, et al. Musculoskeletal symptoms and non-REM sleep disturbance in patients with "fibrositis" syndrome and healthy subjects. Psychosom Med 1975;37:341–51.

[38] Bennett RM, Cook DM, Clark SR, et al. Hypothalamic-pituitary-insulin like growth factor–1 axis dysfunction in patients with fibromyalgia. J Rheumatol 1997;24:1384–9.

[39] Ahles TA, Khan SA, Yunus MG, et al. Psychiatric status of fibromyalgia and rheumatoid arthritis patients and nonpain controls: a blinded comparison of DSM-III diagnoses. Am J Psychiatry 1991;148:1721–6.

[40] Cook DB, Lange G, Ciccone DS, et al. Functional imaging of pain in patients with primary fibromyalgia. J Rheumatol 2004;31(2):364–78.

[41] Gracely RH, Petzke F, Wolf JM, et al. Functional magnetic resonance imaging evidence of augmented pain processing in fibromyalgia. Arthritis Rheum 2002;46(5):1333–43.

[42] Goldenberg DL, Felson DT, Dinerman H. A randomized, controlled trial of amitriptyline and naproxen in the treatment of patients with fibromyalgia. Arthritis Rheum 1986;29: 1371–7.

[43] Russell IJ, Fletcher EM, Michalek JE, et al. Treatment of primary fibrositis/fibromyalgia syndrome with ibuprofen and alprazolam: a double-blind, placebo controlled study. Arthritis Rheum 1991;34:552–60.

[44] Fossaluzza V, DeVita S. Combined therapy with cyclobenzaprine and ibuprofen in primary fibromyalgia syndrome. Int J Clin Pharmacol Res 1992;12:99–102.

[45] Wolfe F, Zhao S, Lane N. Preference for nonsteroidal anti-inflammatory drugs over acetaminophen by rheumatic disease patients: a survey of 1799 patients with osteoarthritis, rheumatoid arthritis, and fibromyalgia. Arthritis Rheum 2000;43:378–85.

[46] Wilder-Smith CH, Hill L, Spargo K, et al. Treatment of severe pain from osteoarthritis with slow-release tramadol or dihydrocodeine in combination with NSAIDs: a randomized study comparing analgesia, antinociception and gastrointestinal effects. Pain 2001;91:23–31.

[47] Roth SH. Efficacy and safety of tramadol HCl in breakthrough musculoskeletal pain attributed to osteoarthritis. J Rheumatol 1998;25:1358–63.

[48] Katz WA. Pharmacology and clinical experience with tramadol in osteoarthritis. Drugs 1996;52(Suppl 3):39–47.
[49] Biasi G, Manca S, Manganelli S, et al. Tramadol in the fibromyalgia syndrome: a controlled clinical trial versus placebo. Int J Clin Pharmacol Res 1998;18(1):13–9.
[50] Schnitzer RJ, Gray WL, Paster RZ, et al. Efficacy of tramadol in treatment of chronic low back pain. J Rheumatol 2000;27:772–8.
[51] Goldenberg D, Mayskiy M, Mossey C, et al. A randomized, double-blind crossover trial of fluoxetine and amitriptyline in the treatment of fibromyalgia. Arthritis Rheum 1996;39: 1852–9.
[52] Bendtsen L, Jensen R. Amitriptyline reduces myofascial tenderness in patients with chronic tension-type headache. Cephalalgia 2000;20:603–10.
[53] Brown BR Jr, Womble J. Cyclobenzaprine in intractable pain syndromes with muscle spasm. JAMA 1978;240:1151–2.
[54] O'Malley PG, Balden E, Tomkins G, et al. Treatment of fibromyalgia with antidepressant: a meta-analysis. J Gen Intern Med 2000;15:659–66.
[55] Bennett R. Fibromyalgia, chronic fatigue syndrome, and myofascial pain. Curr Opin Rheumatol 1998;10:95–103.
[56] Sayar K, Aksu G, Ak I, et al. Venlafaxine treatment of fibromyalgia. Ann Pharmacother 2003;37(11):1561–5.
[57] Arnold LM, Lu Y, Crofford LJ, et al. A double-blind, multicenter trial comparing duloxetine with placebo in the treatment of fibromyalgia patients with or without major depressive disorder. Arthritis Rheum 2004;50(9):2974–84.
[58] Offenbaecher M, Ackenheil M. Current trends in neuropathic pain treatments with special reference to fibromyalgia. CNS Spectr 2005;10(4):285–97.
[59] Davies J. Selective depression of synaptic transmission of spinal neurons in the cat by a new centrally acting muscle relaxant, 5-chloro-4-(2-imidazolin-2-yl-amino)-2, 1, 3-bensothiodazole (DS 103–282). Br J Pharmacol 1982;76:473–81.
[60] Ono H, Mishima A, Ono S, et al. Inhibitory effects of clonidine and tizanidine on release of substance P from slices of rat spinal cord and antagonism by alpha-adrenergic receptor antagonists. Neuropharmacology 1991;30:585–9.
[61] Crofford LJ, Rowbotham MC, Mease PJ, et al. Pregabalin for the treatment of fibromyalgia syndrome: results of a randomized, double-blind, placebo-controlled trial. Arthritis Rheum 2005;52(4):1264–73.
[62] Fragoso YD, Carrazana EJ. Low doses of gabapentin may be helpful in the management of chronic daily headache. Med Gen Med 2000;2(3):E52.
[63] Smith HS, Audette J, Royal MA. Botulinum toxin in pain management of soft tissue syndromes. Clin J Pain 2002;18(6 Suppl):S147–54.
[64] Dodick DW, Mauskop A, Elkind AH, et al, BOTOX CDH. Botulinum toxin type A for the prophylaxis of chronic daily headache: subgroup analysis of patients not receiving other prophylactic medications. A randomized double-blind, placebo-controlled study. Headache 2005;45(4):315–24.
[65] Troost BT. Botulinum toxin type A (Botox) in the treatment of migraine and other headaches. Expert Rev Neurother 2004;4(1):27–31.
[66] Cheshire WP, Abashian SW, Mann JD. Botulinum toxin in the treatment of myofascial pain syndrome. Pain 1994;59:65–9.
[67] Fishman LM, Konnoth C, Rozner B. Botulinum neurotoxin type B and physical therapy in the treatment of piriformis syndrome: a dose-finding study. Am J Phys Med Rehabil 2004; 83(1):42–50.
[68] Fishman LM, Anderson C, Rosner B. BOTOX and physical therapy in the treatment of piriformis syndrome. Am J Phys Med Rehabil 2002;81(12):936–42.
[69] Porta M. A comparative trial of botulinum toxin type A and methylprednisolone for the treatment of myofascial pain syndrome and pain from chronic muscle spasm. Pain 2000; 85:101–5.

[70] Wheeler AH, Goolkasian P, Gretz SS. A randomized, double-blind, prospective pilot study of botulinum toxin injection for refractory, unilateral, cervicothoracic, paraspinal, myofascial pain syndrome. Spine 1998;23:1662–6.
[71] Gobel H, Heinze A, Henize-Kuhn K, et al. [Botulinum toxin A for the treatment of headache disorders and pericranial pain syndromes.] Nervenarzt 2001;72:261–74 [in German].
[72] Aoki KR. Review of a proposed mechanism for the antinociceptive action of botulinum toxin type A. Neurotoxicology 2005;26(5):785–93.
[73] Komiyama O, Kawara M, Arai M, et al. Posture correction as part of behavioural therapy in treatment of myofascial pain with limited opening. J Oral Rehabil 1999;26: 428–35.
[74] Edwards RH. Hypotheses of peripheral and central mechanisms underlying occupational muscle pain and injury. Eur J Appl Physiol Occup Physiol 1988;57:275–81.
[75] Bhatnager V, Drury CG, Schiro SG. Posture, postural discomfort, and performance. Hum Factors 1985;57:189–99.
[76] Crockett DJ, Foreman ME, Alden L, et al. A comparison of treatment modes in the management of myofascial pain dysfunction syndrome. Biofeedback Self Regul 1986;11: 279–91.
[77] Ferraccioli G, Ghirelli L, Scita F, et al. EMG-biofeedback training in fibromyalgia syndrome. J Rheumatol 1987;14:820–5.
[78] Kaplan KH, Goldenberg DL, Galvin-Nadeau M. The impact of a meditation-based stress reduction program on fibromyalgia. Gen Hosp Psychiatry 1993;15:284–9.
[79] Berman BM, Ezza J, Hadhazy V, et al. Is acupuncture effective in the treatment of fibromyalgia? J Fam Pract 1999;48:213–8.
[80] Assefi NP, Sherman KJ, Jacobsen C, et al. A randomized clinical trial of acupuncture compared with sham acupuncture in fibromyalgia. Ann Intern Med 2005;143(1):10–9.
[81] Acupuncture. NIH Consensus statement 1997;15(5):1–34.
[82] Birch S, Jamison RH. Controlled trial of Japanese acupuncture for chronic myofascial neck pain: assessment of specific and nonspecific effects of treatment. Clin J Pain 1998; 14:248–55.
[83] Melzack R, Stillwell DM, Fox EJ. Trigger points and acupuncture points for pain: correlations and implications. Pain 1977;3:3–23.
[84] Gam AN, Warming S, Larsen LH, et al. Treatment of myofascial trigger points with ultrasound combined with massage and exercise: a randomized controlled trial. Pain 1998;77: 73–9.
[85] Hernandez-Reif M, Field T, Krasnegor J, et al. Lower back pain is reduced and range of motion increased after massage therapy. Int J Neurosci 2001;106:131–45.
[86] Kruger LR, Van der Linden WJ, Cleaton-Jones PE. Transcutaneous electrical nerve stimulation in the treatment of myofascial pain dysfunction. S Afr J Surg 1998;36:35–8.
[87] Graff-Radford SB, Reeves JL, Baker RL, et al. Effects of transcutaneous electrical nerve stimulation in the treatment of myofascial pain and trigger point sensitivity. Pain 1989; 37:1–5.
[88] Mannerkorpi K. Exercise in fibromyalgia. Curr Opin Rheumatol 2005;17(2):190–4.
[89] Graff-Radford SB, Reeves JL, Jaeger B. Management of chronic headache and neck pain: effectiveness of altering factors perpetuating myofascial pain. Headache 1987;27:186–90.
[90] Feinberg BI, Feinberg RA. Persistent pain after total knee arthroplasty: treatment with manual therapy and trigger point injections. J Musculoskeletal Pain 1998;6:85–95.
[91] Travell JG, Simons DG. Myofascial pain and dysfunction: the trigger point manual. Baltimore: Williams & Wilkins; 1983.
[92] Hong CZ. Lidocaine injection versus dry needling to myofascial trigger point: the importance of the local twitch response. Am J Phys Med Rehabil 1994;73:256–63.
[93] Childers MK, Simons DG. Botulinum toxin use in myofascial pain syndromes. In: Lennard TA, editor. Pain procedures in clinical practice. 2nd edition. Philadelphia: Hanley & Belfus; 2000. p. 191–202.

[94] Cummings TM, White AR. Needling therapies in the management of myofascial trigger point pain: a systematic review. Arch Phys Med Rehabil 2001;82:986–92.
[95] Baldry PE, Yunus MB, Inanici F. Myofascial pain and fibromyalgia syndromes: a clinical guide to diagnosis and management. Edinburgh: Churchill Livingstone; 2001.
[96] Chu J. Twitch-obtaining intramuscular stimulation: observations in the management of radiculopathic chronic low back pain. J Musculoskeletal Pain 1999;7:131–46.
[97] Gunn CC. The Gunn approach to the treatment of chronic pain: intramuscular stimulation for myofascial pain of radiculopathic origin. 2nd edition. New York: Churchill Livingston; 1996.
[98] Fischer AA, Imamura M. New concepts in the diagnosis and management of musculoskeletal pain. In: Lennard TA, editor. Pain procedures in clinical practice. 2nd edition. Philadelphia: Hanley & Belfus; 2000. p. 213–29.
[99] Cassisi JE, Sypert GW, Lagana L, et al. Pain, disability, and psychological functioning in chronic low back pain subgroups: myofascial versus herniated disk syndrome. Neurosurgery 1993;33:379–85 [discussion: 385–6].
[100] Roth RS, Horowitz K, Bachman JE. Chronic myofascial pain: knowledge of diagnosis and satisfaction with treatment. Arch Phys Med Rehabil 1998;79:966–70.
[101] Heikkila H, Heikkila E, Eisemann M. Predictive factors for the outcome of a multidisciplinary pain rehabilitation programme on sick-leave and life satisfaction in patients with whiplash trauma and other myofascial pain: a follow-up study. Clin Rehabil 1998; 12:487–96.
[102] Wolfe F, Anderson J, Harkness D, et al. Health status and disease severity in fibromyalgia: results of a six-center longitudinal study. Arthritis Rheum 1997;40(9):1571–9.

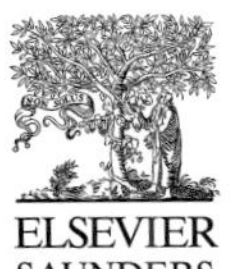
ELSEVIER
SAUNDERS

Phys Med Rehabil Clin N Am
17 (2006) 511–517

PHYSICAL MEDICINE
AND REHABILITATION
CLINICS OF
NORTH AMERICA

Index

Note: Page numbers of article titles are in **boldface** type.

A

B

1047-9651/06/$ - see front matter
doi:10.1016/S1047-9651(06)00024-6

pmr.theclinics.com

C

Q

R

S